Becoming a Supple Leopard

The Ultimate Guide
to Resolving Pain,
Preventing Injury,
and Optimizing
Athletic Performance

Dr. Kelly Starrett

with Glen Cordoza

Victory Belt Publishing Inc.
Las Vegas

First Published in 2013 by Victory Belt Publishing Inc.

ISBN 13: 978-1-936608-58-4

This book is for educational purposes. The publisher and authors of this instructional book are not responsible in any manner whatsoever for any adverse effects arising directly or indirectly as a result of the information provided in this book. If not practiced safely and with caution, working out can be dangerous to you and to others. It is important to consult with a professional fitness instructor before beginning training. It is also very important to consult with a physician prior to training due to the intense and strenuous nature of the techniques in this book.

Printed in The USA

RRD 06-13

TABLE OF CONTENTS

This book is ultimately dedicated to my daughters, Georgia and Caroline.
This book is your primer. Go burn the world to the ground and build a better one. Your secret
mermaid names will always be safe with me.

ACKNOWLEDGMENTS

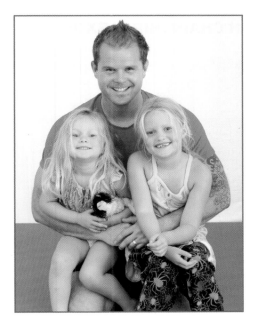

A little over two years ago, I sent back my signed copy of the publishing contract for this book and realized it was time to wrestle what I had in my head onto the printed page. I knew that wouldn't be a walk in the park, but what I really dreaded, even then, was the day I'd have to sit down and begin the impossible task of trying to thank all of the people to whom I owe a debt of gratitude. That day has come.

One thing that many people don't know about me is that I have a strangely accurate memory for interpersonal interaction and events. This means that I can recall most of the feelings, lessons, and experiences that have come to shape the thinking behind *Becoming a Supple Leopard: The Ultimate Guide to Resolving Pain, Preventing Injury, and Optimizing Athletic Performance*. Apparently, I'm not alone. I remember reading a story about what the great American dis-

cus thrower Al Oerter said in his acceptance speech as he was being inducted into the Track and Field Hall of Fame. If memory serves me right, Mr. Oerter said, essentially, that every coach and training partner he'd ever had should have been on the stage accepting the award with him. He made it clear that he could never have achieved his extraordinary career without the tens of thousands of mostly pedestrian hours he and his coaches and training partners had spent together, pushing and refining their training. I feel the same way about this book. Certainly it draws on my personal experience, including my own athletic success and failure. But it's also the synthesis of thousands of conversations and as many, if not more, hours spent learning with and from others in training, competition, coaching, and graduate school. Trying to whittle down all that experience and give proper and adequate thanks is a little overwhelming.

I often say that we are not the first people to have taken a real and thoughtful crack at solving the problems that attend human movement and performance. The difference is, I have had the benefit of living in this age. Technology, in combination with a modern, classical, doctoral level education in physiotherapy, has equipped me to create what I believe is a fresh, new, and integrated model for understanding and interpreting the work of the thousands of brilliant physios and coaches who came before me and who work around me. I had the foresight and good luck to open one of the first fifty CrossFit gyms with my wife, Juliet. It has since provided me with tens of thousands of practical hours in human movement pattern recognition—something I could never have achieved even a decade ago. (*Ursul, we have worm-sign the likes of which even god has never seen…*)[1] I remember reading the seminal textbook *Maitland's Peripheral Manipulation* when I was in the second year of my doctoral program and having my mind blown: Someone had conceived of an idea based on his study and clinical practice and integrated that idea into a cohesive and cogent model. Now, nearly two years into the process of writing this book, I can see the moment I felt like I had something to say, a sort of "concept" inflection point. I hope this book makes a significant contribution to the incredible bodies of work already out there—and those to come.

I should be frank. While it's easy to say with certainty that I can recall thinking I should write this book, it would never—and I mean *never*—have happened without the confluence of two specific events and two very special people. The first of these events is the regular trainer course that I teach for Cross-Fit. Several times a month, I get to stand in front of fifty or so extraordinary coaches and athletes from around the world, each with a different background and story. These coaches and athletes are fierce in their passions and brilliant in their capacity to seek out and integrate better movement practices into their own training. They are a ruthlessly experienced and inquisitive mob and every day that I have the pleasure of teaching them is a bit of a trial by fire. There is no place to hide. Every idea I teach must

withstand clinical validation and must be built on observable, measurable, and repeatable experience. If not, I will be torn to pieces by wild dogs. What the thousands of attendees don't realize, of course, is that they are part of my own, large-scale experiment. I never would have been ready to open my thinking to the larger world without their tacit support over this last half decade.

Event two is the Mobility Project. In the fall of 2010, I made a foolhardy commitment to film a video about position, mobility, and human mechanics every day for a year. I don't know the last time you tried to perform a public creative act for 365 days in a row, but you have to get really competent, quickly. With nearly 1.5 million unique users on the site, the real time feedback is unmatched. There is no place to hide on camera so you'd better be sure in your thinking lest the Internet destroy you and expose you for a fraud.

That said, this book would never have happened without the patience and friendship of Glen Cordoza. For the last eighteen months, Glen forced me to organize and clarify my thinking. He pressed me ruthlessly to explain and simplify the complex processes of my practice and coaching. It would have taken me another, oh, ten years to solidify my thoughts without his constant questioning and unshakeable faith in me. I actually believed that I could pull this book off by myself at one point. Then I realized I didn't even own a camera that wasn't attached to my phone. Sure I had some ideas about human movement and performance, but I sure as hell didn't know how to write a book about it. Where some people have a weekend or go on vacation, I worked on the book with Glen. He has become a confidant, brother, fellow revolutionary, brother to my wife, and uncle to my children. I shudder to think how much Glen has been exposed to my brain. I'm not sure he will ever recover and I know I'll never be able to repay him his effort or friendship.

And then there's Jstar. As I've come to find out, writing any book is an act of will and of hope. It's like planting bulbs in the fall, hoping that you'll be around in the spring to see them bloom. During the long, dark, wet winter, it's really, really difficult to remember that you actually planted the bulbs *and* that they actually might bloom into something beautiful.

---

1 Spoken by the character, Stilgar, in the science fiction novel, *Dune.*

From the first time I turned our home's back office into a scene from the movie *A Beautiful Mind*, my wife Juliet didn't flinch. After a week balancing a life, the gym, my work travel, and our children, Juliet would stoically pick up the additional slack that fell to her when I was "working on the book." The spine of this book should really just read "Starretts." If you are reading this, be sure to remember to email my wife your thanks. Trust me, in a million ways, I could not have written a single word without her steadfast stewardship, cheerleading, counsel, keen eye, and hard work. I'd still be sleeping in a truck and selling Kayaks somewhere in Colorado if Juliet hadn't had the faith to plant a few bulbs for the spring. The first flowers of this book are for her.

There are a few really important coaches who influenced me. I would be remiss if I did not mention Mike Burgener and Mark Rippetoe. They spent a great deal of time with a hungry young kid seeking to understand what they already knew. Coach Rip once answered the phone when I called his gym and talked to me for thirty minutes about how he thought the adductors worked in squatting. To this day, this blows my mind and I always think of his kindness toward me when a young coach comes to me wanting advice or guidance. Coach B is my sensei. He has shown me that I need to be able to coach everyone, and that my thinking has to work for everyone, from children to Olympians. Thank you both.

Greg Glassman and the incredible people behind the scenes at CrossFit have created, supported, and nurtured literally thousands of coaches. I am proud to call myself one of these. Greg created a template that was broad and complete enough to leave room for my own thinking and discovery. I will never be able to repay him, his faith in me, or his incredible generosity. He challenged me to validate what I thought to be true in the hard, cold light of observable, measurable, and repeatable human function. I have often said it, but finding CrossFit and Greg's early writing was like discovering the unified field theory of human performance. I had the good fortune to train at the original CrossFit Santa Cruz when Greg was still coaching every day. His counsel—that the most important research I could do was right there in front of me, in the athletes and coaches I was working with—continues to serve me well. Greg's work has forever changed my life and the lives of my family. His thinking is at the core of this book.

Thanks also go to:

The coaches of SFCF: Tonya, Ty, Roop, Connie, Maggie, Kelsi, Diane, Sean, John, Tuller, Bmack, Erin, Kristin, Courtney, Nate, Boz, Kimmie, Patrick, Debbie, and Carl. I would be nothing without you guys. POD.

Tom and Lisa Wiscombe. They were vital in the production and overall coolness of this work. I'm pretty sure they invented the computational leopard. Their brilliance inspires me.

Janet and Ed. From making the invisible visible, to lagging indicators, your love and support make it possible for this family to work. Thank you.

TJ Murphy: Any creative project of this scale is like a miracle of emergence, serendipity, and machine-like precision. Frankly, I can't imagine pulling this off without your humor, advocacy, and keen brain. It's like a butterfly flapped its wings somewhere and I ended up with you on my team.

Carl Paoli, Brian MacKenzie, John Welbourn, Jill Miller, Mark Bell and Jesse Burdick. Every good coach I know has a few close friends who can call bullshit, open doors, and make the journey worth it for each other. The archetype of the monk-coach—someone working things out by themselves in isolation—is total crap. I am surrounded by some of the best thinkers and coaches on the planet. Don't worry, guys: I'll happily smash your quads for life. Thanks for having my back.

Mom and Don. I knew that I didn't want to kayak forever. Sorry I didn't share that part of the plan with you right away. You were right; grad school was a good choice. Knowing you guys are in my corner is like having a formidable secret weapon.

Kelly Starrett

INTRODUCTION

Often these days, I find myself crammed into an airplane seat on my way across the country to work with athletes, coaches, professional sports teams, CrossFit gyms, corporations, and elite military forces. Inevitably I end up making small talk with the poor soul imprisoned next to me. Soon enough I get the question: "What do you do for work?"

Dozens of answers run through my head.

"I make the best athletes in the world better."

"I work with the government to improve our military's force protection and force resiliency."

"I work with athletes and coaches to help them understand and resolve common and preventable losses of torque, force, wattage, and output."

"I'm trying to change the world's movement-based economy from subsistence tension-hunting to sustainable, high-yield torque farming."

"I'm fomenting revolution. I'm trying to empower people to live more integrated, pain-free, self-actualized lives."

No, I don't mention anything about farming torque or self-actualization, which I'll spend plenty of time on in the pages to come. I keep it simple. "I'm a teacher," I say.

Typically eyes glaze over, and the conversation sputters to a halt. But once in a while, my seatmate is curious enough to ask the obvious follow-up—"What do you teach?"—unaware of the depths of my obsession with human movement and performance, but he soon finds out.

What I teach—and what you will learn in this book—is a multi-function, extraordinarily effective movement and mobility system. Learn, practice, and apply it and you will understand how to move correctly in all situations. And I mean *all*. It will serve you at rest *and* when you are executing a demanding physical feat—say, in the midst of an Olympic competition, or in a strenuous combat or rescue operation.

This is a strength-and-conditioning system that is also diagnostic in nature: It can help you—or your coach—detect movement and positioning errors even as it improves your performance and brings you to the top of your game. My system gives you the tools to dissolve the physical restrictions that prevent you from fully actualizing your potential. With enough practice, you can develop yourself to the point at which your full physical capabilities will be available to you *instantaneously*. You will develop the motor-control and range-of-motion to do *anything* at any time.

You could ultimately become the human equivalent of a *supple leopard,* always poised and ready for action.

You might ask, "What does it mean to become a *supple leopard*?" It's a good question, one that warrants an explanation.

I've long been fascinated with the idea of a leopard: powerful, fast, adaptable, stealthy… badass.

When I was fourteen I watched the movie *Gallipoli* with my dad. It's about two Australian sprinters who go off to fight in Turkey during World War I. There's a memorable scene at the beginning where Archy, a rising track star, is being trained by his uncle Jack. The pep talk goes like this:

Jack: What are your legs?

Archy: Springs. Steel Springs.

Jack: What are they going to do?

Archy: Hurl me down the track.

Jack: How fast can you run?

Archy: As fast as a leopard.

Jack: How fast are you going to run?

Archy: As fast as a leopard!

Jack: Then let's see you do it!

For whatever reason, the "fast as a leopard" mantra stuck with me. But it wasn't until a Navy SEAL buddy of mine said, "You know, Kelly, a leopard never stretches," that this notion of becoming a supple leopard drifted into my consciousness.

Of course a leopard doesn't stretch! A leopard has full physical capacity available at all times. It can attack and defend with full power at any moment. Unlike humans, it doesn't need to prep for movement. It doesn't need to activate its glutes; it doesn't have to foam-roll; it doesn't have to raise its core temperature—it's just ready.

Obviously, we do not share the same physical playing field with leopards. We have to warm-up for strenuous activities and practice and ingrain good movement patterning. But that doesn't mean we can't be working toward the goal of having full physical capabilities available to us instantaneously, or having the motor-control and the range-of-motion to perform any physical feat at any time. Leopards don't have to work at being supple; they naturally are. But people are brutally tight and missing key ranges of motion that prevent them from moving as pliantly and powerfully as a leopard.

Metaphorically speaking, if you want to become a supple leopard, you need to understand how to move correctly in every situation. You also need the tools to deal with stiff and adaptively short tissues that restrict range-of-motion. This is the basis of my Movement and Mobility System.

A New Human-Performance Epoch

Is what I teach radically new? Yes, and then again, no.

I see myself as one of the latest in a long line of teachers concerned with organizing and optimizing movement to maximize physical performance—consistently and without injury.

Certainly, human beings have explored this for eons. In fact, I've seen a thousand-year-old image on a coin that shows a man sitting in full lotus—a posture that creates more stability for the spinal system. More recently, some three hundred and fifty years ago, a famous Japanese swordsman, Miyamoto Musashi, wrote about the importance of keeping your belly firm and your knees and feet in a good position: "Make your combat stance your everyday stance." It is strange yet perfect advice from Musashi's famous text, *The Book of Five Rings*.

What's exciting about being alive today is that we're in the midst of a human-performance epoch. Physical mastery is not limited to the few. As I see it, we are experiencing a quantum leap in the quality, reproducibility, and ubiquity of absolute human physical potential. In fact, if we imagine the peak expression of human potential to be some kind of golden ratio, then the current generation of coaches, athletes, and thinkers have achieved the equivalent of a Fibonacci jump at light speed.

It's crazy. I mean, even my mother is gluten-free and casually brags about her latest deadlift personal record.

What's going on? What's so different about the time in which we live?

What's different is that we've seen a convergence of factors create a new golden age in human physical performance. Four key factors are responsible.

First, the advent of the Internet and modern media has enabled the sharing of ideas globally. Isolated pockets of embodied knowledge are more easily transferred and shared. Ten years ago, finding an Olympic-lifting coach required bloodhound-like determination or luck. Most likely both. Now the clean and snatch—the two core Olympic-lifting movements—are widespread practices.

Second, for the first time in the modern training era, there is an unparalleled cross-discipline exchange among training practices and theories of human movement. For example, our gym, San Francisco CrossFit, is an interdisciplinary melting pot: physiotherapists hang out with elite powerlifters, Olympic-lifting medalists talk to champion gymnasts, and ballet dancers train with elite endurance coaches. This phenomenon is the strength-and-conditioning equivalent of the

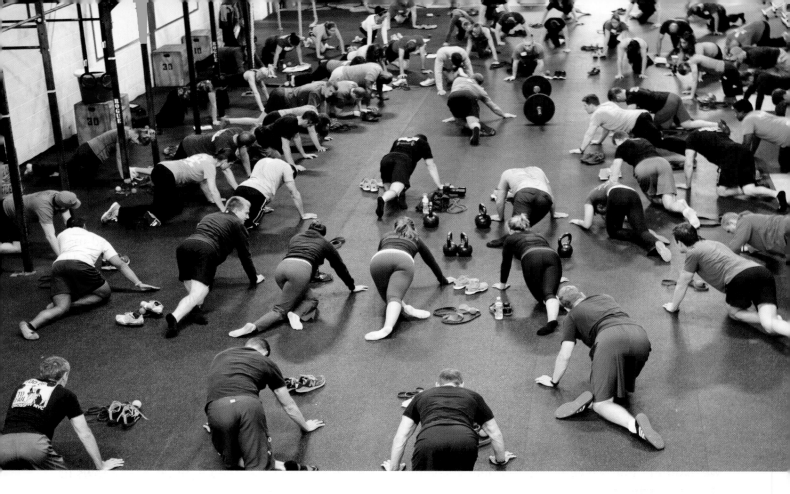

great systems theorist Buckminster Fuller's concept of mutual accommodation: that correctly organized, functionally sound systems are never in opposition. They mutually support one another.

Everyone shares the same basic design and body structure. People's shoulders all work the same way: the principles that govern a stable shoulder position while vaulting in gymnastics are the same in the bench press; how you organize your shoulders to sit in lotus posture while meditating is the same way you organize them when working at your computer. It's just that the same set of problems have been solved from radically different angles and approaches. Until now.

Third, we appear to be living at a time when there is growing interest in the body. While this topic probably merits its own book, there can be no doubt that the accessibility of online and mobile tools that make it possible to measure our behavior—as well as our lifestyle, nutrition, and exercise habits—has shifted the responsibility for keeping our bodies in the best shape possible back where it belongs: on the individual.

Elite and recreational athletes alike can track

and measure nearly any aspect of their performance and biology with little effort and cost. Want to know how that afternoon coffee affects your sleep quality? No problem. Want to fractionate your cholesterol and find out if you are eating too much bacon? No problem (although I'm pretty sure that it's impossible to eat too much bacon). Whether people are tracking their own blood chemistry or daily step totals, or trying to get to the root of their own knee pain, there has been an enormous shift in consciousness, leading to a greater sense of self-control. Eating, sleeping, and moving correctly are not gimmicks or fads. The dam has burst and the personal biological revolution is here.

It's a brave new world. We don't have to wait decades or endure multiple knee surgeries and heart attacks to find out that we're running poorly, eating poorly, sleeping poorly, and training poorly. Peter Drucker—world-renowned management consultant, educator, and author—was right, "What gets measured, gets managed."

The fourth factor contributing to this golden age is the evolution of strength-and-conditioning. People have been lifting heavy weights, moving quickly, and working very hard to real effect for some time. The difference now is that a good strength-and-conditioning program *has all of the elements of human movement covered.* That is, an intelligently structured strength-and-conditioning program gives the athlete full range-of-motion in his joints, limbs, and tissues; the motor-control to express those ranges; and the ability to do so under actual physical load, metabolic demand, cardio-respiratory demand, speed, and stress. Couple this complete physical paradigm (the CrossFit model holds that people should look and train like Olympic-lifting-sprinter-gymnasts, for example) with the number of people now using a common language of movements and movement paradigms, and you have the largest-scale model experiment in human movement in the history of the world.

Let's put this in perspective. In the seven years our gym, San Francisco CrossFit, has been open, we estimate that we've facilitated nearly seventy thousand athlete training sessions. The sheer volume of pattern recognition this is capable of generating is staggering and could take a clinician or a coach a lifetime to accumulate. Now multiply this by thousands of locations, across hundreds of sports platforms, and suddenly a simple strength-and-conditioning system also becomes the world's most potent diagnostic tool with unmatched test and retest capabilities. This accumulated wisdom is what has given rise to my system. The gym is suddenly the laboratory.

We are able to eliminate correlates for human movement and performance and replace them with actual human movement. You don't have to demonstrate an active straight-leg raise (a common physical-therapist tool for assessing hamstring range-of-motion); you just need to demonstrate that you can pick something up off the ground while keeping your spine organized and flat (in other words, a deadlift). This is how you bring it down to the bare essentials.

Realize what a huge shift in thinking this is.

Our previous model of strength-and-conditioning was predicated on the fact that if you were just stronger and fitter, you'd be a better ath-

lete and better at your chosen sport. Clearly, that's not true. In fact, anterior cruciate ligament (ACL) injury rates in children continue to increase. Running injury rates are estimated to be as high as 70 percent in some studies. And therein lies the problem.

In the past, it has been difficult to understand the nuances of poor technique and biomechanics as expressed by athletes. Anecdotally, basketball is the most dangerous sport a middle-aged man can play. Why do middle-aged guys so readily tear their Achilles playing pickup B-ball? Because it's hard to see the underlying poor movement patterns while they're playing. They're changing shapes, transitioning from one position to another at high speeds.

To prevent these injuries, we need a tool to make the invisible visible. We need to bring athletes into the lab (i.e., the gym) to assess their movement patterns before the catastrophe occurs—an ACL tear, herniated disk, or torn rotator cuff. In addition, we need a model that allows us to identify the problem, be it motor-control or biomechanical in origin.

By consistently and systematically exposing athletes to the rigors of full-range movements and optimal human motor-control, we're able to quickly identify force leaks, torque dumps, bad technique, motor inefficiency, poorly integrated movement patterns; holes in strength, speed, and metabolic conditioning; and restrictions in mobility. Best of all, the tool we use to detect and prevent injury is the same tool needed to improve an athlete's performance. The middle-aged "tore my heel cord" syndrome is a lot less likely to happen if an athlete's ankle is regularly exposed to full ranges of motion in movements like pistols or overhead squats (see page 111).

But there's even more to it than that. This complete and modern strength-and-conditioning system has not only become the *most complete* way to systematically test and retest athletic performance, and to diagnose movement inefficiencies and dysfunction; it has also created a formal, universal language of human movement. In short, if you understand the principles that govern full-range strength-and-conditioning exercises and can apply them in this low-risk environment (like a gym), you understand and can apply them to the activities and positions of life, sports, dance, combat, and play.

Take the squat for example. Squatting isn't just a movement performed in the gym; it's how human beings lower their center of gravity. A full-range squat (with hips below the knee crease) with loads overhead, in the front of the torso, on the back, or on one leg pretty much covers the human range of squatting activities. If you understand the principles of this formal movement training language, then you are better prepared to express a more informal or applicable form of human movement everywhere else. You can start to connect the dots between the safe, stable positions practiced in the gym to the movements you perform outside the gym. For example, if you understand how to organize your spine and stabilize your hips and shoulders correctly while performing a deadlift or clean, you have a ubiquitous model for picking something off the ground. If you understand how to create a braced-neutral trunk and generate torque off of a bar when performing a pull-up, you will have no problem applying the same principles when climbing a tree.

This is the rub: If you only ever climb trees, it may be impossible to know if you are working in the safest and most efficient positions—with a stable shoulder and stable trunk—unless you also do formal pull-ups. In other words, it's a lot harder to identify whether someone is moving in a safe, stable position when climbing a tree than when performing a pull-up in the gym, even though both activities abide by the same fundamental movement principles. So in addition to being a lab in which to identify, diagnose, and treat poor movement practices, the gym is a safe and controlled environment in which we can teach and layer these ubiquitous concepts with accelerated learning capabilities and reduced potential for injury.

Moreover, the idea of creating a common movement language based on formal strength-and-conditioning principles is why there can suddenly be so much interdisciplinary,

movement-based discussion and collaboration. We are able to move beyond "people should train in gymnastics," to "people should train in gymnastics because the handstand position easily teaches and exposes shoulder stability and organization and has the same finish position and shoulder demands as the jerk." The commonality and universality of "formal" human movement is easily understood by coach and athlete alike, and it is easy to track and test changes in positional quality by measuring the very thing we are chasing in the gym anyway—performance. This is precisely why we keep track of work output, wattage, poundage, reps, and time.

Brilliant people have spent their entire lives developing systems that help us understand how and why humans move the way they move and have the ailments they do. Do these systems work? Of course they do. They work to varying degrees and with varying application. Should we discard them? No, of course not. But there is a significant disconnect between our older models of human movement and our current understanding about how to best maximize human physical potential.

Here's a real-life example. Recently I was on a working vacation to Australia with my wife and two daughters. We booked a few days at a beautiful spa along Australia's west coast. My wife, Juliet, noticed that there was a free yoga class the following morning at 8 a.m. and thought it would be amusing for me to attend. I showed up ten minutes before the hour as I was instructed but found that I was the last person to arrive. The instructor sighed in resignation when she saw 225-pound me walk into her yoga class "late." (There were already fifteen or so intense I-do-yoga–looking women there; I was the only man.)

In a fake-pleasant voice, she asked me if I'd ever done yoga. I said I had, which was true: I'd done a lot of yoga when I was much younger. Not five minutes into the session she started making very complimentary comments about the abilities of the "bloke" in the back row. "Great job back there!" "Wow!" And the more effusive and surprised the instructor became, the more I became the hated target of all the skinny women struggling with the postures.

At the end of class, the instructor rushed right up and apologized for not recognizing that I was obviously an advanced practitioner. (I mean clearly I'm a beginner, but I was loads better than everyone else, and I do lift weights and perform gymnastics.) When she asked me where I practiced, I laughed a little and said that I didn't. In my nicest voice I said that I actually hadn't done yoga in over ten years. She was a little taken aback: I could clearly perform the movements in her class, but didn't actually practice. So she had to ask, "What do you do?"

I said I was a teacher.

HOW TO USE THIS BOOK

To help you navigate this book, it's important that you understand the basic construct and function of my Movement and Mobility System.

There are three movement principles: midline stabilization and organization (spinal mechanics), one-joint rule, and laws of torque. Think of the movement principles as the master blueprint for creating safe and stable positions for all human movements. You will learn about these in chapters 2, 3, and 4. If you practice them in the order presented, you will know how to stabilize your spine in a braced, well-organized position; how to maintain good posture during loaded, dynamic movements; and how to create stability in your joints to generate maximum force, power, and speed. Then you will have the necessary foundation to properly execute the strength-and-conditioning exercises in chapter 5.

Realize that you can immediately apply the movement principles to the actions of sports and life. Once you understand position as a skill and the underpinnings of stability, you can start to bring consciousness to your position in all situations, whether you're trapped behind a desk at work, picking up your child, carrying groceries, or playing volleyball. But mastering the movement principles takes practice. And you need to be able to identify restrictions in range-of-motion and motor-control dysfunction so that you can isolate and solve your unique problems. That's why the movement principles are practiced in a safe, controlled environment (the gym) using fundamental (transferable) strength-and-conditioning movements.

In chapter 5, "Movement Hierarchy," you will learn how to properly execute functional full-range strength-and-conditioning movements—squatting, pulling, and pressing iterations—as well as how to identify and correct common movement errors. Once you understand and can apply the movement principles to functional movements, you will have no problem using those skills to correct errors and optimize movement efficiency for all of your movements.

The key is to prioritize position and movement first. Most of you will probably want to skip right to the mobilization techniques later in the book. And if you have a tight muscle or a painful joint that needs to be dealt with, by all means go there. (See chapter 7, "The Systems.") But know that you will never get to the bottom of your pain and dysfunction if you don't correct the movement or position that is causing the problem. It's like treating a symptom without addressing the disease. The problem will still be there.

Note: The evolution of the Movement and Mobility System continues to progress at an exponential rate. New ways of improving performance and torturing athletes are being developed every day in the San Francisco CrossFit laboratory. For the latest and most up-to-date mobilizations, go to MobilityWOD.com.

CHAPTER 1
THE MOVEMENT AND MOBILITY SYSTEM

How do you know you have some sort of musculoskeletal problem? More specifically, how do you know when what you are doing or how you are doing it is wrong? Typically, the average athlete uses a set of cues like pain, swelling, loss of range-of-motion, decreased force, or numbness and tingling. The medical community calls these "pathognomonic" signs or cues. The conversation with yourself begins something like this: "When I run lately, my knee hurts. I wonder what's wrong with my knee?" While typical, there are many errors in this line of thought.

The first problem is that pain and the other symptoms of injury are all lagging indicators. For example, swelling might indicate tissue overuse or strain from poor mechanics. But swelling is an after-the-fact sign. The tissue damage has already occurred. It's too late to go back. It's helpful to have a diagnostic tool, something that will highlight your dysfunction and let you know something is wrong, but only if it is applicable before the fact.

Imagine having to blow up your car engine to know if you should add oil. Or a soldier having to wait for his weapon to jam in the middle of a firefight before he knows if he should perform some preventative maintenance. That would be ridicu-

lous, right? Of course. But in general terms, this is how modern sports medicine operates. We wait until something is broken, sometimes horribly so, before we expect our physician or physiotherapist to fix it. This paradigm keeps orthopedic surgeons very busy.

You can imagine what the doctor thinks when you come into his office with a hole in your kneecap from years of poor movement practices and overly tight tissues. Seriously? That bone in your knee was designed to last 110 years. You managed to wear a hole in it in twenty (true story). Imagine waiting until you are suffering from unrelenting back pain and having your leg go numb to find out that you used poor spinal mechanics carrying that 100-pound pack as a young marine (true story).

It's like this: Our bodies are set up to go through millions of movement cycles. Every time you squat, bend over, or walk in a compromised position, you're burning through those cycles at an accelerated rate. Think of turning on and off the lights in your house. That light switch is set up for tens of thousands of cycles. Well, your body is set up for millions of cycles. Seriously, millions! So by the time you've worn a hole in your kneecap, herniated your disk, or torn your labrum, chances are good that you've expended millions of cycles. In other words, your tissues and joints didn't just wear out; your body put up with your crappy positions and movements for the equivalent of millions of cycles. Everyone is different—genetics, training volume, and other lifestyle factors have a profound impact—but if you learn to move the way the body is designed to move, there's less stress on the system, reducing the number of cycles you burn through.

The second issue is that the human animal is set up for survival. Your central nervous system (CNS) controls the sensory and mechanical information for the entire body. It's not an accident that the pain and movement pathways in the brainstem are one and the same. If a child bangs her finger, the first thing she does is to start moving it around. Why? She can no longer hear the pain signal along with the movement signal. This is a very elegant system to keep people moving and surviving because it literally relegates those pesky pain signals to background noise, which you can't hear until you stop moving. Put another way, movement (sensory input) overrides the pain signal so that you can continue moving, exercising, and training. No wonder your shoulder starts to throb when you lie down and go to sleep. Your brain is no longer receiving any movement signal input. All your brain gets now is full-blown pain.

Now imagine training like an athlete your whole life. You've spent countless hours ignoring the horrible pain signals your body is send-

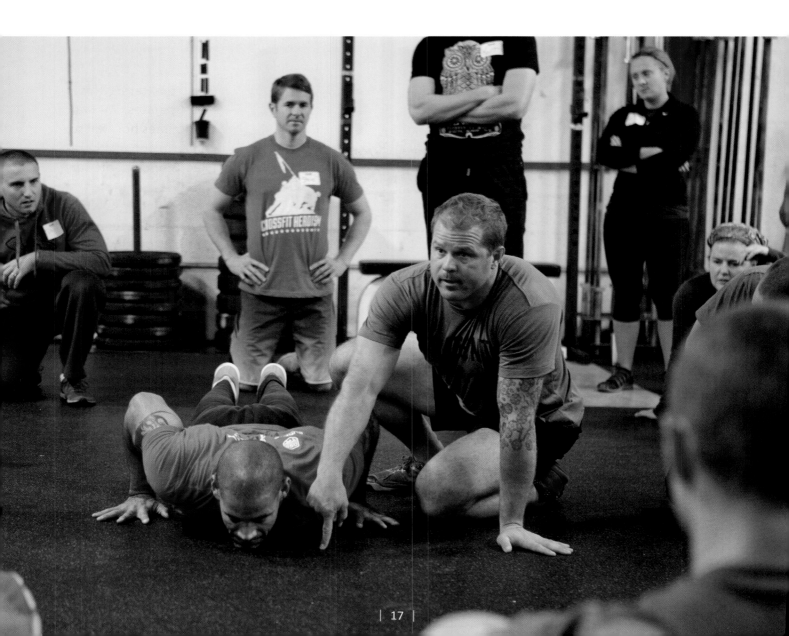

ing while you train and compete. There is little chance that you can actually hear the pain of tissue injury failure amid all that movement and other pain noise. Pain doesn't actually work during periods of high movement load and peak output demand. Add stress into the equation, and it's a recipe for disaster. If you've ever been in a fight, you know that one of the great secrets of fighting is that you probably won't feel any immediate pain. If you talk to professional fighters, they'll tell you that they feel violent impacts and concussion but don't immediately feel pain. Humans are designed to be able to take the hit, keep fighting, and deal with the consequences later. And there are certainly consequences to getting haymakered in the face.

In actuality, exercise presents a similar scenario. What you can count on is an absolute assuredness that when you start to lose position and compromise your tissues—like rounding your back during a deadlift—you may not feel it at the time, especially if you're under competition stress. However, just as a fighter feels the abuse from combat after his adrenaline has worn off, an athlete's back will scream in pain when he cools down from a workout where he did twenty improperly executed deadlifts. Just as you could say that the more skilled fighter usually suffers the least amount of damage and as a result doesn't feel as much—if any—pain after battle, the better you are at deadlifting, the less likely you are to tweak your back.

The third problem with our current thinking is that it continues to be based on a model that prioritizes task completion above everything else. It's a sort of one-or-zero, task-done-or-not, weight-lifted-or-not, distance-swam-or-not, mentality. This is like saying: "I deadlifted 500-pounds, but I herniated a disk," or "I finished a marathon, but now I have plantar fasciitis and wore a hole in my knee." Imagine this sort of ethic spilling over into the other aspects of your life: "Hey, I made you some toast! But I burned down the house."

Hang out at the end of any local marathon and you'll notice a significant number of finishers who are obviously suffering. They look as if they were hit by cars and stricken by disease. Yes,

you say, but they finished. And this is true. Being task-completion obsessed certainly has its place, like in the Olympic finals, a world championship, the Super Bowl, or a military mission. But even then, there may be a heavy price to pay. Couple this task-priority blindness with an overly simplified system of a pain's indicators and it's easy to understand how athletes can dig themselves into some pretty deep holes.

Many athletes go about their business this way for decades, spending their genetic inheritance, getting their daily workout done without pain, until one day it's game over. You can lift with a rounded back and sit in a chair in a slouched position, until one day you can't. So how do you keep people from harming themselves? You need a set of leading indicators—a set of observable, measurable, and repeatable diagnostic tools that allow you to predict potential problems before they manifest as a recognizable disorder. The good news is that we already possess this information. It's called positioning.

It's About Performance

Human movement, and by extension the body's positions within those movements, is really just a combination of biomechanics and movement technique. By exposing people to a broad palette of movements, by making people express body control through full, normal ranges of motion, we are able to expose holes and inefficiencies in their motor-control and mobility. We can make the invisible visible.

This means that while we are training for a stronger set of legs, or a bigger set of lungs, we are simultaneously thinking in terms of diagnostics. The deadlift is no longer just a matter of picking up something heavy from the floor. Rather, it becomes a dynamic question: Does the athlete have the capacity to keep his spine efficiently braced and stable and express full posterior-chain range-of-motion while picking up something and breathing hard in a stressful environment? We don't need to develop an entirely new set of correlate or diagnostic movements to understand what is happening when people lift something off the ground. Rather, we simply need to see and understand what's happening during the movement he is performing. That means you not only have to understand why the movement is performed, but also how to do it correctly.

Repurposing training so that it also serves as a diagnostic tool is useful on many other fronts as well. First, it's efficient. Systematically and effectively assessing and screening for movement problems in athletes can be an enormous moving target at best and a colossal exercise in misplaced precision at worst. Any system or set of tools that helps us better understand what is going on under the hood is a good thing. Here's the key: Any good assessment tool, even one that's built on movement correlates rather than actual movement, needs to be easily scalable, meaning that the movement or exercise can be adjusted and applied to all athletes. It needs to be topical, addressing the issues that the coach is seeing that day, with that set of athletes, with those movements. Ultimately, it has to be able to render changes that both the coach and the athlete can observe, measure, and repeat. Over time, this daily combination of training and assessment frees the coach and athlete to work through and discover problems systematically.

What you have to remember is that human movement is complex and nuanced. Marrying the diagnostic process to the training process ensures that no stone will go unturned. However, we can't train every movement or energy system an athlete may use in a single training session. Nor do we need to assess and address every deficiency in the athlete in a single day. It's a lifelong process of identifying problems, fixing them, and then exposing more holes in the athletic profile with more challenging stimulus. It's a never-ending cycle of correcting problems and finding new ones. This is how we become better athletes.

This model, based on the movements and training of the day, has the added benefit of being psychologically manageable in scope and practice. Anyone can fix one problem at a time. But the typical list of dysfunction for the average athlete is just that, a list. The most important thing we can do is to get the athlete to train and address the problems along the way. Small, consistent positional interventions don't create extreme, additional time demands on the athlete or the coach. The priority remains training, not resolving what is probably a laundry list of dysfunction in one training session.

I have yet to meet an athlete with perfect motor-control, mobility, and biomechanical efficiency. Hell, most of the really successful athletes I know are dumping huge amounts of torque, bleeding horrendous amounts of force, and missing key corners in their range-of-motion. Yet they are still the best in the world. A ten- or fifteen-minute intervention performed on the spot, within the context of the current training, is manageable and sustainable. The modern training session is a little miracle. It's a frantic, compressed session of teaching, nutritional and lifestyle counseling, strength work, skill work, metabolic conditioning, and mobility work. Layering complex, time-demanding, full body diagnostic movements and interventions on top of a cramped training session, especially if you're training several athletes at once, will only make you throw your hands up and revert to a wait-till-they-break model. But if a coach is able to program a few specific fixes for the demands of the day's movements, then the coach wins and the athlete is able to embody the connection between mobilization and improved positioning. Athletes are both greedy and smart—greedy in that they will do whatever it takes to get better in the shortest amount of time possible, and smart in that they will absolutely repeat specific practices and interventions that improve their performance or take away their pain.

The second benefit of using training exercises as a diagnostic tool is that it shifts the issues of lost or poor positioning from the realm of injury prevention to the realm of performance. This has twofold implication. The first is that it diverts the athlete's focus from task completion. "Well, I didn't get hurt, my knees aren't in pain, and I have an Olympic gold medal, so why should I care about injury prevention?" But, if we focus on output, the athlete is in a constant state of chasing performance, of eking out small changes in position, efficiency, work output, poundage, and wattage. Our goal isn't just to make the best athletes in the world. Our goal is to make the best athletes in the world *better*.

These are the metrics that matter, because functioning well is never a force-production or a work-output compromise. We don't have to make the binary choice between safety and a world record, sacrificing one for the other. If we chase performance first, we get injury prevention in the bargain. If we obsess over the reasons behind poor positioning, we get better mechanical advantage, improved leverage, and more efficient force production. For example, improved hip mechanics may mean a change in the total range-of-motion of the athlete's hip, but when it translates into a world-record squat, it actually means a little more to the athlete. When we are able to improve a rower's thoracic extension, she will definitely sit taller on the seat and have better shoulder control. But when she notices greater wattage output and decreased times, she is a believer and will reproduce the phenomenon herself.

Using the training movements of the day as an instantaneous and ongoing diagnostic screening tool serves athletic development in other ways as well. For example, assessing an athlete for mechanical dysfunction with common screening processes is primarily a snapshot of that athlete on that day. It's not uncommon to run into athletes who have recently acquired tissue stiffness after a brutal training micro-cycle, tournament, or prolonged mission. Programming diagnostic/mobility work based on a well-rounded strength-and-conditioning program's daily movement is a roving, built-in, periodized system. Nothing is missed as long as an athlete is performing movements that express full range-of-motion and motor-control within those ranges. This leads to another useful change in the conceptual framework of what the gym can and should be.

The Gym Is Your Lab ✔

The modern strength-and-conditioning center should be considered a human-performance laboratory. The goal of both the coach and the athlete should be to exceed any strength, speed, or metabolic demand the athlete might need in life, sport, or shift on the SWAT team. It should also be the place where the coach and athlete hunt out every positional inefficiency, every poor mechanical tendency, and every default or compensatory movement pattern. Where else can the athlete safely expose his movement and tissue dysfunctions? The training center/lab is a controlled environment where the coach and athlete can safely and systematically layer skill progressions while simultaneously addressing mechanical and range-of-motion issues.

The hallmark of any good strength-and-conditioning program is twofold: to consistently and routinely challenge both the strength and fitness components of an athlete's constitution, and to express motor-control under a wide variety of demands and situations. For example, most movement screens, quick-movement tests, or range-of-motion tests are performed statically and without any external load. The problem is that these tests don't even come close to replicating real-life demands, much less those of a sport or combat mission. But if the paradigm is altered, and if the strength-and-conditioning program continuously challenges an athlete's position with the additional stresses of actual load, metabolic demand, speed, and competition, there is little doubt that the athlete's conditioned tendencies, default motor patterns, and true physical self will be revealed.

Let's use a simple example to help illustrate my point. We regularly see athletes who can correctly perform an overhead squat with a PVC pipe. This is the most challenging squat iteration because it has high hip and ankle demands: The athlete must keep his torso absolutely upright and his shoulders stable while the load is locked out overhead. But what if we take that same person and have him or her run 400 meters, then overhead squat anything heavier than a barbell for more than a few repetitions, all while competing against someone else? We end up with a totally different athlete. And all we did was add a little bit of volume, intensity, stress, and metabolic demand to the overhead squat. Very quickly, and very safely, we make the invisible visible.

The point is that the athlete who flashes the quick test will sometimes fall apart under real-life working conditions. We just have to adjust load, volume, and intensity to match the abilities and capacities of the athlete. We do this not only to expose holes in the athlete's movement profile, but also to make her stronger, faster, more explosive, and a more capable human being. In other words, if you're coaching an athlete who has perfect form and fast times, you need to up the weight, volume, and metabolic demands, as well as introduce movements that require a higher degree of motor-control and mobility. We should be seeking thresholds where our athletes begin to breakdown, and use that not only as an assessment and diagnostic tool, but also as a way to make the athlete better.

Coaches have always done this in the gym, but typically only by challenging the athlete with load and sometimes with repetition. It's not an accident that some of the best strength coaches on the planet will regularly advocate for a twenty-plus-rep squat set, or a maximal fifteen-rep set of overhead squats. There are great athletes who can buffer their movement dysfunctions—meaning that they can hide their mobility restrictions and poor technique—for short periods of time, but regularly lose effective positioning when they begin to fatigue even a little. But if an athlete has the mobility and motor-control to maintain a stable spine, hips, and knees during a brutal working couplet of heavy front squats and running, then that athlete is more likely to be able to reproduce that efficient mechanical positioning when it matters the most (say, in the last 500 meters of the Olympic rowing final).

As I said, the gym is the lab. It's practically impossible for a coach to follow around hundreds of athletes while they're engaged in their actual sport in order to spot movement errors. That coach would not only have to be a world-class expert in hundreds of sports and have perfect timing—catching the athlete when he or she just happens to break down—he would also need the skill set to correct those faults within the context of that particular sport.

Fortunately, strength-and-conditioning coaches don't have to be an expert in every training modality to identify and fix problems that are specific to an athlete's chosen sport. All they need to do is re-purpose the training movements so that they also serve as diagnostic tools. That coach will be able to observe and highlight every aspect of an athlete's movement quality and fix the suboptimal pieces.

This coach/athlete/test/retest–centric model moves the strength-and-conditioning program to the heart of athletic development and the heart of any human-performance/resiliency model. A program that is organized around challenging an athlete's movement capacities with load, speed, cardiorespiratory and metabolic demand, and stress leaves very few body and capacity dysfunction stones unturned. For example, we regularly work with world-class athletes who cannot perform the most basic and light deadlifting, squatting, or pushups without horribly dysfunctional movement. It's not surprising that these same athletes have difficulty maintaining decent spinal or shoulder positioning at the end of a race. If an athlete understands the principles of, say, midline stabilization and shoulder-torque development—both of which are covered in this book—he will be able to apply those principles to another set of movement demands. Running is just maintaining a braced and neutral spine while falling forward and extending the hip. And rowing looks an awful lot like performing a light deadlift while breathing really, really hard. For the strength coach, this is invaluable insight.

The role of the coach is to prepare the athlete physically for the demands of his sport (even if this sport is life or combat), and serve as the athlete's chief movement and mobility diagnostician. The goal of every lab/gym is to ready the athlete for new skill and task acquisition. The athlete who has few mobility restrictions and understands and has been training in principle-based movement is literally a blank canvas for the coach. It doesn't matter if you've never wrestled or played volleyball before: if you understand how to get organized—how to stabilize your trunk and create torque in your extremities—you enter the playing field with a distinct advantage.

Remember, classical strength-and-conditioning movements (gymnastics, Olympic lifting, powerlifting, sprinting, etc.) are the vocabulary of the human movement language. Sport doesn't really look exactly like squatting and benching. But if we connect the dots for our athletes, drawing their attention to the principles inherent in these movements, they can apply those principles to the new set of variables that is their sport. I can't tell you how many calls we get from coaches who want to thank us for preparing athletes for optimal coaching.

Think about it like this: If a person understands grammar and spelling, then he can write a sentence. If a football player understands how to create shoulder torque off a barbell or pull-up bar, he'll be able to find the stable and effective shoulder position needed to tackle another player. Conversely, if the coach observes that the athlete loses effective shoulder stability in the bottom of a bench press, that pattern will probably present as a more vulnerable and less effective shoulder position during tackling.

You Are an Amazing, Adaptable, Healing Machine

The human being has an immense capacity to heal itself. At any age, and in nearly any state, the human animal is capable of an incredible amount of tissue repair and remodeling. Clearly torn ACLs don't magically reattach, and herniated lumbar disks are slow to heal, but the human body will take a ton of abuse for a really long time before it finally gives up the fight.

For example, I was in an elevator in Las Vegas a few years ago with another coach with whom I was teaching a course on human performance at a local gym. On the way down, the elevator stopped and a woman got on. This woman was at least as wide as she was tall. She was holding one of those very long, fifty-plus-ounce beer cups with a big straw, carrying a bag of pastries, and smoking. The best part was, she apparently felt great! She was stoked and actually flirted with the

two of us during our short time together! When she got out, we both looked at each other in awe. I think I spoke first, "Well, that proves one thing. Human beings are very hard to kill."

This is the problem: Our bodies will put up with our silly movement and lifestyle choices because they have a freakish amount of functional tolerance built in. We shouldn't, however, make the classic error of confusing this miraculous genetic inheritance with a tacit rationalization for eating, sleeping, or moving however we please. This incredible mountain of a woman illustrates a larger point: Most of the typical musculoskeletal dysfunction that people and athletes deal with is really just preventable disease.

When thinking about movement dysfunction, it's useful to classify pain and injury in four categories, which I've organized here according to frequency of occurrence:

That which accounts for 2 percent of movement dysfunction in a typical gym:

1. Pathology (something serious is going on with your system)

2. Catastrophic injury (you got hit by a car)

Pathology

This category is in the realm of traditional medicine, and any good practitioner/coach is thinking on this level during any conversation with an athlete: "I don't think it's just back pain you're experiencing. It sounds like you have the makings of a kidney infection." Or: "I don't think you're overtrained. Based on that bright red ring around that suspicious bite on your arm, you may need to get checked out for Lyme disease." These are both real-life examples and why a good clinician always asks about changes in bladder or bowel function, unaccounted-for weight loss or gain, night sweats, dizziness, fever, nausea, or vomiting—just to make sure that "knee pain" isn't "knee cancer." We tell our coaches that if something doesn't fit about the way athletes are talking about their musculoskeletal issues, they should always punt them to their physician. Pathology is dealt with through traditional medicine and honestly accounts for about a whopping 1 percent *or less* of the typical problems we see in the gym.

Catastrophic Injury

This category includes getting hit by a car, jumping downwind out of an airplane at night and landing on a stump, or having a three hundred pound lineman roll into your knee. This is where modern sports medicine excels. Bad things are going to happen to soldiers and athletes working to their limits in their respective fields. Reconstruction and injury-management capabilities are at an all-time high. Fortunately, except for wounded warriors, this category also falls into the 1 percent bucket.

So if we have accounted for roughly 2 percent of the typical movement dysfunction we catch in the gym, where do the other 98 percent reside? Simple, they reside within the preventable-disease categories of overtension and open-circuit faulting.

That which accounts for 98 percent of all the dysfunction we see in the typical athlete:

3. Overtension (missing range-of-motion)

4. Open-circuit faults (moving in a bad position)

Overtension

We regularly observe athletes who lack significant ranges of motion. For example, it's not uncommon to see an Olympic medalist missing 50 percent or more range-of-motion in the anterior-chain system of the hips and quadriceps. Imagine having dinner with a good friend and noticing that he can't bend his elbow past 90-degrees.

"What's wrong with your elbow?" you'd ask.

"Oh, nothing," he'd say. "I just set the bench press world record. But my neck and wrist kill me every time I eat."

This example would be silly except that it is not unusual. In general, though, it occurs in less socially crippling joint/tissue systems like the an-

kle, shoulder, and hip. And don't just think flexion (bending) and extension (straightening). Full range-of-motion has to include your body's rotational capacities as well. Move your hand to your face as if you are going to eat. Is there resistance in this range-of-motion? There shouldn't be. Your limbs and joints should get stiff near end-range and then suddenly stop. They should not be limited in range nor be excessively stiff through full range-of-motion. Either symptom is a simple sign that your tissue-based mechanical system is overtensioned. Put simply, you're missing normal ranges of motion as a result of your tight tissues.

In nearly every athlete we evaluate for compensated mechanics or for injured and painful tissues, we find an obvious and significant restriction in the joints or tissues immediately above or below the site of the dysfunction. Achilles tendinopathy? Weird that your calf is brutally short and stiff and that your ankle has no dorsiflexion. What? You've worn a hole in your kneecap and have chondromalacia? I'll bet that your hip extension is limited and that you don't have full range-of-motion in the tissue of your upper leg. To put it simply: If you have ankle pain, chances are good that your calves are tight and are pulling on your ankle, limiting your range-of-motion. If you have knee pain, chances are good that your quads, hips, hamstrings, and calves (all the musculature that connects to your knee) are brutally tight. It's no mystery why you have pain: You can't get into the correct positions or move with good form because you're missing key ranges of motion. Mitigating overtensioned systems using mobilization techniques feeds "slack" to the "injured" site, reducing localized joint pain by improving the efficiency of the system.

Here's an analogy: A tight hinge on a door will have a pile of dust underneath it. So if the tissues surrounding your knee—quads and calves—are tight, you will literally have a pile of meniscus dust underneath it. The brutally stiff tissues upstream and downstream of the joint cause a mechanical deformation that affects how the joint moves and operates.

It's important to note that when we have traditionally thought of overtensioned tissues pairing, like "hamstrings and back pain,"[1] we have typically laid the lion's share of culpability on the "short muscle" aspect of the system. But it's not this simple. Muscle "length" is a far more complex phenomenon comprising, among other things, intramuscular stiffness, neurodynamics, motor-control, hip and joint mechanics, and even hydration. What does ultimately matter, however, is that if the system is overtensioned, it needs to be remedied—by addressing position and range-of-motion restrictions.

Open-Circuit Faults

This category encompasses most of the serious athletic trauma in the world of strength-and-conditioning. Injuries like ACL tears, flexion-related disk herniations, torn biceps tendons, labral tears of the hip and shoulder, and torn Achilles tendons belong in this category. Your body is a simple mechanical system composed of "wet" biological tissues. It operates best when it is able to create ideal, stable positions before it generates freakish outputs of power.

In fact, most people are familiar with the maxim that functional movement begins in a wave of contraction from the core to sleeve, from trunk to periphery, from axial skeleton to peripheral skeleton. This principle is a good example of the body operating best when all of its circuits are closed—spine stable and braced, hip stable, shoulder stable, ankle not collapsed, etc.—before movement is initiated. The problem is that the body will always be able to generate force, even in poor positions. This is not unlike being able to temporarily get away with driving your car with no oil in the engine or with a flat tire. Sure, you can do it; it just gets expensive. Your body will always default to a "secondary" or "second order" system of stabilization.

Here's an example: Children with cerebral palsy have damaged motor-control systems in their brains. They are cognitively intact; they just have aspects of movement that aren't well controlled in the brain itself. Yet these children are able to ambulate despite this. Their bodies are clever enough to default to a collapsed arch and ankle, internally rotated and valgus knee, internally rotated and impinged hip, and overextended lumbar spine. These kids are literally able to leverage their tissues into secondary positions of stability that turn out to be quite functional—until they wear out. These positions should look familiar to anyone watching a heavy front squat gone wrong. If you don't or can't create a stable position from which to generate force, your body will provide one for you. You don't need to address your ankle or hip range-of-motion; your body will address it by turning your feet out. You don't need to work on restoring anterior hip range-of-motion; your body will overextend at the lumbar spine.

Open-Circuit Faults Include:

▸ Rounded back

▸ Shoulders rolled forward

▸ Overextended lumbar spine

▸ Feet turned out

▸ Head tilted up or down

▸ Elbows flared out

Herein lies the problem: We have confused functionality with physiology. Positions that have served us functionally—like jumping and landing with feet like a duck's—quickly become a liability when speed, load, or fatigue is introduced. Sure, you can lift heavy loads with a rounded back (default spine-stability position) for a long, long time, but at some point your tissues will fail, resulting is some kind of injury. Eventually those "off label" tissue uses with which you exercised and moved so freely will expire.

The implications of this concept are incredible. Most of the ACL injuries in the world are … *preventable*, especially in children. Most of the

---

[1] Coaches and physical therapists have chalked back pain up to having tight hamstrings for ages. Although tight hamstrings contribute to back pain, it's more than likely only part of the problem. It's a system of systems. Position, movement mechanics, and other tight musculature—psoas, hip flexors, quads, to name a few—all play a role.

shoulder dislocations we see are ... *preventable*. Most of the herniated disks we see are ... *preventable*. Remember, your tissues are designed to last 110 years. You just have to know what the stable, tissue-saving, catastrophe-avoiding positions are. And, you have to practice them. A lot.

You Cannot Make Basic Adaptation Errors

As I said earlier, I will teach you how to use the safest and most effective positions for your body so that you can optimize performance and resolve pain and dysfunction. But before moving on to the actual diagnostics, movement, and mobilizations, it's important for you to understand that lifestyle errors have a direct impact on how well or how poorly you move. Let's address these now and set the foundation for your success.

We cannot make basic errors in our lifestyles and expect our bodies to be able to absorb the consequences when we are working in a performance-biased paradigm. For example, it is possible to make fundamental errors in hydration, nutrition, sleep, and stress and not suffer any direct impact on our elliptical biceps training. However, every athlete at the top of his game can make direct correlations between the errors listed above and his potential for creating significant decreases in performance outputs. Being dehydrated by even 2 percent can cause a decrease in VO$_2$ output of 5 percent to 10 percent. Less than six hours of sleep? Say hello to elevated blood-glucose levels (think pre-diabetes). Stressed out? Forget about getting a healthy adaptation response to that crushingly difficult workout—you will simply get crushed.

The less obvious implication of lifestyle maladaptation is on the athlete's tissues. Connective tissue, menisci, spinal disks, fascia, articular cartilages, tendons, and ligaments all suffer from the immediate and downstream effects of unhealthy lifestyle choices. Managing and optimizing the lifestyle aspects of sports performance are certainly beyond the scope of this book, but I would be remiss if I did not mention that we regularly observe significant changes in an athlete's mobility (and ultimately position) when he begins to address and correct these vital aspects.

Adaptation Errors Include:

▶ No warm-up or cool down

▶ Sleep deprivation

▶ Dehydration

▶ Poor nutrition

▶ Prolonged sitting

▶ Chronic inflammation

▶ Stress

▶ Insulin insensitivity

It's easy get overwhelmed when you consider how complicated human movement can be and how many different aspects of your life directly affect mechanics and tissue health. But underlying all of this beautifully complex technology is a simple truth: Your body has an amazing capacity to deal with your poor mechanics. It also has an extraordinary capacity to self-correct with just a little input.

All human beings should be able to perform basic maintenance on their bodies. It is both a human right and a responsibility to understand how your body works.

CHAPTER 2
MIDLINE STABILIZATION AND ORGANIZATION
(SPINAL MECHANICS)

Throughout history, advanced thinkers have harped on the importance of tightening the body, bracing the abdomen, and stabilizing the trunk. The "core to extremity" concept is not a new idea. If you don't organize your spine optimally, you can't stabilize and transmit force to the primary engines of your hips and shoulders. This results in staggering losses of stability, force, and power—all of which could be otherwise channeled into fusion-reactor-hot athletic performance.

Yet the spine remains the weak link. In my physical therapy practice, I see trunk-related errors and weaknesses among the world's best athletes. A stable, well-organized spine is the key to moving safely and effectively *and* maximizing power output and force production. So why do so many athletes regularly commit fundamental spinal sins that impede performance and invite injury?

There are a few reasons. For starters, many athletes focus on completing the lift or movement with little or no regard for good form. Speed is often part of this equation, too. Consider an athlete craning his head back to reach his chin over a bar during a pull-up. After all, it's still possible to generate huge amounts of force from a bad position without immediate, overt negative consequences. I've seen athletes lift enormous loads from rounded and overextended positions and

walk away unharmed, grinning from ear to ear. This isn't always bad, and by that I mean that it may be a *conscious* choice by a professional athlete who has measured what he stands to gain against the cost. One example: the powerlifter who chooses to round his back to break the deadlift world record. He knows damn well he's flirting with potential injury, but he's willing to take the risk. Another example? The Major League pitcher throwing fastballs at 100 mph is less concerned with his elbow than with a multi-million-dollar contract. Again, these are conscious choices.

For most athletes, however, the risk is not worth it. Moving incorrectly, especially in a training environment, not only increases susceptibility to injury, it develops and reinforces faulty body mechanics that will exact payment during more complex movements. Patterns repeated in practice will be revealed at game time. Rounding your back for a deadlift will ensure that you tackle with a flexed spine. Your dysfunctional, overextended spine, pushup position will transfer to overextension in your running. Sure, there is a strength stimulus of sorts, but—and this is a critical message I want you to hear—sacrificing good form will cannibalize your potential benefits. Hear this too: You may get away with poor form at first, but poor mechanics—whether rounding your shoulders in a deadlift or slumping in your computer

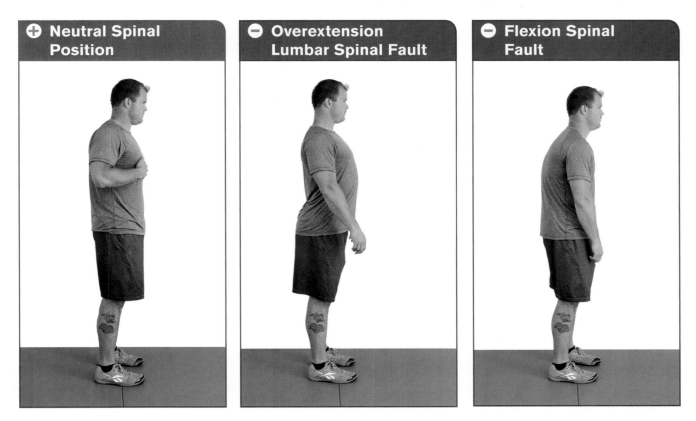

⊕ Neutral Spinal Position

⊖ Overextension Lumbar Spinal Fault

⊖ Flexion Spinal Fault

chair—will ultimately come down hard in the form of pain and injury.

Athletes who aren't aware of these fundamental truths will compromise form by default when training and competing. Of course, they'd never do this if they immediately felt the consequences of their actions, but often they don't. As I've said, you can lift with a rounded back, run like crap, and sit at your computer with your neck and shoulders rounded for a long time … until you can't. That's when your body offers up some hard truths—that you've been moving incorrectly or that you've been hanging out in bad positions. And it doesn't just whisper in your ear; it crams the message down your throat by zapping your ability to generate force and opening the floodgates to pain.

Another problem that keeps athletes from prioritizing midline stabilization or organizing the spine properly is the practice-makes-perfect paradigm, which coaches unfortunately reinforce. Fact is, we do a *great* job celebrating the completion of fifty pushups, but we haven't done a good job of identifying loss of good spinal positioning for our athletes. If you accomplished such a task with a back that looks like a snake that's been hit

by a car, you've just taught yourself to generate pressing force from that broken spinal position. And exercise is only the half of it. If you sit at a computer all day with a rounded back, it shouldn't come as a big shock to you that you can't brace your spine in a good position and stabilize your shoulders during loaded athletic movements.

Then again, athletes aren't completely to blame. Many simply lack a model for bracing their spine (not to mention the fact that most chairs are designed for aesthetics not function). While trainers will talk obsessively about core strength, posture, and bracing, they seldom teach athletes how to organize and brace their spine as an independent sequence. Instead, they attempt to ingrain midline stabilization in athletes as they practice complex movements. This is like teaching a child how to ride a bike and juggle at the same time. The child might get the juggling part down, but there is a good chance he will crash that bike into the nearest mailbox. When midline stabilization isn't taught by itself, the result is often poor bracing strategies. And poor bracing strategies ultimately lead to a host of biomechanical compromises.

Three Reasons for Bracing Your Spine

There is a step-by-step blueprint for stabilizing your spine: It's called the "bracing sequence." But before I delve into that, you should understand the reasons for prioritizing spinal mechanics over everything else.

First, learning how to brace your spine in a good position eliminates one of the greatest threats to the human animal: injury to your central nervous system (CNS). If you injure the meniscus in your knee, you can still soldier on—you can still run, still fight. It might not be all that pleasurable, but you can go on with your life. If you herniate a disk or injure a facet joint, on the other hand, it's game over: The whole human mechanical system shuts down. You are unable to run, lift, move quickly, reproduce, have fun—you can't do jack squat. And it is not a minor interruption; potential injuries to your spine are a hard bell to unring. There will be a long, brutally slow healing process on the docket. In my practice, if an athlete has a little spinal tweak, it's a minimum of two days to get that athlete back into training. And that's for a minor positional fault. We regularly get calls from athletes who have missed a week or two after a minor spine tweak. This is two weeks of preparation (not to mention two weeks of less-than-optimal life experience) missed because of a simple and preventable trunk-related error. Still think that that extra back squat with an overextended lumbar spine was worth it?

Second, a disorganized spine will lead to mechanical compromises. For example, I regularly run into athletes who look as if they have horribly restricted posterior-chain tissues—specifically their hamstrings. Old school thinking would have us fix the problem by stretching those stiff cables running down the backs of the legs. While this may in fact improve hamstring flexibility, it doesn't alleviate the back pain. What we've found is that if we simply organize an athlete's spine into a braced, stable position, range-of-motion improves by upwards of 50 percent. This is why we prioritize mid-line stabilization and good movement mechanics over mobilization techniques, because what often looks like tight musculature is really just the body

protecting the nervous system. So before we have someone smash the crap out of his hamstrings, we make sure his spine is in a good position.

Third, when you lose spinal positioning—head, ribcage, or pelvic fault—you potentially shut down force production and lose the ability to stabilize your hips and shoulders. That's right, your shoulder and knee pain could stem from your trunk instability.

To clarify this, think of your trunk and spine as a chassis for the primary engines of your hips and shoulders. If your spine is in a bad position, creating a safe, functionally stable hip, knee, ankle, or shoulder position is impossible. Again, that's why we fix spinal positioning before we go after the poor mechanics or tissue restrictions at the shoulders or hips: You'll never fix those big engines if the chassis is broken.

So it doesn't matter what is going on at your shoulder, elbow, knee, or ankle—whether it is a motor-control or mobility issue: If your spine is out of whack you're never going to be able to fix the problem.

The Bracing Sequence

To reiterate, people default into mechanically unstable spinal positions for three reasons:

1. They have a task-completion, get-the-job-done mindset.

2. They've ingrained poor positions and movement patterns in their training and day-to-day life.

3. They don't have a reproducible, all-encompassing bracing strategy that transfers to the majority of movements.

The bottom line is that you need to have a conscious plan for bracing your spine in a neutral position, a step-by-step template that will give you the same results every single time. That way, when you're tired, scared, or under stress, your default motor pattern is the same: you revert back to the same mechanically stable, neutrally braced spinal position.

Bracing Sequence

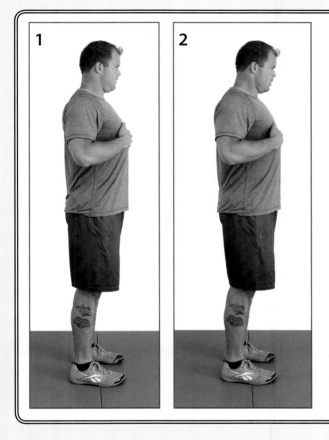

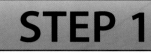

STEP 1

Squeeze your butt as hard as you can.

The first thing you need to do is set your pelvis in a neutral position. To accomplish this, position your feet directly under your hips—keeping your feet parallel to each other—screw your feet into the ground and squeeze your butt as hard as you can. Don't think about tilting your pelvis. Just squeeze your butt. You will always end up in the right position because it's your butt—those glutes were engineered specifically for your pelvis and spine. A lot of people mistakenly think they can get tight by simply engaging their abdomen. Although the musculature of your trunk stabilizes your spine, it's nearly impossible to use your abdominals to control the position of your pelvis. For that reason, you have to use your butt to set the position.

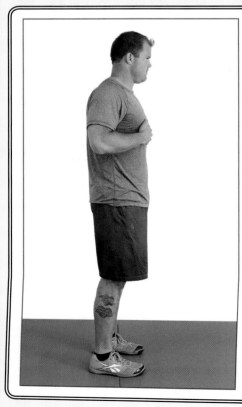

STEP 2

Pull your ribcage down.

Next, pull your lower ribs in, balancing your ribcage over your pelvis. Imagine that your pelvis and ribcage are two bowls filled to the brim with liquid. The idea is to keep your pelvis and ribcage neutral so that liquid doesn't spill out either end. If you overextend, water pours out the front of your pelvis and out the back of your ribcage. If you round forward into flexion, water pours out the back of your pelvis and out the front of your ribcage. Although this analogy only applies to standing perfectly upright in a braced-neutral position—you can still be in a braced-neutral position and hinge forward or lean back—the idea is to get your ribcage and pelvis aligned.

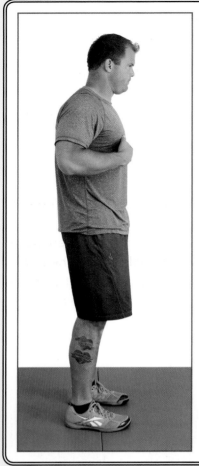

STEP 3

Get your belly tight.

The next step is to lock your pelvis and ribcage in place with your abdominals. You can't move with your butt squeezed so you need to lock in the position by engaging your abs. Think about it like this: Glutes set position, abs brace position. And you need at least 20 percent tension to set and maintain a braced-neutral spinal position. To correctly execute this step, continue squeezing your glutes, take in a big breath of air, and then exhale. As you let the air out, engage your abs and get your belly tight. Think about shrink-wrapping your spine with your abdomen by pulling your bellybutton to your spine. It's not sucking in or hollowing; it's not even drawing in; it's stiffening in place as you exhale. As the musculature of your trunk compresses toward your midline, you create a higher intra-abdominal pressure around your spine, creating an even more rigid lever. Another way to approach this step is to think about lifting your pelvic floor, which is expressed with the common cue sphincter to bellybutton. With your spine neutral, butt squeezed, and your belly tight (stiffening as you exhale), now you can breathe into that tight space or already compressed spinal system as if you were putting compressed air into a steel tank. You don't make the tank tight around the air; you put air into the rigid tank (see "Breathing Mechanics," page 39).

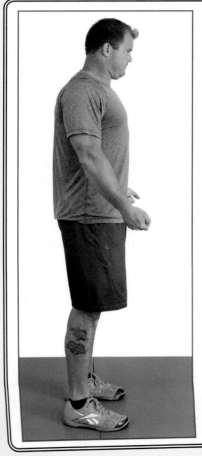

STEP 4

**Set your head in a neutral position and
screw your shoulders into a stable position.**

Lastly, center your head over your shoulders, and gaze forward. Think about aligning your ears over your shoulders, hips, and ankles. As you do this, draw the heads of your arm bones back, spreading your collarbones wide, and release your shoulders down. Keep your thumbs pointed forward and think about aligning. Note: You don't need to squeeze your shoulder blades together; just feel the tips of your shoulder blades reaching toward your hips. This puts you in a stable position and represents a stable shoulder position.

Go through this load-order sequence, burning the checklist into your motor program, so that you can reproduce the same stable position in any situation or environment. This takes time. In the beginning, it might take 20 to 30 percent of your mental RAM just to keep your shoulders in a stable, externally rotated position, your abs on tension, and your back flat. You have to cultivate the mindset that anything that is not a braced-neutral spinal position is probably going to kill you.

To bring awareness to the bracing sequence, I developed a simple and effective method to help coaches and athletes highlight spinal positioning. I call it the two-hand rule.

The Two-Hand Rule

This is a technique to help people see and feel the difference between a braced-neutral position and a broken position, like when they're rounded forward or overextended.

Here's how it works: Take one thumb and put it on your sternum—keeping your hand splayed, palm facing down—and pin your other thumb on your pubic bone, creating two parallel planes. The key is to keep your hands on the same horizontal plane as your ribcage and pelvis so that any deviation from neutral will reflect in a change in hand position. If your hands move apart, you're overextended. If your hands move together, you're rounded forward.

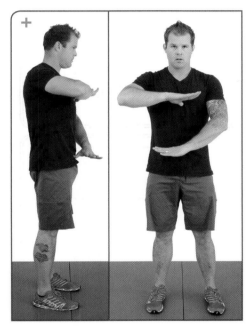

You can apply the two-hand rule to everyday life positions like standing, sitting, and lying down. It can also be used with basic body weight movements like squatting, walking, or running.

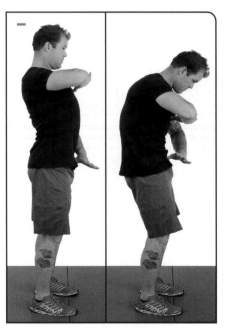

Although we should think of the spine as one contiguous stable structure with the same nervous system running through it, dividing it into parts is a convenient way to spot spinal faults. This is why the two-hand rule is so effective: it brings a heightened sense of awareness to these reference points—pelvis and ribcage—so that you can start to identify where you or your athlete is losing form.

There's just one problem with this model. We miss a key reference point, which is every bit as important as the pelvis and ribcage—the head. In fact, it would be very useful if we had a third hand because there are three main parts to the spinal system: the head (cervical spine), ribcage (thoracic spine), and pelvis (lumbar spine). If any one of these pieces is out of alignment, it's difficult to create optimal positioning.

When using the two-hand rule to bring awareness to the bracing sequence and spotting spinal faults, don't forget that your head is an essential factor: if your head is out of position—meaning that it's tilted forward or back—you compromise spinal position and lose the ability to stabilize the structures of your primary engines. The Tony Blauer test is a perfect example of this.

Pelvic Floor Dysfunction

Whenever you're in an overextended position, your pelvic floor turns off, which can unleash problems galore, especially among women. For example, one of the things that happens when women jump and land, or more commonly when they're doing double unders—meaning passing a rope under the feet twice per jump when jumping rope—is that they have trouble controlling their bladder. (And this is one of the problems with doing pike double unders.) Fixing this problem is really simple: squeeze your butt to set your pelvis in a neutral position, and then get your belly tight to brace the position. What you'll find is that a lot of the issues caused by pelvic floor dysfunction spontaneously resolve once your pelvis is locked into a neutral position.

➕ JUMPING WITH A NEUTRAL SPINE

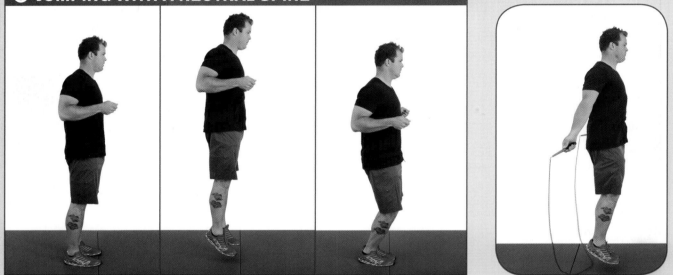

Whether you're performing double unders or jumping up and down, you want to go through the bracing sequence, keep your shoulders back, and maintain abdominal tension to keep you pelvis locked in a neutral position.

➖ LUMBAR OVEREXTENSION SPINAL FAULT

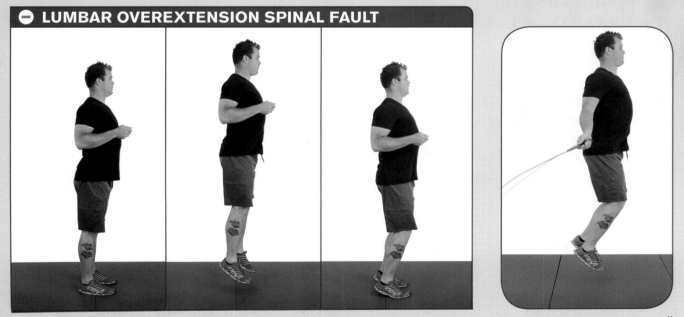

If your butt and abs are offline, maintaining a neutral spinal position is nearly impossible to manage. You will automatically default into an overextended position. This is a mechanism for low back pain and a host of other problems.

TONY BLAUER TEST

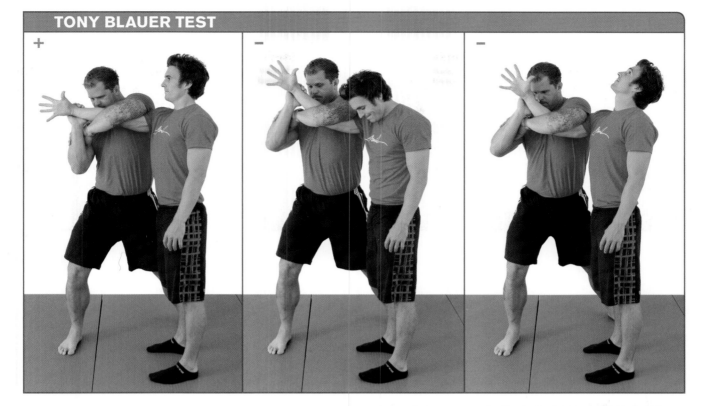

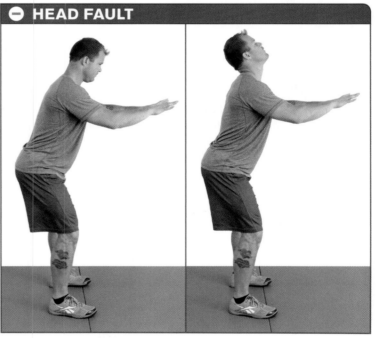

HEAD FAULT

I've established a figure four lock on Carl's right arm. With his arm straight, spine neutral, fingers splayed, and shoulder externally rotated, I can't bend his arm. But the moment he looks up or down, or deviates from a neutral head position, his arm bends instantaneously. This drill really helps to illuminate the fact that if you break a neutral head position, it throws a kink in the entire system and destabilizes the structures downstream, making it impossible to maintain an integrated position. The same thing occurs during a squat. The moment you throw your head back, you immediately default into an overextended position.

As you can see, the moment an athlete deviates from a neutral head position, you lose stability and the flow of potential force with it. And this is not limited solely to the head. Anytime you see one or two vertebral segments hinge or express greater degrees of motion in relation to the rest of the spine—whether it's the head, ribcage, or pelvis—creating a stable carriage is nearly impossible. This is what I refer to as a local-extension or local-flexion spinal fault.

⊖ LOCAL EXTENSION AND FLEXION SPINAL FAULTS

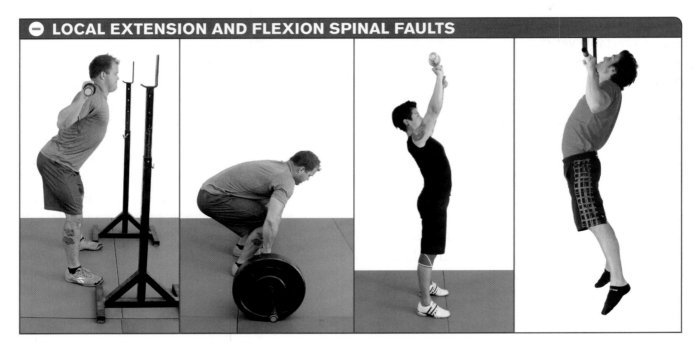

If you overextend at your lumbar spine as you initiate a squat, round your back while picking something off the ground, tilt your ribcage back as your press a weight overhead, or crane your head back to raise your chin over the bar during a pull-up, you're committing a local extension fault that compromises your entire biomechanical system. (To learn how to correct these faults, see chapter 5, "Movement Hierarchy.")

This is why we have to look at the spine as a continuum. If you're trying to generate force and one section of your spine is wobbling back and forth, you're doomed. Not only will you leak power, but you'll also risk creating significant spinal shear forces across your nervous system and the structures of your spine. You're opening the door to destructive forces—in the short run, it can shut down force production, and in the long run, it may result in spondylolisthesis, herniated discs, pars fractures, and stenosis.

Braced-Neutral Standing Position

Now that you have a model for organizing your spine in a neutral position and can spot local extension faults, you can start to apply the bracing sequence to fundamental positions like standing and sitting. Whether you're at work, chatting with a friend in the grocery store, or standing at attention, your basic setup is always the same: feet straight, back flat, belly tight, head neutral, and shoulders externally rotated in a stable position.

Don't be that guy or gal who stands with arms crossed, shoulders rolled forward, back slouched, feet angled out, etc. Besides destroying your squat and running mechanics, it's not sexy.

⊕ IDEAL STANDING POSITION

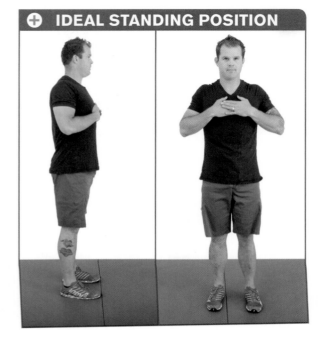

As you can see from the photos, I prefer to place my hands on my chest because it puts my shoulders in a comfortable yet stable position, which is what you might consider my active standing position. This is just a personal preference. With my hands up and in front of my body, I'm ready to do pretty much anything: I can defend, attack, text, whatever. But let me be clear: I'm not advocating that you stand around with your hands on your chest. It's just one example of an effective standing position that gives you movement options, which is especially important if you're military or law enforcement personnel. You can position your arms any way you want as long as they are in an externally rotated, stable position: if your shoulders are internally rotated (rolled forward) it puts strain on the system, pulling you into a flexed position.

The other issue here is that standing with your butt squeezed all day and keeping your abs tight for prolonged periods of time is impossible. At some point, your muscles will fatigue, causing you to default into a weakened position. (No wonder your back is cooked after standing all day!) The easiest way to take a load off your lumbar spine and reduce trunk tension is to prop your foot up on something. You still want to maintain a moderate amount of tension, with the glute of your grounded leg activated, but placing your foot on a bar or a short stool will reduce the amount of tension required to keep your pelvis in a neutral position. You can also lean your butt against a bar stool to give your legs a bit of a rest. The idea is to vary your position often to avoid fatigue, focusing on staying in a braced-neutral position while you transition from one position to another. If you're typing, just bend your arms to about 90-degrees, and then flip your palms down, rotating from your elbows.

The takeaway is this: Standing is a technique in and of itself. Just because you have a workstation that enables you to stand doesn't make you immune to muscle stiffness and back pain. Sure, you open up your hips and turn on the musculature of your legs, but it's not a cure-all. You need to practice the bracing sequence and remain conscious of your position at all times.

CAPTAIN MORGAN POSE

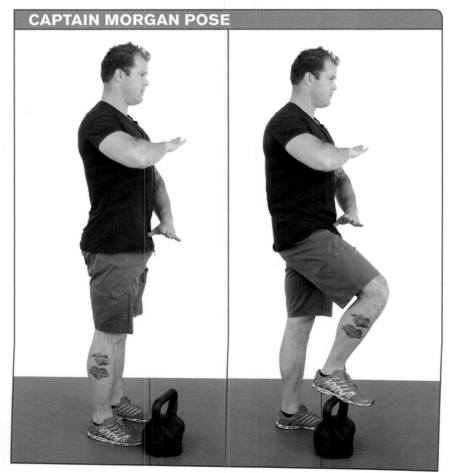

Stabilizing Your Head And Jaw Positioning

People will do some crazy things with their jaws in an attempt to stabilize their head and neck system. For example, if someone is surprised or getting ready to take a punch, he'll clinch his jaw tight.

What you have to remember is that your jaw is a large open circuit right in the middle of a complex and very important kinetic chain. To avoid defaulting to a compensated head or neck position (i.e., Olympic-lifter yawn), you need a strategy for setting your jaw in a good position.

The general recommendation is this: Relax your face, pin your tongue to the roof of your mouth, jamming it behind your teeth, and close your jaw. This will allow you to create tension in your jaw without clinching, opening your mouth, shortening your neck flexors, or compromising breathing mechanics. It's that simple. There are even companies that build specific mouthguards to help facilitate this!

Braced-Neutral Sitting Position

I have a saying: Sitting is death. Sure, sitting causes muscle tightness, but that's not all. Long periods of sitting devour your potential for peak athletic performance. This is even truer for those who spend seven to nine hours a day sitting in compromised positions, in chairs designed primarily for aesthetics, not function. It's no wonder you feel like a broken-down mess and experience back pain, shoulder pain, hip pain, and carpal tunnel agony after sitting on a plane, in a car, or at your desk at work. You've forced yourself into a toxic position that feasts on athletic potential.

The trouble is, you can't avoid sitting. It's an unfortunate construct of modern society. So the question is: How do you avoid or at least reduce the havoc wreaked by extended periods of sitting?

For starters, learn how to sit. Sitting—like standing—is one of the most technically challenging things we do. Yet most of us are clueless when it comes to sitting well. In order to stabilize your spine in a neutral position, you have to get organized while standing by following the bracing sequence. (Note: A basic understanding of how to box-squat—see page 94—also plays a key role in organizing yourself to sit.) Once seated, you need to keep at least 20 percent tension in your abs to maintain a rigid spine.

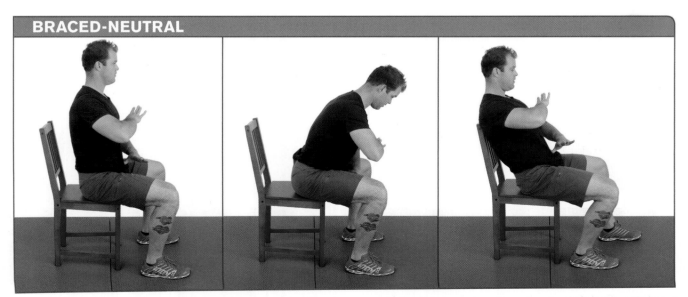

BRACED-NEUTRAL

You're not limited to just sitting perfectly upright: You can still lean forward, or lean back while maintaining a braced-neutral spine.

And herein lies the problem: Keeping your abs engaged at 20 percent is extremely taxing. All the research indicates that it's not muscular strength, but muscular endurance, that dictates loss of spinal position. (Muscular strength is like doing a one-rep-max back squat, while muscular endurance is like doing a thirty-rep back squat.) This is why so many people tweak their backs at the end of a run or workout. This also helps explain why most people collapse into a horribly rounded or overextended position after only a couple of minutes. It's more comfortable and doesn't require any work. Maintaining a stable position, on the other hand, takes extreme focus and abdominal endurance.

The best way to avoid defaulting into a bad position is to stand up and get reorganized every ten to fifteen minutes. It's almost impossible to remain in a good position for anything longer than that. I know—this is a huge pain in the ass and not always possible. But if you want to heal your body and reach the performance goals you're entitled to, you have to do the work. You have to make sacrifices. So pony up!

Another helpful strategy is to change your position as often as possible. What you have to remember is that you don't need to stay locked in a sitting position all the time. You can kneel in front of the computer to open up your hips while answering emails, go for a walk while talking on the phone, or even stretch while sitting at your desk. The key is to avoid correcting your posture once you're already seated.

The moment you sit down, your glutes go on vacation. This not only places additional stress on your spine, but also makes it difficult to stabilize your pelvis in a neutral position. So if you fail to address the bracing sequence before you sit down, don't keep your belly tight, or round or overextend your spine once seated, fixing your position from your chair is difficult. For example, say you flop down into your favorite armchair for Super Bowl Sunday and slouch. After the pre-game, you become aware of how bad your posture is (or just become uncomfortable) and try to fix it by flattening your back. Although it may seem as if you're rectifying the problem, all you're doing is going from a flexed position to an overextended one.

PELVIC GIMMBLE

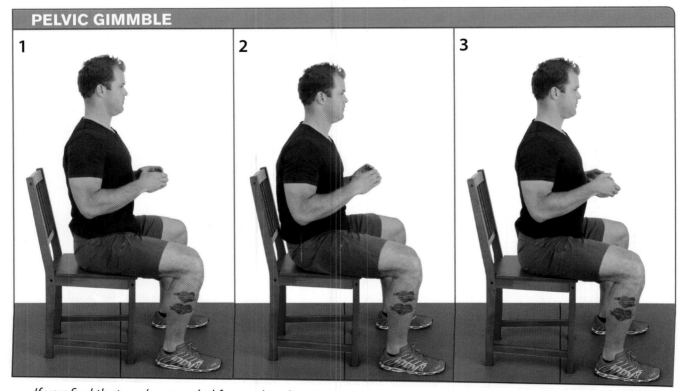

If you find that you've rounded forward and try to correct that by straightening your back, you'll probably just end up in an overextended position. Instead, stand up, run through the bracing sequence, and then sit back down, keeping your back flat and belly tight.

The same thing happens during a squat (see butt wink fault, page 91) when athletes fail to brace from the top position. It's a big thumbs down.

In addition to getting up and changing your position, you need to work on restoring function to the tissues that become adaptively short and tight after long periods of sitting. As a rule, you should mobilize for four minutes for every thirty minutes of sitting. For example, you could do the couch stretch—a brutal hip opener you can find on page 331—for two minutes on each side every half hour. The idea is to tackle the areas that become restricted, specifically your glutes, psoas and other hip flexors, thoracic spine, hamstrings, and quads (to mention a few). Think of it as a mobilization penalty based on sitting time.

Realize that these are just ideas to get you thinking. It doesn't matter how much you mobilize, stand up, or change your position, or what kind of chair, keyboard, or mouse you have: if you're hanging out in a position that's compromising your posture, you will continue to experience the same consequences. That said, getting an ergonomic chair or using some kind of lumbar support (which is particularly useful during long car rides) will definitely give your lower back a break and put you into a more conducive posture.

Abdominal Tension

As I've mentioned, your abs should have some tone all the time. The minimum tension to maintain a braced-neutral spine for basic standing and sitting positions is about 20 percent of your peak stiffness. However, the moment you add dynamic movement or axial load (a force compressing on your spine), you need to increase abdominal tension or trunk stiffness to avoid rounding or flexing your back. For example, if you're running around the block or doing pushups, you might need about 40 percent trunk stiffness to maintain a good spinal position. But if you're going for a max deadlift, you will need 100 percent abdominal tension.

But perhaps you can't relate to numbers like 20 percent or 40 percent. You might find it helpful to rate abdominal tension on a scale from 1 to 10—with one being little to no tension, ten being max tension. On this scale:

▶ Sitting in a chair requires a 2 (20 percent).

▶ Pushups or running around the block requires a 4 (40 percent).

▶ Max back squat, deadlift, or a 50-meter sprint requires a full 10 (100 percent).

In short, the tension necessary to maintain a braced, well-organized spine largely depends on the action and load on your spine. What you need to understand is how and when to cycle up to peak stiffness based on the demands of your exercise or activity. A cobra doesn't cruise around with its head up and hood flared out all the time: It hits peak tension when it's getting ready to strike. Similarly, you don't want to walk around with trunk stiffness at a 10 or attempt a high rep, heavy back squat with abdominal tension at a 2. Knowing how much tension you need to preserve a braced-neutral position is a skill that requires a ton of practice. The better you are at this, the less energy and thought you have to put in to managing abdominal tension. It becomes instinctual.

Belly-Whack Test

As with the two-hand rule, the belly-whack test is another way to help bring consciousness to a braced-neutral position and the 20 percent constant-tension concept. It's simple: You should always have enough abdominal tone to take a whack to the belly. We do this at our gym and around the house. If you've got a spongy middle, you get caught right away.

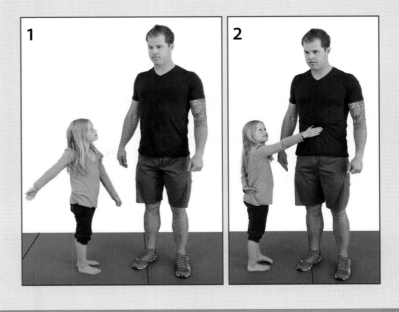

Breathing Mechanics

One more thing: As I discussed in the bracing sequence, to create a braced-neutral position you have to breathe in through your diaphragm, then engage your abs or stiffen your trunk as you exhale. Maintaining this diaphragmatic breathing pattern is, however, extremely difficult in positions that require high tension or an enormous load. What usually happens when people don't have a bracing strategy or a model for getting into a braced-neutral position is that they inhale and the hold their breathe with their lungs full of air, which is not only ineffective, but costly.

If you lie on your back and put your hand on your stomach, you should feel your belly rise and descend as you inhale and exhale. This is diaphragmatic breathing. When you're braced correctly, you will automatically default to this breathing pattern.

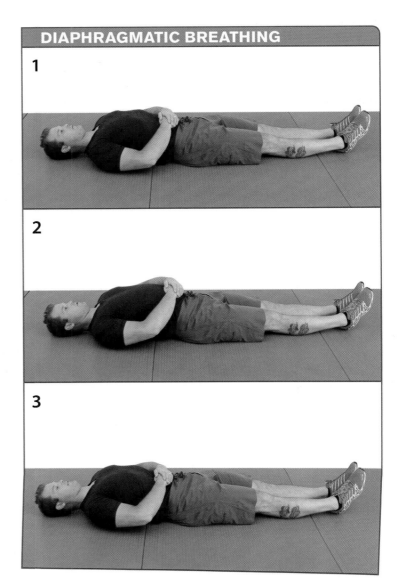

DIAPHRAGMATIC BREATHING

⊖ CHEST AND NECK BREATHING FAULT

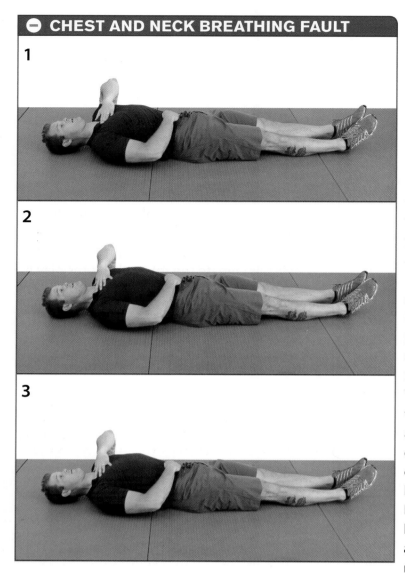

1

2

3

If you're keeping your belly tight, but not diaphragmatic breathing, your breath will be confined to your chest and neck.

Imagine taking in a huge breath and then stiffening your trunk with all that air trapped inside. Do you think you could perform a high-rep back squat while keeping your spine rigid? Better yet, could you take a punch to the belly? Not a chance in hell. It's like this: You can use your diaphragm to stabilize your trunk, but the moment you have to breathe, you surrender your spinal position. So it might work for a max-effort deadlift, but you're doomed after your first rep or the moment you have to breathe. You can imagine how this bracing strategy will play out when you do anything highly aerobic. With your diaphragm jammed down to stabilize your spine, you have only one breathing option, and that is to breathe using only your neck and chest. Now you're reduced to taking very shallow breaths, which will restrict respiration and make it difficult for you to create and maintain stability. It is perilously incorrect.

This is why it's so important to do, say, high-rep back squats and lift heavy objects while under cardiorespiratory stress. In addition to challenging your capacity to maintain a rigid position while breathing hard, it mimics the realities of the real-life scenarios we face as athletes, soldiers, and firefighters. Having said that, let me caution those of you who are coaches: It's best to stick to low-risk tests when you teach these concepts to novice athletes. One good way to find out whether an athlete can breathe while maintaining a rigid spine is to have him perform the active straight-leg test (which follows). Make sure he can get braced and breathe through his diaphragm before you introduce more complex, heavily loaded movements.

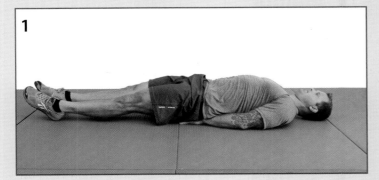

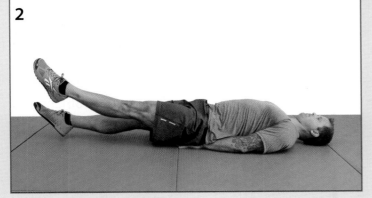

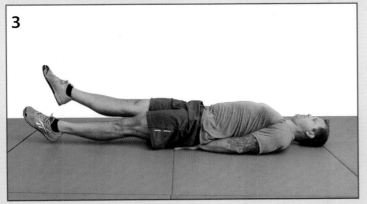

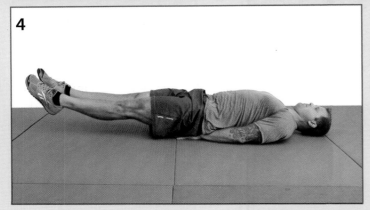

Active Straight-Leg Test

To correctly execute this test, lie on the ground and go through the bracing sequence on page 29. Next, lift one leg off the ground at a time (you can use the two-hand-rule principle), and then both legs. You will notice that with each subsequent step, you have to increase the level of tension in your glutes and abs in order to maintain a neutral spinal position. Again, this is an excellent way to test the fluency of your bracing strategy.

In addition, the active straight-leg test really helps illuminate the role your glutes play in keeping a neutral spinal position: if you lie on your back and raise your legs off the ground with your butt offline, you will immediately default into an overextended position.

1. Lie on your back. Squeeze your butt, pull your legs together, and point your toes. Then take in a big breath and get your belly tight as you exhale. Think about stiffening your belly around your spine as you let out air. An important distinction worth noting here is I'm not telling you to push your low back into the ground. The key is to squeeze your butt and then engage your abs to lock in a neutral spinal position.

2. Keeping your toes pointed, legs straight, and your lower back flush with the ground, raise your left leg. It's important to note that by pointing your toes, it makes it easier to activate your glutes.

3. Next, raise your opposite leg off the ground. Again, there should be no change in spinal position.

4. To increase stabilization demand, raise both legs off the ground.

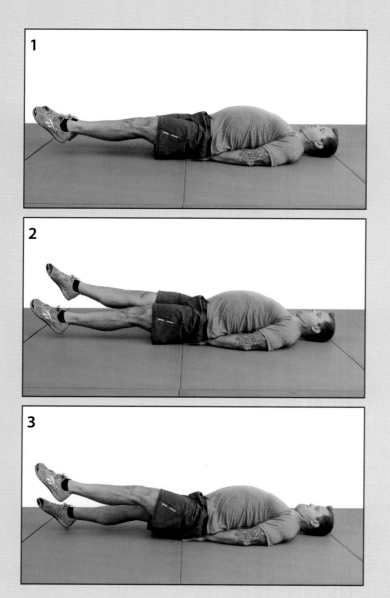

Spinal-Flinch Fault

If there is a change in spinal position—whether it's a global arch, an anterior pelvic tilt, or a ribcage spinal flinch (in which the ribcage tilts back)—chances are good that you failed to squeeze your butt and tighten your belly. If that happens, readdress the bracing sequence.

Now, it's important to understand that if you're bracing correctly—meaning that your belly is tight and your spine is neutral—you don't need to put a conscious effort into breathing through your diaphragm. It's a self-regulating system. Breathing through your diaphragm is the most effective way to preserve a stable position, plain and simple.

For example, if you watch elite gymnasts in moments of peak tension or strongmen under enormous loads, they will take short, concise breaths through their diaphragm—diaphragmatic gasps—and reconstitute trunk stiffness every time they exhale. They never lose spinal stiffness, disengage their abdomen, or stop breathing through their diaphragm. Rather, they keep their trunk stiff while continuing to breathe into that compressed system: take a short breath in, exhale into tension, take a short breath in, and exhale into tension, all while keeping the belly tight. It's important to note that when you're in full kickass mode, you will inevitably use your sternum and chest to help facilitate breathing, but as long as you prioritize bracing and diaphragmatic breathing, your body will take care of the rest.

The same pattern applies to all sports: When we restore position, we restore function. When we improve position, we improve function.

CHAPTER 3
ONE-JOINT RULE

When I teach seminars to a new group of athletes, coach someone for the first time, or rehab an athlete coming off an injury, I always start with the bracing sequence (page 29). It's the first and most important step in rebuilding and ingraining functional motor patterns, optimizing movement efficiency, maximizing force production, and preventing injury.

The problem is not necessarily getting athletes to prioritize spinal mechanics. Rather, it is getting them to preserve a stable, well-organized trunk during complex, loaded athletic movements. In fact, most athletes grasp the midline-stabilization/spinal-mechanics concept and have no trouble applying the bracing sequence to fundamental static positions. It's not until you ask them to change shapes while maintaining a neutral spinal—hinge from their hips, move from their shoulders, or set up in an unfamiliar position—that the glaring flaws in their bracing strategy become apparent.

The majority of human movements—specifically formal training exercises—require you to create and maintain spinal stiffness through a full range-of-motion. In other words, you should be able to lower into the bottom of the squat, press a barbell overhead, and set up for a deadlift without defaulting into a broken spinal position (characterized by spinal flexion or extension fault). And this is where a lot of athletes start to have problems. Either they can't keep their spine rigid at the end-range positions because they are missing range-of-motion, or they don't have the motor-control to preserve spinal stiffness through range. Think of the athlete setting up for a deadlift who can't help rounding his shoulders. If he's missing range-of-motion in his hamstrings as he hinges from his hips (he's reached his end-range position), he will have to compensate by rounding forward to grab the bar. Conversely, if he doesn't have the strength or doesn't know how to perform the lift correctly (motor-control), chances are that he will default into a rounded position. This is why it's helpful to show athletes the bracing sequence, and then challenge their organizational strategy with basic movements.

There are two really easy ways to do this. The first is to have them raise their arms overhead—either from the standing position or while lying down—and the second is to have them bend over and touch their toes.

The former expresses movement through their shoulders, while the latter requires them to hinge from their hips. If they default into an overextended or rounded position, it's a clear indication that they made a setup or movement error.

OVERHEAD TEST

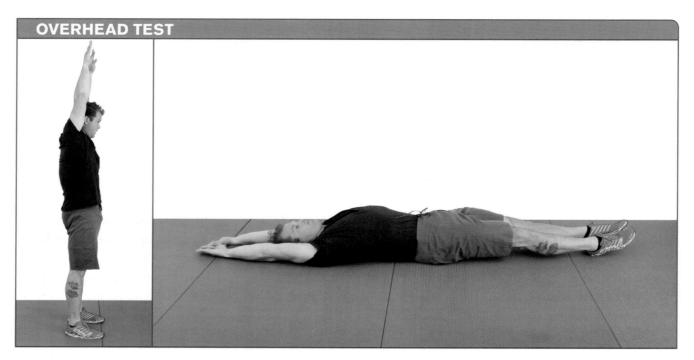

HIP HINGE TEST

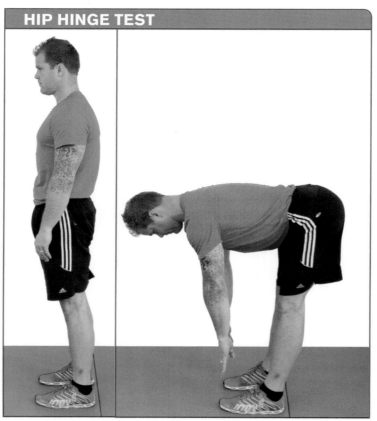

Remember, your spine is not meant to handle loaded flexed or extended positions. The musculature is designed to create stiffness so that you can effectively transmit energy to the primary engines of your hips and shoulders. If you don't preserve trunk stiffness while moving from your hips and shoulders, you will lose power and force. This is the basis of the one-joint rule: you should see flexion and extension movement happen only at the hips and shoulders, not your spine.

It's important to realize that your hips and shoulders function in much the same way—hence the one-joint rule. They are both ball-in-socket joints; they both have a ton of rotational capacity; and both are designed to handle freakish amounts of flexion and extension load.

Consider men's rings gymnastics. The athlete locks out his wrists and elbows and then moves his shoulders in all directions while keeping his whole body stiff.

Although the parameters are simple, the degree of shoulder strength, trunk stability, and motor-control required is mind-boggling. That's why only a few people in the world can pull off a legitimate iron cross.

When thinking about it like this, you can see how the one-joint rule is really just an extension of the two-hand-rule principle. That is, if you see flexion or extension anywhere in the spine, it's an error. This gives coaches a really easy template for spotting spinal faults. Anytime you see an athlete's spine change shape during a movement, you automatically know that: a) he didn't set up correctly, or b) he doesn't have the motor-control or mobility to get into or maintain the correct position.

No doubt, managing an organized spine during loaded athletic movements is very difficult. Keeping your back flat during a heavy deadlift, overhead press, or squat is no joke. It takes humongous motor-control and a keen understanding of how these systems work.

And here's the rub: It doesn't matter how strong you are; if you're a big, floppy mess or your technique is not up to par, you will leak power, bleed force, and dump torque from the system.

PUSHUP

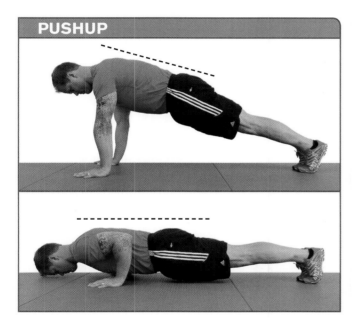

The majority of human movements require that you keep your spine in a neutral position through the entire range-of-motion. If you are performing a pushup, for example, movement should occur in the shoulders and elbows, not in the spine.

If you are performing the squat, movement should occur in your hips and knees. Again, there should be no movement in your spinal system.

SQUAT

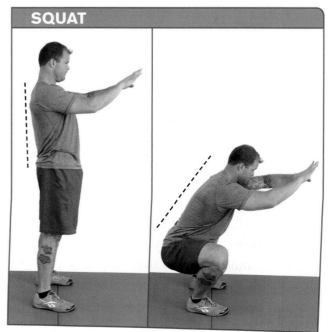

Braced Spinal Extension and Flexion

A braced-neutral spine is always ideal for the majority of human movements—squatting, pulling, running, jumping, and so forth. However, there are situations when assuming a flat-back position is impossible. For example, if you have to lift a keg, a massive stone, or a super heavy, awkward object, good luck trying to get into anything but a braced-rounded or braced-extended position. Is it ideal? No way. It is technically a compromised position, but it's the only position that works in these circumstances. And you need to be able to pick up heavy, awkward objects and not mess up your back. It's part of being a fully functional human being.

To avoid injury and optimize position, it is critical that you pay attention to the details. When you lift something from a braced-flexed or braced-extended position, you have to brace in that arched position and maintain that position through the full range of the movement. And this is where people get confused. Braced flexion or extension is characterized with a greater global arch, usually in the thoracic spine. Arching does not represent a loss of position; arching is bracing against your neutral spine.

All the same rules apply. You're still *not* changing your spinal position under load or during the movement, and you're *not* committing a local extension fault (see page 34). Rather, your spine is braced and stable in a slightly flexed or extended thoracic arched position at the start, and you maintain that fixed shape throughout range. The thoracic spine is able to handle braced flexion loads better than the lumbar spine.

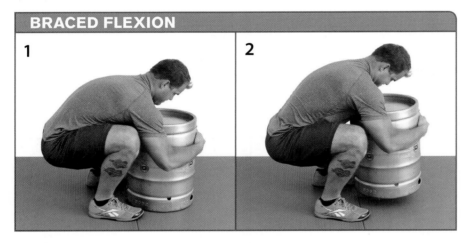

BRACED FLEXION

1

2

If you examine the photos, you'll notice that there is a global arch in my upper back. I get braced against the object and maintain that position as I lift the keg off the ground. The same rules apply to extension. If you have to load something onto your chest and then lift it overhead, focus on keeping your butt squeezed to stabilize your lower back and maintain the deviation away from a perfectly setup spine.

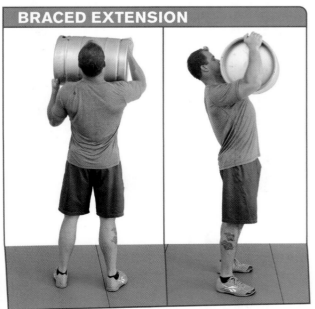

BRACED EXTENSION

Global Spinal Extension and Flexion

There are other situations that require an athlete to flex and extend into globally arched positions. After all, you can't move around with your spine stiff and straight all the time. In order to perform the dynamic actions of sport, you need to be able to create flexion and extension throughout the entire system. Imagine a volleyball player's spike, a tennis player's serve, or a pitcher throwing a 100 mph fastball. In all these movements, the athletes are essentially using the spine as a whip, creating a global opening and closing, or flexing and extending, throughout the entire spinal system.

As with braced extension and braced flexion, these positions are expressed as a continuum of flexion and extension throughout the entire spine. There is rarely axial load on your spine, and you're not flexing or extending at a single joint (committing a local extension fault). So when someone tumbles, summersaults, or does a back flip, we're seeing a global arch, which is very challenging. This is why doing the cobra pose in yoga is so difficult—it entails extending to create a global arch. It's no wonder that most people extend at only one or two segments of their lumbar or cervical spine. It's easier.

Although it's difficult to teach these globally extended and flexed, dynamic, violent, stable, high-speed positions, there are things that you can do in the gym to help develop motor-control and highlight the mobility dysfunction that may prevent you from getting into the ideal positions when it matters most. This is why it's useful to implement movements like the kipping pull-up (page 171): it not only teaches you how to create dynamic, globally arched positions, but it also ensures full range-of-motion in your spine. Even having someone swing from the bar can be used as a diagnostic. If you can't get into these large global shapes, you should ask a very important question: What's going on?

GLOBAL FLEXION

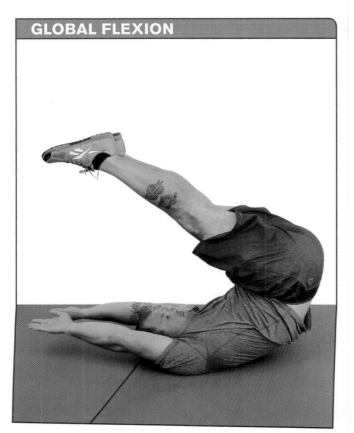

GLOBAL FLEXION AND EXTENSION

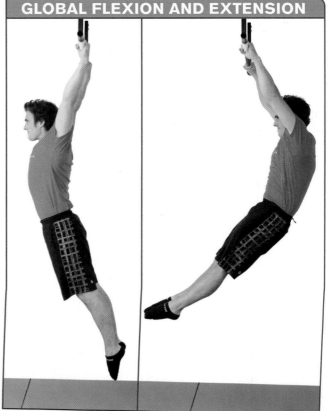

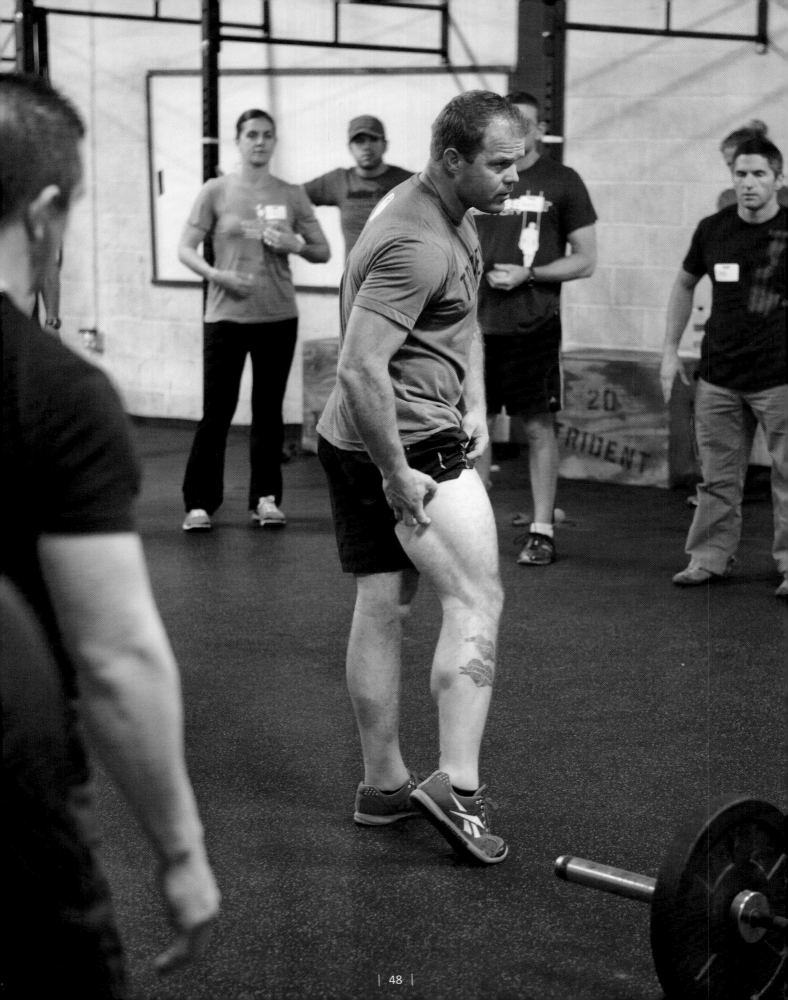

CHAPTER 4
LAWS OF TORQUE

TORQUE: Something that produces or tends to produce torsion or rotation; the moment of a force or system of forces tending to cause rotation.

Watch a video of a powerlifter setting up underneath a bar loaded with 800-pounds to perform a squat. Although he might look as if he has the raw power capacity of a class 8 tow truck, you will notice that his form is precise. He hinges from the hips, keeps his abs tight and his back as flat as humanly possible. He doesn't lose position, wobble, or make compensations. The primal expression on his face and his monstrous body might suggest that he is capable of just about any superhuman lifting feat, but he knows that things can go terribly wrong in an instant, and with 800-pounds perched on his shoulders, not completing the lift could be the least of his worries. In order to move such a staggering amount of weight, he must channel the strongman's magic ingredient—torque. It must flow through him like a supercharged magnetic field.

There is no getting around the laws of torque. This principle of movement is bedrock to all safe, high-yield athletic movements.

Torque gives the powerlifter the ability to minimize the variability in movement. If there is no torque, there will be instability. And if there is instability, things get ugly quickly. The ankles and knees will collapse inward, the hips will wobble, the spine will bend, and the shoulders will round into an unstable position. It's a recipe for disaster.

Although the idea of torque has long been part of the lifting and athletic movement conversation, it hasn't been so identified, nor, to my knowledge, has anyone drawn on physics to explain its benefits. Even Pavel Tsatsouline—a top fitness instructor who is commonly referred to as the "king of the kettlebells"—wrote about screwing your hands into the ground and spreading the floor with your feet in his book *Power to the People! And coaches still use these cues, but no one calls it what it is.*

We're not going to mince words. We're calling this "strongman's magic ingredient" by its proper name: torque. Consider it a new weapon to think about, practice with, and master so that you can grab more and more performance as you apply it to anything and everything athletic. While we're at it, let's add something else to the strength-and-conditioning conversation by explaining "why" we do it in the first place.

Again, it all boils down to stability.

Let me be clear: Global stability is achieved by creating an organized, stable framework for your carriage, by hinging from your primary engines, and by generating a torsion force through your extremities. In other words, midline stabilization and torque are two parts of a unifying system that work in conjunction with each other. If you don't have an organized carriage, you can't generate torque or transmit force to your primary engines. Conversely, if you don't generate enough torque, you can't stabilize your trunk in a good position.

Strength-and-Conditioning Movement Cues

Universal cues for creating a stable hip position:

▶ Screw your feet into the ground.

▶ Spin your feet as if they are on dinner plates.

▶ Spread the floor.

▶ Shove your knees out.

Universal cues for creating a stable shoulder position:

▶ Break (bend) the bar.

▶ Keep your elbows in.

▶ Armpits forward (when pressing overhead).

▶ Elbow pits forward (when doing a pushup).

These common strength-and-conditioning cues remind us of two things: 1) that our bodies are set up for rotation, and 2) that we need to generate a rotational force in order to create stable positions from which to move.

ONE JOINT BODY

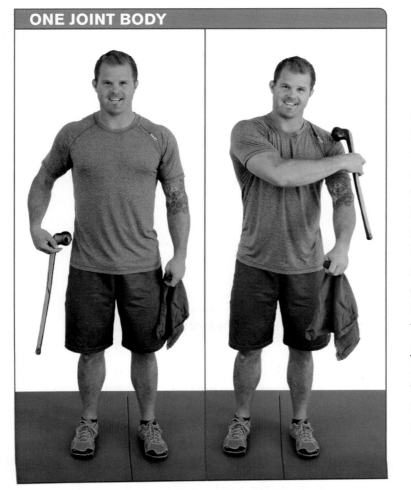

As I mentioned in the "One-Joint Rule" chapter, your hips and shoulders are ball-in-socket joints that are very similar in design and function. This is why the cues for creating a stable shoulder are essentially the same as those for creating a stable hip. Screwing your feet into the ground stabilizes your hips, while screwing your hands into the ground stabilizes your shoulders. Exactly why do we need to generate a rotational force to create stability in our primary engines? It's simple. There is slack within these ball-in-socket joints that allows for full movement of the limb. To make your joint stable, you need to wind up, twist, and spiral your limb into your hip or shoulder socket. Put simply, you need to generate torque.

I'm using an African shillelagh (club) as a model for both the femur and humerus.

CAPSULAR SLACK

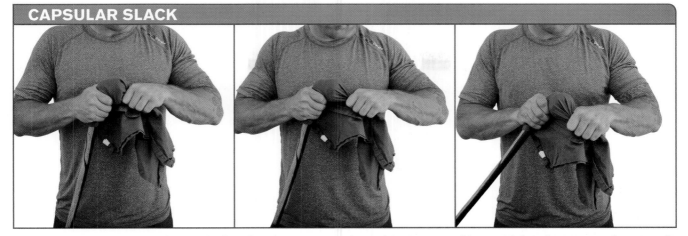

When there is zero torque, there is slack within the joint capsule, making it impossible to stabilize the joint in a functionally stable position.

Here is a simple example to help you understand how this works. If you examine the photos, you'll notice that I've wrapped a rag around the head of a club, and bundled up the loose cloth in my opposite hand. While the rag is wrapped snuggly around the head of the club, there is still space around the head, which means it can be pulled and manipulated in different directions—that also means there can be no torque (rotation). Now imagine that the club is the head of your femur (upper-leg bone) or humerus (upper-arm bone), and the rag is the joint capsule. As long as there is slack in that rag or joint capsule, your shoulders, hips, and downstream joints will never get into tight, stable positions. The results are—you guessed it—huge losses in power and increased risk of injury.

CAPSULAR STABILITY

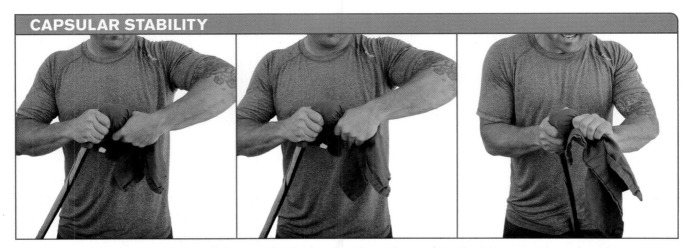

When you add rotation, it takes up all the capsular slack within the socket, making the joint very tight and stable.

When you add rotation, it takes up all the capsular slack within the socket, making the joint very tight and stable. The point is that these attachments are set up to create torsional stability. This is why it's so important to have full rotational range-of-motion in your primary engines. In fact, you can probably get away with missing a little bit of flexion and extension range-of-motion, but if you're missing rotation at the hip and shoulder, your body will default into structurally stable yet inefficient positions in terms of biomechanics. For example, when your shoulders roll forward, your shoulder joint is stable, but you're in a compromised position. Creating a rotational force to stabilize the joint is not limited to your hips and shoulders; it applies to your ankles, knees, elbows, and wrists.

Let's examine the structure of your anterior cruciate ligament (ACL). Your ACL attaches to your femur and tibia (lower-leg bone) and is one of the major ligaments that cross your knee. Its role is to prevent independent rotation of your tibia in relation to your femur. Now it's important to note that although your shoulders and hips function in much the same way, your arms have independent rotation capacities at the elbow (fundamental movements like feeding and grabbing would be difficult without this feature). Your knee does not: you can't internally and externally rotate at your knee as you can at your elbow.

The takeaway is that the right kind of rotation will set your knee into a more stable position, dramatically reducing your potential for injury. But the wrong kind of rotation will put your knee into a disastrous position, increasing the odds of injury sooner or later.

To illustrate how this works, cross your right middle finger over your index finger. (Note, this is a crude model of how your ACL crosses through your knee joint.)

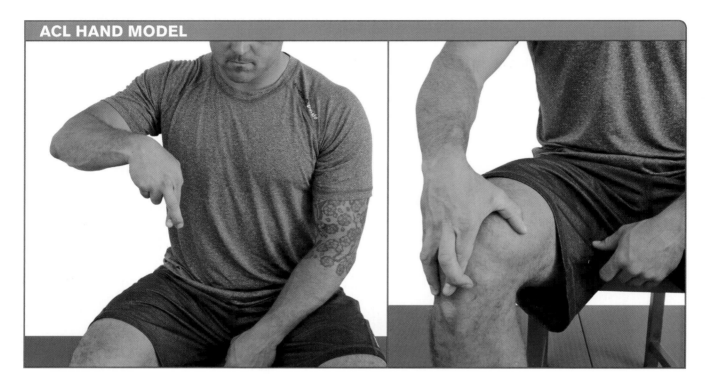

ACL HAND MODEL

Next, wrap your left hand around your fingers and externally rotate your right hand—creating force that tightens your fingers. If you internally rotate your hand, your fingers loosen and come apart. The former is the stable position for your knee, the latter the unstable one. It is this unstable position that can cause the ACL to tear.

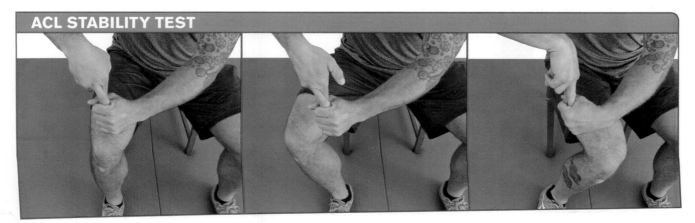

ACL STABILITY TEST

As I mentioned before, if you don't get into a well-organized stable position, your body will create tension in the system somewhere else. This is what I refer to as "tension-hunting." When you start tension-hunting, you create an open circuit that your body closes down immediately by defaulting into a bad position. This looks like a spinal fault, elbows flaring out, or feet and knees collapsing inward. Your body recognizes instability as a liability, and it would rather close that open circuit down in the wrong way than leave you all loosey-goosey.

The Two Laws of Torque

Now that you understand how a well-organized carriage, torque, and global organization relate to one another, we can start to talk about the two laws of torque.

▶ **Law #1:** To create stability when your legs or arms are in flexion, you need to generate an external rotation force.

• **Examples:** Squat/pulling positions, overhead press, front rack.

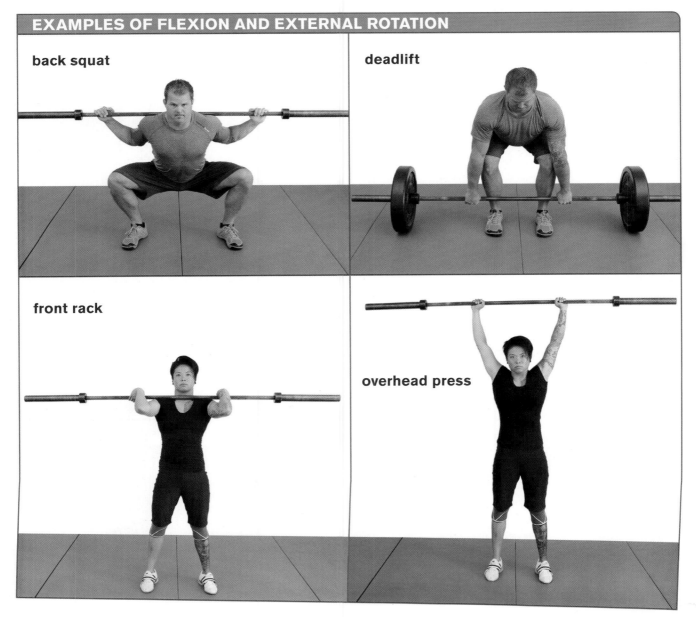

EXAMPLES OF FLEXION AND EXTERNAL ROTATION

back squat

deadlift

front rack

overhead press

Flexion and external rotation cover the broad spectrum of human movements. Squatting, pressing, and pulling all involve flexion and require external rotation to create stability. Turning the key in the ignition, screwing in a light bulb, opening a door, and drawing a bow are all examples of external rotation. This is why being a lefty sucks when you have to screw or unscrew something. (Internally rotating with your left hand to tighten a screw is a weak movement.)

Most torque-related strength-and-conditioning cues involve creating an external rotation force—like screwing your feet or hands into the ground or breaking the bar.

▶ **Law #2:** To create stability when your legs or arms are in extension, you need to generate an internal-rotation force.

• **Examples:** Split-jerk, jumping.

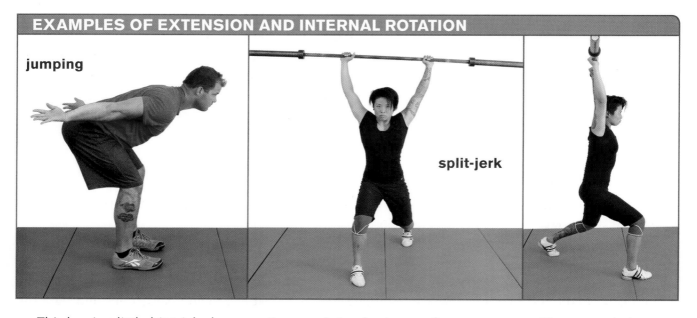

EXAMPLES OF EXTENSION AND INTERNAL ROTATION

jumping

split-jerk

This law is a little bit tricky because it comes into play in very few movements. The most obvious example is when you swing your arms back while jumping, or when your leg tracks behind your body while walking, running, or doing a split-jerk.

Another example is when a boxer or fighter throws a cross—a straight punch with the rear hand. Technically proficient fighters will screw (internally rotate) their rear foot into the ground as they rotate their hips and shoulders. With their ankle, knee, and hip in the most stable position possible, they can effectively harness the energy traveling through the kinetic chain, maximizing the power of the strike.

The second rule sometimes confuses people because there are movements in which your shoulders are in extension but your arms are in flexion—bent at the elbows. The dip, bench press, pushup, and the arm swing in running, are all examples of this. To stabilize your shoulders during these movements, you need to generate an external rotation force.

Think of it like this: If your arms are straight—elbows locked out (extension)—behind your body, you create an internal-rotation force. If they are bent (flexion), you generate an external rotation force.

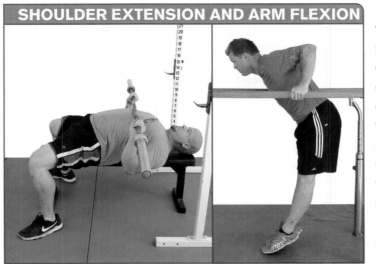

SHOULDER EXTENSION AND ARM FLEXION

Although the anatomical terms of motion are important and you should understand what they mean, they do not perfectly describe movement in planes of motion. For example, if I try to explain what your shoulders are doing during a press using academic terms—flexion, extension, abduction, external rotation, internal rotation—chances are good that you won't know what the heck I'm talking about. More importantly, I can capture only a piece of what is happening. (Planes of motion don't tell you anything about midline stability, for example.) But if I say bench press, pushup, overhead press, squat, deadlift, or clean, you can start to make the connection because it's the formal language of how people move.

Squatting is just an expression of flexion and external rotation. Breaking the bar with your hands as you set up for a bench press is really just creating external rotation torque off the barbell to stabilize your shoulders, elbows, and wrists. Screwing your feet into the ground and shoving your knees out during a squat is really just a mechanism for generating stability in your hip, knee, and ankle. It's the same reoccurring theme again and again. And it's a language that we all speak and that we can all understand.

Torque Tests

The two laws of torque give you a general blueprint for generating stable positions for the primary engines of your body.

(In "Movement Hierarchy," Chapter 5, I'll apply these laws to a broad spectrum of functional movements. But first, let's test this movement principle using two universally transferable movements so that you can better understand how torque works.)

In this section I use the pushup to illustrate how to create stability in your shoulders, and I use the squat to demonstrate how to create stability in your hips. It's important to realize that these two bodyweight movements are more than just training exercises. They are master blueprints that translate to all human movements. For example, if you understand how to set up for a pushup, you have a model for stabilizing your shoulders for anything that requires pressing or pulling. In the same way, if you understand how to squat correctly, you have a universal model for creating torque and stability at your hip, knee, and ankle.

In the following pages, I'll provide you with a series of tests so that you can develop the connection between midline stabilization and torque and also understand how your setup or start position dictates your capacity to move optimally.

Shoulder-Stability Torque Tests

When I teach the rules of torque in my seminars, I typically start at the shoulder and use the pushup as my diagnostic movement. By putting people into the top of the pushup, I very clearly, very safely, and very effectively illuminate the two central tenants of stability. People immediately realize that if they're disorganized at the trunk, they can't get organized at the shoulder. Conversely, if their shoulders are rolling forward or they can't lock out their elbows, they struggle to achieve a flat back.

Pushup Butt-Acuity Test

The pushup butt-acuity test is the first application of midline stabilization and torque that I introduce to athletes. To correctly perform this test, simply get into the pushup start position by making your hands as parallel as possible—positioning your hands underneath your shoulders—and pinning your feet together.

Next, go through the bracing sequence: Squeeze your butt, align your ribcage over your pelvis, and get your belly tight. The key is to make sure that your wrists, elbows, and shoulders are aligned and that your feet are together. A lot of people mistakenly spread their feet apart, not realizing that they're just cheating range-of-motion. This makes it difficult to engage the glutes and stabilize the trunk.

After you establish a well-organized pushup start position, the next step is to disengage your glutes and then try to maintain a flat back. If you can sequence multiple full-range pushups, you'll probably need to do five to ten pushups—one set with your butt online and the others with it offline—to get the desired effect.

What you will find is that the latter setup (glutes offline) is not nearly as stable because there's a domino effect: if you glutes are disengaged you can't organize your spine in a good position. This turns into a great opening diagnostic test because it gives you two really important pieces of information: 1) when your butt is offline, you're susceptible to spinal faults; and 2) a broken midline places additional strain on your shoulders. The difference is shocking.

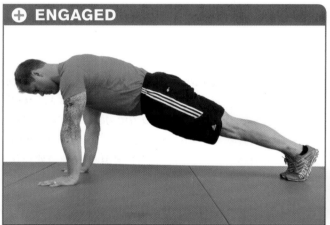 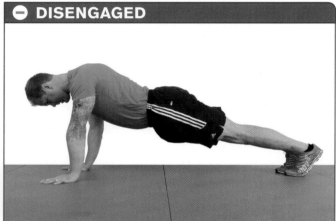

⊕ ENGAGED   **⊖ DISENGAGED**

When your butt is squeezed, it's easier to keep your back flat.   When you disengage your glutes, it's harder to preserve a neutral spinal position, especially as you start sequencing together multiple pushups.

Open-Hand Torque Test

The second test uses one of the most common strength-and-conditioning cues as it relates specifically to the pushup: screwing your hands into the ground.

This is how people really start to understand how important torque is in stabilizing the trunk. With the pits of your elbows forward and the heads of your shoulders externally rotated, it's much easier to keep your back flat. Moreover, this test also teaches you about the connection between hand position and the amount of torque you can generate.

After you perform the torque test with your hands parallel (or as straight as you can get them), the next step is to start spinning your hands out—keep turning your hands out until you reach the limits of your external rotation. You do this while trying to cultivate torque and keeping your back flat in each position. What you will realize is that the more you turn out your hands, the harder it is to create torque and stabilize your trunk. Once you get to 45-degrees or farther, cultivating torque is simply untenable.

At this point, your shoulders start to sag and your spine bends because you're in such a low-torque environment. If you turn your hands out as if you were doing a planche (a difficult gymnastics move in which the entire body is held parallel to the ground—like a high pushup without using the feet), it becomes even harder to keep the trunk stiff and stable. To maintain this position with zero torque is very difficult, and explains why doing a planche pushup, even when your feet are on the ground, is so difficult. Not only does it take extreme mobility, but also extreme strength.

The takeaway is this: In order to create a stable platform for your shoulders and thoracic spine, you have to create torque through your hands. If you put your hands in a position in which you can't create torque, it's hard to stabilize and generate force. Remember, we're not just talking about the pushup; we're talking about the entire gamut of pressing and pulling exercises. Adopting an open-hand position (hands turned out) in the pushup just ensures that you will adopt the same hand position when you block, push a car, do a burpee, you name it.

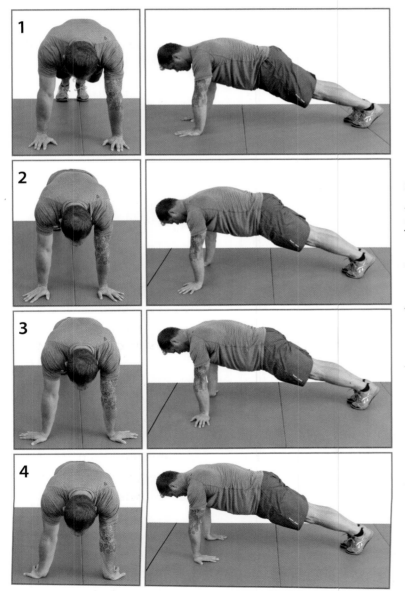

Get into the pushup start position. With your fingers pointed straight head (fingers splayed), screw your hands into the ground. Next, turn your hands out slightly and try to generate torque. What you will find is that you can't create nearly as much torque with your hands turned out. As you turn your hands out farther, you will completely lose the ability to cultivate torque, making it a supreme challenge to stabilize your shoulders and trunk. And if you turn your hands completely backward, you can't create any torque at all.

Note: *Screwing your hands into the ground creates external rotation in your shoulders, but physically externally rotating your hands steals your ability to generate torque.*

Ring-Pushup Torque Test

If you really want to look under the hood of shoulder stabilization, have an athlete do pushups on the rings. His understanding of bracing and torque, or his lack thereof, instantly becomes clear: You can see if he's in a good position or bad position because it's so much harder to stabilize the shoulders and trunk on the rings.

The ring-pushup start position also teaches you that you need to torque early and often. It's difficult to reclaim torque at the bottom of a pushup, in the compression phase, particularly on the rings—you have to arrive with torque. This is why coaches cue athletes to break the bar at the top of the bench press: It optimizes shoulder position when they lower the bar to their chest.

This test helps you understand that if you set yourself up in a good position with adequate torque and an organized trunk, chances are good that you will perform the movement with perfect technique. And it turns out that if you set up properly, a lot of the midrange problems and discomfort that people experience—shoulder pain during a pushup or low back pain during a squat—disappear.

Note: Unlike in the regular pushup where you have a base of support and can screw your hands into the ground to create external rotation, with the ring-pushup, you have to actually physically externally rotate your hands. Your right thumb should be at 1 o'clock and your left thumb at 11 o'clock.

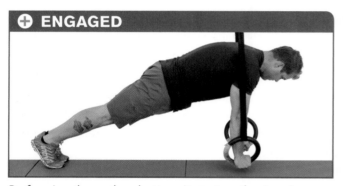

⊕ ENGAGED

Performing the pushup butt acuity test on the rings is an entirely different ball game than doing it from the ground. The stabilization demands are much higher, making it a great diagnostic tool for stronger athletes. To begin, get into a good pushup position, squeezing your butt, engaging your abdominals, and getting your back flat.

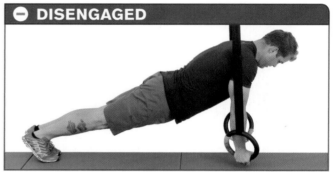

⊖ DISENGAGED

The moment you disengage your glutes, you will immediately feel your hips sag, pulling you into an overextended position.

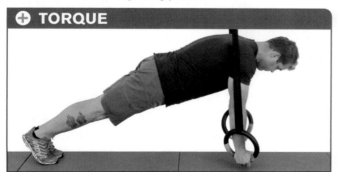

⊕ TORQUE

To create torque, you still have to generate an external rotation force. But unlike performing pushups from the ground, cultivating torque on the rings is a lot harder. To put your shoulders in a good position, you have to turn your hands out so that your thumbs are pointing away from your body. Your right thumb should be at 1 o'clock and your left thumb at 11 o'clock.

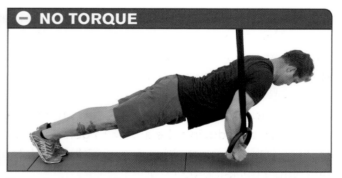

⊖ NO TORQUE

If you don't externally rotate your hands, you can't create torque. And when you can't create torque, you can't organize your spine, your elbows flare out, and your shoulders default into a rounded position.

Torque and Midline Tension

If your torque and midline tension levels aren't in sync, or your midline stabilization strategy is weak, your spine will sag the moment you start applying an external rotation force. Let's say, for example, that you set up for a pushup with your trunk tension a 2 out of 10 and you try to apply torque through your hands at a rate of 5: Your spine will respond by overextending. You need to apply just enough torque to maintain a flat back. For body-weight movements, you don't need that much torque or to keep your belly that tight to maintain good form, but as you increase load or add speed, you have to increase both torque and trunk tension to match the demand of the movement.

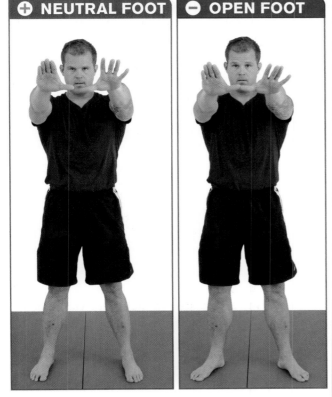

⊕ NEUTRAL FOOT **⊖ OPEN FOOT**

Hip-Stability Torque Tests

Like the pushup, the squat has a broad range of applications. If you understand how to create torque while squatting, you have a global hip-stability model that is germane to the vast majority of movements. In addition, the squat really illustrates that your set-up—specifically your foot position, or stance—dictates your ability to generate torque upstream: in your ankles, knees, hips, spine, and shoulders.

Remember, your joints need to be in a position to facilitate rotational force before you start moving. As the squat torque tests will prove, a straight foot or neutral foot position is ideal for generating maximum torque.

The trouble is that there has been a historical disconnection between foot position and stabilization through torque. For years coaches have taught athletes to turn their feet out—like a duck's—when they squat, which opens up some room in the hip joint and allows athletes to drive their knees out farther and lower more easily into the bottom of the squat.

What coaches and athletes have failed to realize is that you can create room in the hip joint through external rotation torque: by positioning your feet straight (parallel), screwing your feet into the ground, and shoving your knees out. Although this requires more mobility, it allows you to maximize torque and still free the head of your femur.

However, most people don't have the range-of-motion required to perform a full-range, butt-to-ankle squat. Turning the feet out allows them to get the job done. But that quick fix comes at a cost. In addition to reducing the ability to generate torque, it instills dysfunctional movement patterns that carry over to other activities. Squat with a duck-footed stance and you will stand, walk, jump, land, and pull with a duck-footed stance.

And what do you think will happen when you go for a one-rep max back squat? Or spontaneously receive weight in the bottom of the squat during an Olympic lift? Or plant to change directions in a basketball game? This is what will happen: You're going to express the same movement pattern that has been ingrained in your motor program and you're going to dramatically increase your potential for injury. This is the same as rounding your back when you deadlift. Or even better, smoking a pack of cigarettes. It's not a problem until it becomes a problem. And once it is a problem, correcting it is that much harder.

Let's take a closer look at what happens when the feet are turned out. Most importantly, it makes it difficult to generate torque and stabilize your body. What often happens as a result is that your ankles collapse and your knees spiral inward, creating a valgus—twisting and shearing—force across your joints. This is how athletes dump torque and lose force through their hips, and it is the primary culprit in ACL tears.

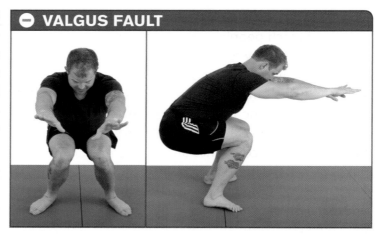

VALGUS FAULT

When I teach neutral foot position as it relates to the squat, I say that you can squat in any position as long as you can create arches in both feet. If your foot sustains an arch, you will be able to generate sufficient torque. It just so happens that straight, neutral feet is the best position for achieving this ideal arch. The more you turn out your feet, the more likely that your arches will collapse. Simple.

For example, if an athlete lowers into a squat but reaches the end of his ankle range-of-motion before he completes the exercise—meaning that he can't flex any deeper as he moves into the bottom position—he has to start tension-hunting by collapsing inward. Although this will make his ankle structurally stable, it compromises the integrity of his joints. He is in effect, just depending on his ligaments and tissues to support him. To ensure optimal positioning of the ankle joint, you need to create an arch in your foot, which is expressed through external rotation torque.

Here's the deal: While athletes can get away with squatting with their feet turned out when working with body-weight and low volume, the moment they increase weight, speed, or volume, the house of cards collapses.

As with the shoulder-torque tests, the goal of the subsequent demonstrations is to drive home the relationship between torque and midline stability, as well as to illustrate why a neutral foot position is ideal for maximizing torque.

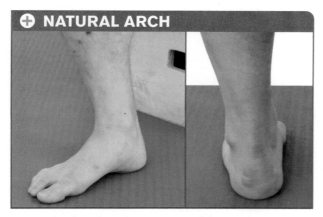

NATURAL ARCH

Your arch is largely a phenomenon of this mechanical system—bones, ligaments, tendons, and connective tissues—derived from the external rotation of your hip. Heel aligned with the Achilles (straight) is ideal, or heel cord matching the calf. If your feet are straight and you externally rotate at the hip, your feet will come into a natural arch. You can lift more weight and you can jump with more force. Oh, and it also happens to be the safest position from which to move.

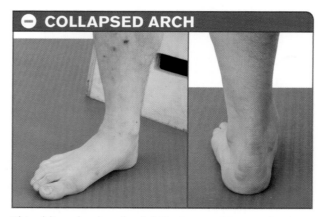

COLLAPSED ARCH

This oblique load on the Achilles is one of the mechanisms for Achilles rupture, Achilles tendinopathy, and ACL tears. One of the ways you can mitigate off axial oblique loads on the Achilles is to get the foot into a straighter position.

Open Foot Torque Test

When I teach people about creating a stable hip position, I start with the open foot torque test because it's really easy to make the connection between a neutral foot position and torque.

To correctly execute this test, stand with your feet directly under your hips, or roughly shoulder-width apart, go through the bracing sequence, and then screw your feet into the ground as if you were trying to spread the floor apart: create as much external rotation force as possible and squeeze your butt as hard as you can without letting your big toe come off the ground. When you externally rotate at the hip, your feet come into an arch—connective tissue contracts, bones are aligned properly, and the muscles are activated—which is the ideal positioning for your feet.

After you carry out the torque test with your feet straight, turn your feet out about 30-degrees and repeat the process. What you will experience is that you can't cultivate the same amount of torque, your foot won't come into an arch, and you can't activate your glutes to the same degree.

Now it's important to mention that you can turn your feet out slightly—maybe between 15 and 30 degrees—and still generate a sufficient amount of torque. However, as you venture into the 45-degree range, there is no torque to be had. The drop off rate in foot position is radical.

Let me be clear: The more parallel your feet, the more stable your position. You can turn your feet out slightly and still create torque, not as much, but some torque. It might not matter so much during body-weight squats or low-intensity exercise, but once you add a metabolic demand or load, your inability to generate torque will result in a biomechanical compromise of some kind. And you must know by now that a biomechanical compromise is like a green light to injury.

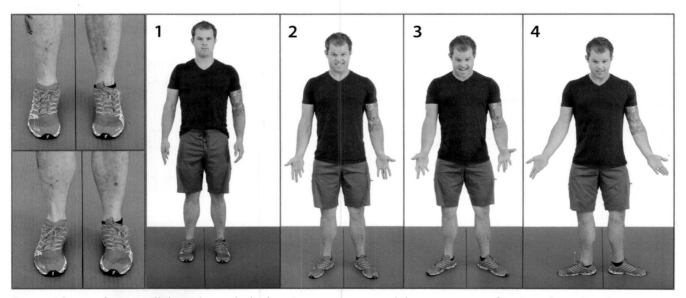

Start with your feet parallel, go through the bracing sequence, and then screw your feet into the ground, creating an external rotation force. You'll notice that your shoes curve. This is your feet coming into an arch. Next, turn your feet out slightly and repeat the process. As your feet venture outward, you'll notice that you can't generate torque, create an arch, or activate your glutes.

You Won't Get Drafted if You Have Collapsed Arches ...

While playing for the NFL, my good friend John Welbourn, founder of CrossFit Football, had his feet observed by a podiatrist 31 times. Why was he checked 31 times? Because a navicular drop, or collapsed arch, is a great predictor of ACL tears.

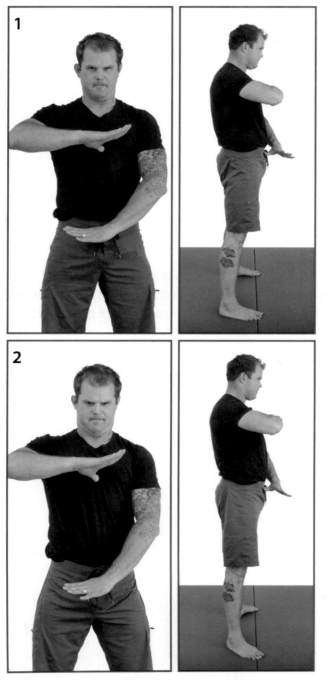

Butt-Acuity Test

The butt-acuity test helps elucidate the relationship between a straight-foot stance and your ability to activate your glutes. With your feet parallel, you can maximize torque and squeeze your butt to stabilize your pelvis in a neutral position. However, if you turn your feet out, you not only lose the ability to generate torque, but also you can't engage your glutes, which creates an unstable pelvic position.

As you experienced during the pushup, if you fail to create torque through your hands or you're in a position in which you can't generate a rotational force, your ribcage tilts. A similar thing happens during the squat, but instead of your ribcage, your pelvis tilts. If you have zero torque, you have to create stability some other way. In the squat it's created by the pelvis moving forward, which is really the mirror action of your ribcage tilting back.

This explains why so many people overextend when they squat and why people experience so much horrible low back pain. In a low-torque environment—meaning their body can't generate any stability—they default to bone-on-bone stability, which is the lumbar-spine-overextension fault.

To begin, go through the bracing sequence with your feet as straight as possible, squeezing your butt as hard as you can. Next, turn your feet out and do the same thing. What you'll notice is that you can't activate your glutes to stabilize your pelvis, which creates an unstable spine.

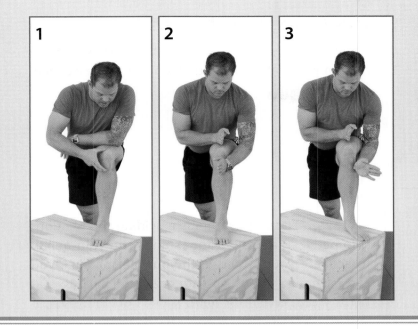

Patellar Alignment

To generate the most force and to avoid knee pain, your kneecap and the insertion of the quad ligament on your shin need to be as perpendicular as possible. When you turn your feet out, the quad ligament gets pulled off axis. That's what my hand positions illustrate. With your foot straight, your kneecap tracks straight up and down over your quad, which is optimal.

Base of Support test

Another problem with turning your feet out is that you limit your base of support. You go from the full length of your foot to about half, compromising forward and backward balance and stability. If you squat with skis on your feet, for example, you would never fall over forward or backward. But if you turn your feet out, you instantly lose that balance and stability.

This is another reason that you see athletes' knees tracking inward. It's not just because they have zero torque; it's because they have zero forward and backward stability. In fact, when your feet are straight, your knees don't track as far inward even when you fail to create torque (see torqueless squat test, page 67). This loss of stability becomes an even bigger issue when you Olympic lift.

For example, say you receive a snatch a little bit out in front or behind your body. With your feet straight, you can adjust your position because you have a large base of support. But if your feet are turned out, regaining your balance is difficult.

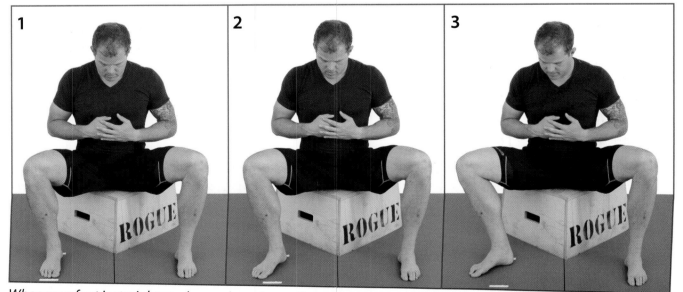

When your foot is straight you have a large base of support. When you turn your foot out, however, you lose around 30 percent of the length of your foot.

Monster-Walk Test

The monster walk is a common warm-up exercise in which you put a band above your knees and walk sideways while in a quarter or half squat. What's interesting is that people don't walk with their feet angled out when they do this drill; their feet are always straight. Why is that? Because it is impossible to keep your knees from collapsing inward as you walk laterally. To remain stable, you have to maintain a position that gives you the most stability, which is accomplished by keeping your feet straight.

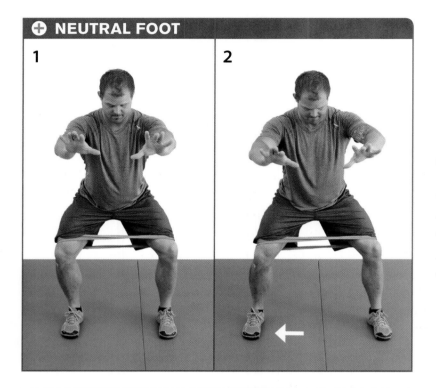

⊕ NEUTRAL FOOT

1   **2**

Wrap a band just above your knees, parallel your feet, and then reach your hamstrings and hips back, lowering into a quarter squat. Because your feet are straight, you can generate more torque and drive your knees out farther, giving you more balance and stability as you sidestep.

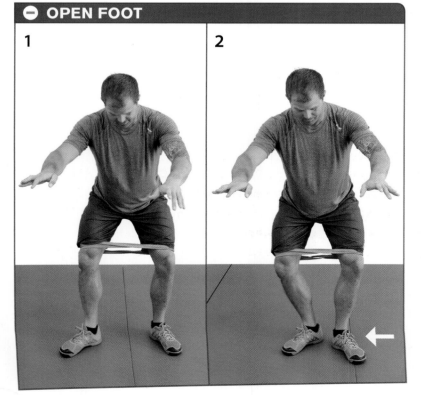

⊖ OPEN FOOT

1   **2**

When you attempt this exercise with an open foot stance, you can't generate enough torque to drive your knees out. The band literally pulls your knees together. This makes it difficult to get into a stable position and maintain balance as you sidestep.

Monster-Squat Test

Squatting with a band wrapped around your knees is another illuminating test. Again, when your feet are straight, it's easier to generate torque and drive your knees out. The moment you adopt a duck stance and squat, on the other hand, it becomes a lot harder to drive your knees out. It just feels like a less stable, weak position. And the band does a really good job of highlighting that fact.

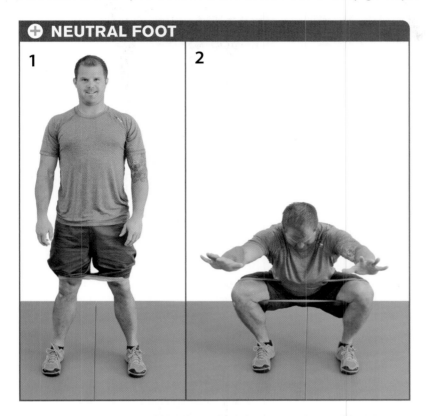

With your feet parallel, it's easier to counter the pressure of the band and squat in a good position.

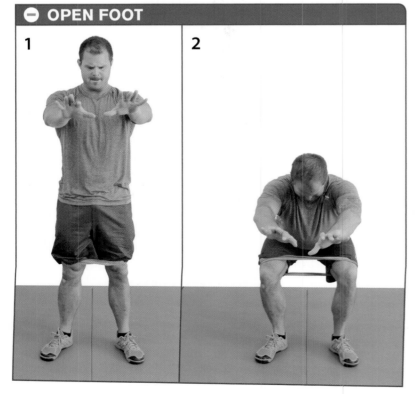

When you squat from an open foot stance, you can't generate sufficient torque and drive your knees out to counter the band's resistance.

Stable Foot Position Test

This test helps to illustrate that with your feet straight, you don't need to drive your knees out that far to achieve ankle stability. However, the more you turn your foot out, the farther out you have to drive your knees to achieve that natural arch and stable ankle position, which at a certain point becomes unattainable.

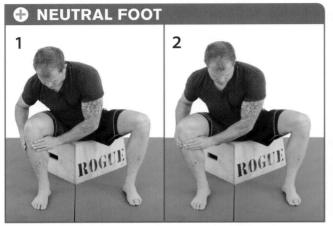

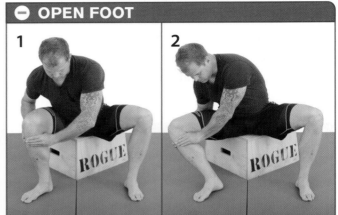

Place your foot in a neutral position and then drive your knee out. Notice that I have to push my knee out only slightly to create a natural arch.

Next, turn your foot out and then drive your knee out until your foot comes into an arch. As you can see from the photo, you have to drive your knee out a lot farther to achieve that arch.

External Rotation Test

This test illustrates the amount of external rotation you can create at your hip with your feet parallel, as well as how limited the range-of-motion in your hip is with your feet turned out.

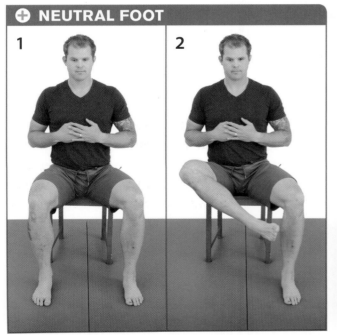

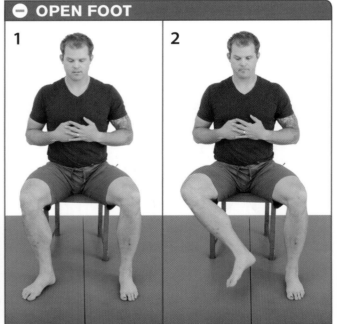

Sit in a chair, position your feet straight, and pull your foot toward your opposite hip. This is an expression of hip external rotation.

Next, turn your foot out and do the same thing. What you will find is that you can't lift your foot as high or create as much external rotation at your hip.

Torqueless-Squat Test (Ankle-Collapse Test)

Keeping your feet straight limits end-range valgus collapse, while turning the feet out increases valgus collapse. You can test this in one of two ways: Either squat with your feet straight and then with them turned out without creating any torque, or sit on a chair and simply drive your knee inward with your foot straight and then again with your foot turned out. The latter test is much easier, but you should try both to see how they feel and then imagine being in these positions under a seriously heavy load or while sprinting down a field and then changing directions.

The bottom line is you need to be able to survive a bad position, just in case the load is too heavy or you make a mechanical or motor-control error. It happens. But if you're in a good position, you can at least mitigate the negative outcome.

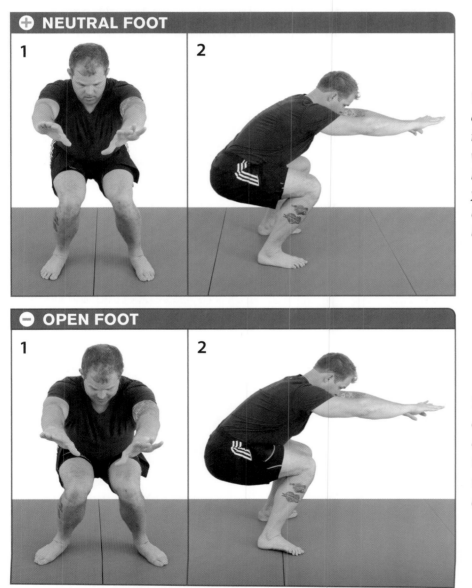

⊕ NEUTRAL FOOT

1
2

When your feet are straight, you can kind of mitigate the valgus force on your ankle and knee when you fail to create torque during a squat. It's also easier to keep your shins vertical and maintain balance because you have a larger base of support.

⊖ OPEN FOOT

1
2

With your feet turned out, your ankles collapse to a much greater degree. Get into this position, and the sketchiness of this valgus force will become immediately apparent.

Ankle-Collapse Test

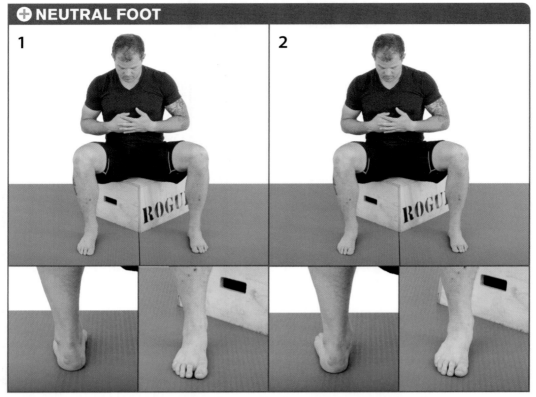

Sit in a chair with your toes pointed forward and try to collapse your arches.

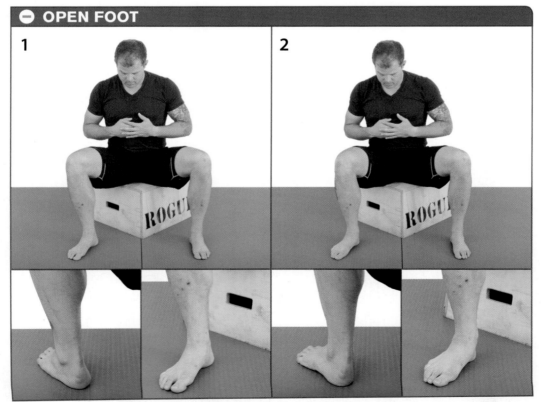

Next, turn your foot out and collapse your arch. As you can see from the photos, it's a much more dramatic collapse.

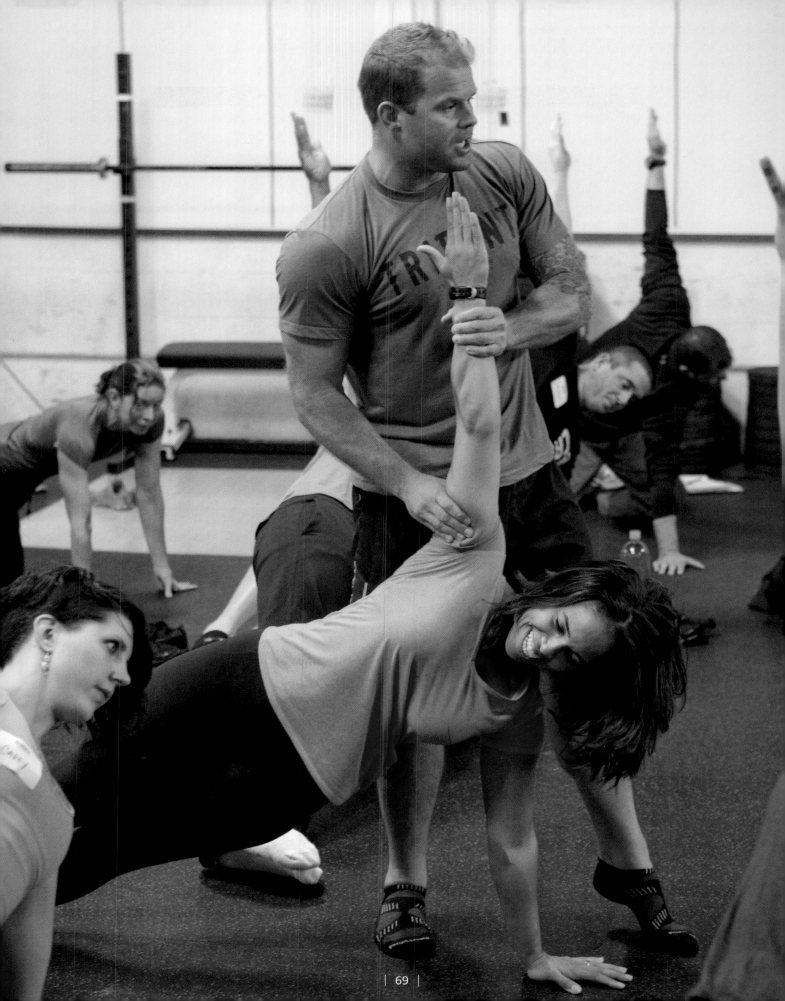

CHAPTER 5
MOVEMENT HIERARCHY

I'm betting that this is you and that this is what you want:

You want to move efficiently. You want to produce more force. You want to maximize power output. You also want to resolve pain and injury issues, or even better, prevent them.

To do all this—as I said earlier—you need to focus on three movement principles: midline stabilization and organization, one joint body, and the laws of torque. Let's consider two questions first:

✓ Can you brace your spine in a stable, well-organized position?

✓ Do you understand how to load and create torque through the primary engines of your hips and shoulders?

Simple concepts, right? The hard part is putting them to work in a safe and controlled environment like the gym so that you can go out and apply them where it matters the most, in play, dance, sports, training, or combat.

As I've already mentioned, learning a strength-and-conditioning system gives you a universal language for human movement. That is, if you're fluent in full-range functional movements—squatting, pressing, pulling, etc.—you have universal models for moving safely and effectively.

For example, if you understand the principles that govern a deadlift, you have embodied the knowledge to safely and efficiently pick anything up off the ground. If you can correctly perform a push-press or squat, you understand how to jump and land with your torso upright—like when you rebound a basketball—without destroying your knees. If you can stabilize your shoulders during a pull-up, you will have no trouble creating that same stable shoulder position while climbing a tree or rock wall.

But here's the crux of the problem: Just because you can complete or perform functional movements in the gym doesn't mean you can apply them somewhere else. You can do a pull-up in the gym, for example, but that doesn't mean you can climb a tree. However, if you understand what is going on when you do a pull-up, it's easy to climb a tree because you already know how to create torque and trunk stability. So as long as you understand how the movement principles work and you develop reproducible motor-control patterns, you have a model for reconstituting organized, stable, and efficient positions in any environment. Whether you're wind surfing, shooting, fighting, dancing, or playing football, you have a transferable template for moving that is both safe and effective.

But human movement is complex. To ingrain functional movement patterns that have universal application, you need an all-encompassing strength-and-conditioning blueprint that translates to all forms of human movement. In addition, you need a model for identifying and resolving dysfunctional movement patterns, unstable positions, and range-of-motion restrictions that kill athletic performance and increase potential for injury and pain.

The movement hierarchy serves as this blueprint. It's a way to categorize movement so that you have a model for:

- Rehabbing an athlete after surgery or injury.
- Layering movements and skill progressions.
- Understanding movement complexity.
- Illuminating movement errors.
- Identifying mobility restrictions.

Skill Progressions and Movement Complexity

Your brain is wired for movement, not musculature. It doesn't think quads; it doesn't think hamstrings. It thinks movement. However, we still need to teach people how to move because, as I said, human movement is complex. We teach kids how to brush their teeth, even though putting the hand to the face is a natural movement. And we teach athletes how to run, deadlift, and squat with proper technique, even though running, squatting, and picking something off the ground is innate. The trick is teaching and layering movements and skill progressions in a way that shortens the learning curve, accelerates athletic performance, and highlights weaknesses in movement and mobility.

When I first started thinking about skill progressions and movement complexity, I looked at it through a rehabilitation lens. I asked myself, *How do I rebuild functional movement patterns after injury or surgery?* More specifically, how do I layer movement progressions within the framework of strength-and-conditioning that will instill good, transferable motor-control patterning?

Here's what I did: First, I introduced the three movement principles. I then applied them to basic, scalable full-range movements like squatting, deadlifting, pushups, pull-ups and so forth.

If an athlete showed physical competency with the basic movements, I would start to challenge the stability of his positions by adding load and metabolic demand, and then by introducing more upright positions. For example, if I had an athlete who could back squat with good form, I might introduce the front squat or overhead squat, or simply have him run around the block—to get his heart rate up—and then perform multiple back squat repetitions.

Default Movement

As I've said before, the positions that you assume at work or while going about your life will impact the way you move in the gym: If you walk around with your back overextended, chances are good that you will default into that same position while squatting. The environment also affects movement efficiency. For example, last year I noticed that my oldest daughter's first grade classmates started to heel-strike (landing on your heel is less than optimal when running and can lead to a ton of problems). They didn't seem to do this in kindergarten. What happened?

Well, they had been wearing cushioned shoes and sitting in a chair long enough to create an adaptation, and it turned into their default movement pattern. This is why it's so important and difficult to get to the root of movement issues, and take the time to reverse engineer patterns that have been hardwired over years of conditioning. If you sit in a chair, you have to spend extra time working on your posture. If you wear high heels, you have to focus on your foot position and calf mobility. Remember, biomechanical pathologies are treatable at any time or stage of development. But it takes time, consciousness, and a ton of practice. It starts with understanding the movement principles and then practicing and applying them to every facet of your life.

The final step was to challenge the athlete's motor-control and test his mobility. I did this by adding a speed element and layering transitional movements like Olympic lifts and burpees. What I realized is that by systematically layering movements, I could not only rehab an injured athlete, but also progress movements—from basic to more advanced exercises—for the novice or elite athlete. This basic template not only allowed me to ingrain good (and transferable) movement patterning, but also to illuminate common movement faults and limitations in range-of-motion.

I'll use the squat as an example. Say you're teaching an athlete how to squat and you notice that his knees cave in (valgus knee fault, page 88) as he moves into the bottom position. This fault tells you that either he doesn't understand how to correctly perform the squat—to create torque by screwing his feet into the ground or driving his knees out—or he is unable to get into the correct position because he's missing range-of-motion somewhere. It's also an indication that he will exhibit this same fault during more complex, heavier-loaded movements: if an athlete rolls his knees in during a body-weight squat, chances are good that this same fault will rear its ugly head when he jumps and lands. It's no wonder so many middle-aged men get injured playing basketball!

The idea is to identify movement faults and mobility restrictions in an environment where the athlete's chances of getting hurt are minimized. To make continual improvements, you need to be

Movement Mobility Template

Whether it's a valgus knee fault or another movement error, the template for teaching and correcting dysfunctional positions and movement patterns is the same: Prioritize technique (motor-control) first, and then if the athlete can't physically get into a good position, use mobility to improve position and function.

► **Technique:** Always address motor-control first. Make sure you understand how to correctly perform the movement and get into the right position without making a load sequencing error (i.e., failing to brace or create torque).

► **Mobility:** If you are physically unable to assume a stable position because you are missing range-of-motion (i.e., you can't drive your knees out because your quads are tight), then address mobility, targeting the areas that are restricting your movement.

In the technique portion of this chapter, I highlight common faults associated with specific training movements. To improve your understanding of how this template works, I offer tips on how to correct the motor-control error. I also offer mobility prescriptions. If you're an athlete, having a coach help you spot and correct these fundamental faults is ideal.

It's important to note that the mobility prescriptions offered are vague due to the complex nature of tissue restriction. Every athlete is different and has unique issues that contribute to a limited range-of-motion. It's a system of systems. Your tight quads might prevent you from getting your knees out, but the cause could also be your tacked-down heel cords, tight hamstrings, or brutally stiff adductors (to mention a few possibilities). For these reasons, the mobilization target areas, which refer to subsection contained within the Systems chapter, are simply to get you moving in the right direction. It will take time and a ton of experimenting to get to the bottom of your mobility restrictions. If there are several target areas listed, the best approach is to systematically address the areas that might be limiting your range-of-motion using the test and retest model. To learn more about how to treat range-of-motion restrictions, visit chapter 7, "The Systems," which starts on page 204.

able to scale, progress, and constantly test that athlete's motor-control and mobility. To do that, the coach and the athlete needs to understand "how" to correctly perform the movement, as well as "why" some movements are more complex than others. Imagine having someone perform snatches early in their ACL surgery rehab. That would be silly, if not surreal. Similarly, you wouldn't show someone a full snatch without first introducing an overhead squat and snatch balance.

Whether you're rehabbing someone, progressing a beginner, or coaching an elite athlete, the movement hierarchy is a universally applicable template that allows you to systematically highlight motor-control and range-of-motion issues,

as well as safely and effectively challenge the athlete with movement stimulus aimed at improving performance and eradicating pain.

I've broken down movements into three categories based on stabilization and speed demands. It's important to realize that the movements featured in this chapter just scratch the surface of transferable training exercises that you can and should implement. My goal is to provide you with the key ingredients so that you can start to connect the dots between the movement principles covered in this book and the full-range strength-and-conditioning movements that are performed in the gym/lab.

Category 1 Movements

Category 1 movements represent basic squatting, pressing, and pulling techniques: air squat, back squat, front squat, overhead squat, pushup, bench press, overhead press, and deadlift.

Movements that fall into this category have relatively low speed demands, express normal or full ranges of motion, and closely resemble the actions of daily life, like picking something up off the ground. Category 1 movements allow you to create and maintain torque through the full range of the movement. For these reasons, category 1 movements—specifically the squat, deadlift, pushup, and strict-press—serve two primary purposes. First, they enable you to start to layer and instill good movement practices into motor programs. Second, they serve as the primary diagnostic tools for assessing motor-control and mobility dysfunction.

All of these exercises share a common sequence: They start in a position of high stability (PHS)—meaning a braced-neutral position that can maximize torque in the hips and/or shoulders—and maintain that stable position throughout the entire range-of-motion.

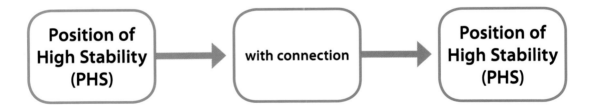

- ▶ **Position of High Stability (PHS):** A braced, well-organized position that allows you to create and maintain maximum stability through your hips and shoulders.
- ▶ **Connection:** Maintaining a torsion force through the entire range-of-motion.

Let's use the air squat to discuss this. You begin in a PHS (top position), lower your body into a squat (bottom position), and finish the movement in the same PHS (top position). You go from one shape, to another shape, back into the original shape. Because your feet remain in contact with the ground throughout the entire movement, you can maintain a torsion force through the entire range of the movement. It is this torsion force that keeps you *connected* to the movement.

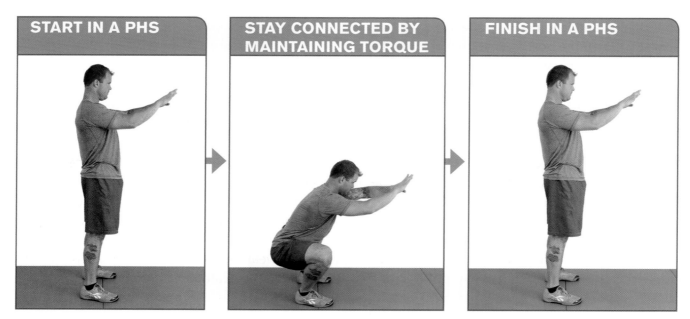

Category 2 Movements

As with category 1 movements, category 2 movements take you from a PHS to a PHS. But instead of maintaining torque throughout the entire range of the movement, you insert a speed element—jumping and landing, wall ball, snatch balance, running, rowing, etc.—between beginning and end.

| Position of High Stability (PHS) | → | remove connection with speed | → | Position of High Stability (PHS) |

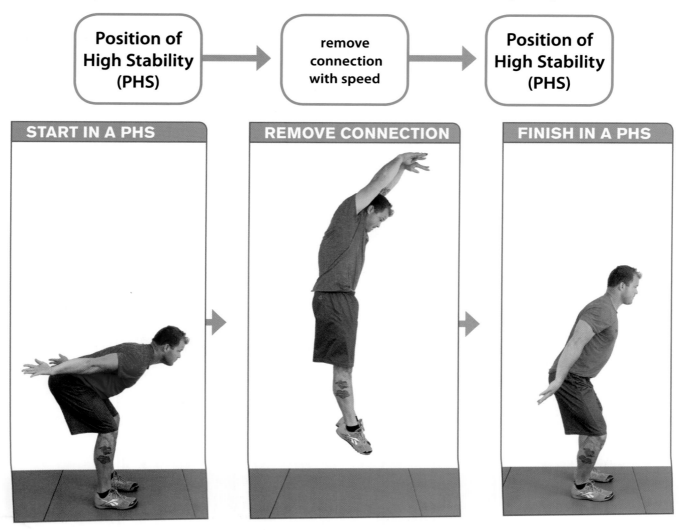

Jumping and landing is a perfect example of this. You start in a PHS, you remove connection (torque) as you jump off the box, and then you have to spontaneously stabilize your spine, screw your feet into the ground, and drive your knees out to finish in a PHS. You still start and finish in the same position, but by removing your torsion force and adding speed—jumping in the air—you increase the motor-control and mobility demands of the movement.

What you will find is that it is a lot harder to hide weaknesses as you progress into category 2 movements.

People can disguise their movement dysfunction and mobility restrictions behind the veil of category 1 movements, so you have to constantly challenge their motor-control and range-of-motion capacities. For example, you might find that you can perform, say, a squat with good form, but the moment you take that squat position to an elevated platform and jump off it, everything unravels: feet turn out, ankles collapse, knees cave inward, lumbar spine overextends.

To improve as an athlete, you have to work very hard to find weaknesses in your movement profile. It's not enough to move fast, lift heavy, or perform high-repetitions within category 1. As you move closer to the actions of sports, you need to be able to spontaneously arrive in a safe and stable position. Your tissues are not normal unless they're capable of moving quickly while remaining stable at end-range.

Category 3 Movements

Category 3 movements closely resemble the actions of sports. This means changing direction: going from a pull to a push/press, cutting, jumping and then landing in a different position, etc. The formal definition of a category 3 movement is to start in one position, remove the connection (torque), and arrive in a completely different position. Put another way, an athlete needs to be able to spontaneously generate stability while changing position or direction.

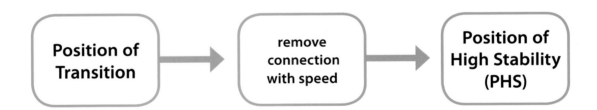

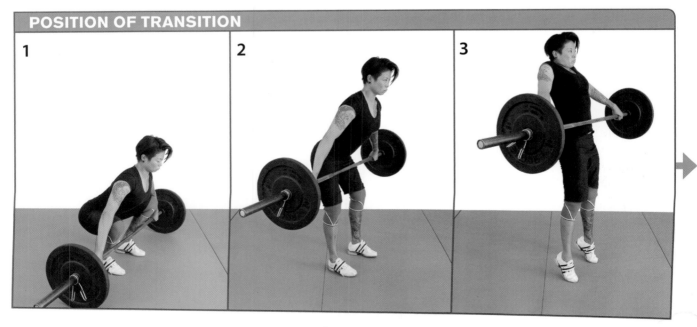

POSITION OF TRANSITION

1   2   3

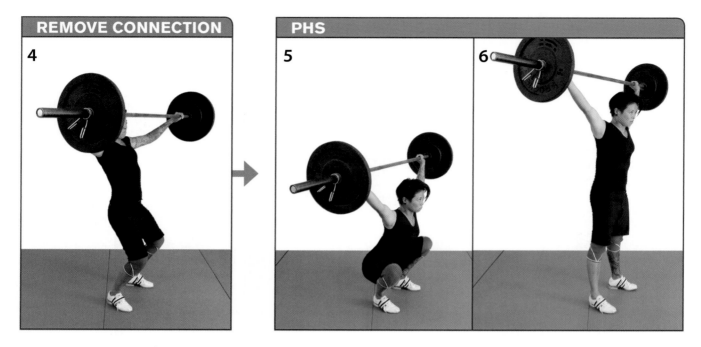

One of the most difficult and easily recognizable category 3 movements performed in the gym is the snatch. As you can see from the photos, you start in a pulling position, open your hips into full extension, and then drop into the bottom of the squat with your arms overhead. As the bar travels upward, there is a moment of weightlessness when you lose torque with the ground and the bar: This is the position of transition and where you lose connection (you momentarily lose torque). Receiving the weight in the bottom of the overhead squat is your PHS. You go from one shape, which is a position of transition (a pulling position), remove the connection, and then arrive in a completely different shape, in the over-head squat, or PHS.

As with category 2 movements, when you expose athletes or you start implementing these full-range movements, technique falls apart. The simple fact is that these changes of direction are very challenging. You can't disguise poor movement patterns or limited ranges of motion. And that's the goal. Remember, to ensure continual growth, you need to hunt down all your motor-control and mobility issues, expose them, and then work on fixing them.

The bottom line is that you need to train category 1 movements like power lifts (squat, deadlift, bench press) to layer the fundamental movement principles. But if you want to improve athleticism and really highlight an athlete's understanding of midline stabilization and torque, you need to expose her to category 3 movements like Olympic lifts.

Upright-Torso Demands

The orientation or verticality of your torso is another way to categorize complex movements within the framework of the movement hierarchy. It's really simple: The more upright the torso, the more motor-control, range-of-motion, and stabilization required to carry out the movement.

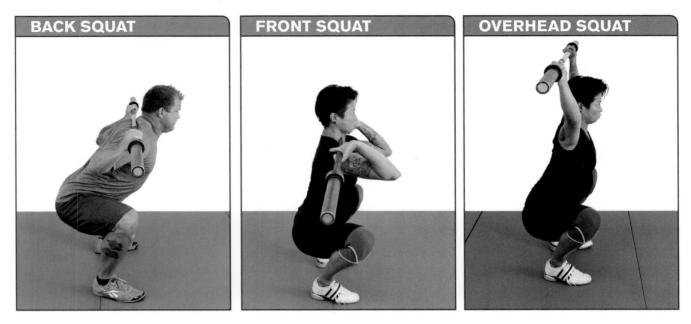

BACK SQUAT FRONT SQUAT OVERHEAD SQUAT

The squat variations present perhaps the best examples of how an upright torso increases the difficulty of a movement. For instance, the back squat is the simplest of the variants because it has relatively low upright-torso demands. You can tilt your torso slightly forward, giving your hips, hamstrings, and ankles some room to breathe. But if you increase the verticality of your torso in the form of a front squat, right away you will start to see weaknesses in your athletic profile. You will have a much harder time keeping your back flat, your knees out, and your shins perpendicular. The overhead squat is the toughest of the squat iterations because you have to keep your torso perfectly upright to avoid defaulting into an unfavorable position.

Although each squat variation requires you to stabilize the barbell and organize your shoulders in a different position, the orientation of your torso adds to the difficulty of the lift. Even having an athlete do a high-bar back squat (squat with the torso upright) in place of a low-bar back squat (squat with the torso tilted forward) creates new challenges in terms of motor-control and mobility.

When I teach my Movement and Mobility Seminars, I highlight this concept by asking those in attendance to go through a three-squat series.

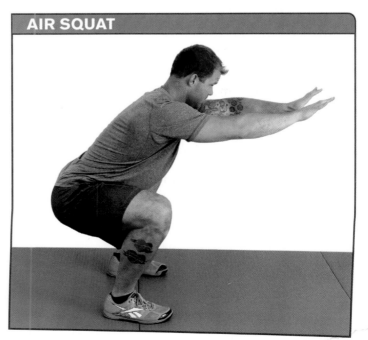

AIR SQUAT

First, I ask them to perform a body-weight squat. I never specify what kind of squat, just that they squat with their back flat and shins vertical. Without fail, everyone always shows me a close iteration of an unweighted back squat because it's the easiest of all the squats as you can tilt your torso forward and descend into the bottom position without compromising form.

Next, I'll ask them to put their hands behind their heads, which forces their torsos into a more upright position, and squat again. This is the equivalent of going from a back squat to a front squat. At this point, people will start to struggle to keep their backs flat and shins vertical. To stay integrated, they have to increase tension in their trunk and drive their knees out a little bit farther to correctly execute the movement, resulting in a lot more faults.

The last thing I'll ask them to do is squat with their arms locked overhead, which is essentially an unweighted overhead squat. And this is where people start defaulting into some pretty wonky positions to keep their torsos upright, shins vertical, and arms overhead. Obviously, you can still tilt your torso forward while keeping your hands overhead. However, to get the most out of this exercise, you need to increase the verticality of your torso with each subsequent squat.

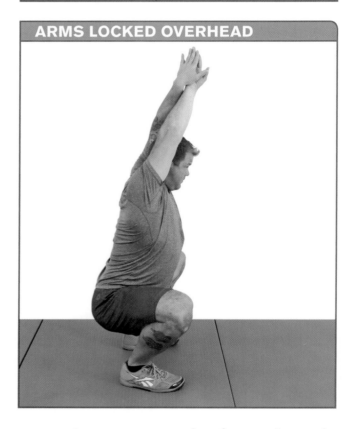

HANDS BEHIND HEAD

ARMS LOCKED OVERHEAD

This three-squat series turns into a really simple category 1 movement template for spotting problems and challenging the athlete with higher degrees of motor-control and mobility.

Whether you're layering on exercises to rehab an athlete post-injury or after surgery, or trying to expose restrictions in a beginner or elite athlete's mobility and technique, skill progressions and movement complexity become easy if you understand the upright-torso demands principle and the movement hierarchy. You should be able to identify basic universal shapes of stability. You should also be able to spot movement faults and understand what it is happening and know how to fix it. Finally, you should be able to teach and incorporate transferable, full-range strength-and-conditioning movements in a way that instills good movement patterning for athletes of all ability levels.

MWOD FIGHT CLUB DRILL

The goal is to equip you with the knowledge to correct movement faults and address your own range-of-motion problems. However, that doesn't mean you do it alone; having someone analyze your movement and keep you honest is key. You're way more likely to pay attention to your foot position when you stand and your posture when you sit if someone else is holding you accountable. You need a coach, and you need a training partner, people who understand this material and will call you out when you're hanging out in lousy positions or moving poorly. You need someone who will offer tips on how to correct the problem and help prescribe specific mobility remedies based on your issues. I call this the MWOD Fight Club Drill. The idea is to make an agreement—whether it is with your coach, training partner, kid, significant other, etc.—to always be in a good position. You can't run, and you can't hide.

CATEGORY 1 MOVEMENTS

Position of High Stability (PHS)	with connection	Position of High Stability (PHS)

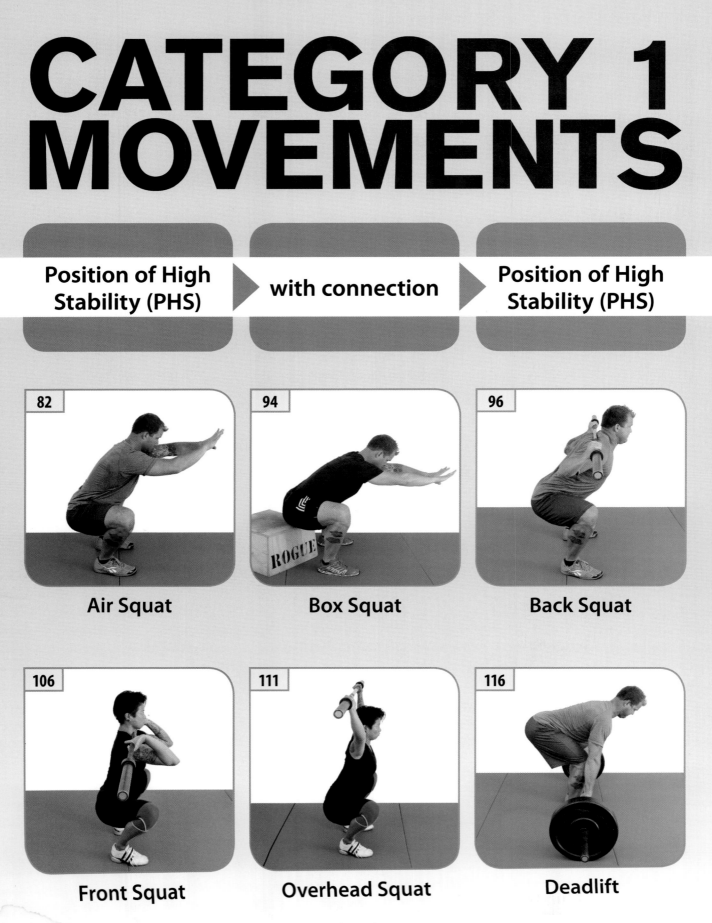

82 Air Squat

94 Box Squat

96 Back Squat

106 Front Squat

111 Overhead Squat

116 Deadlift

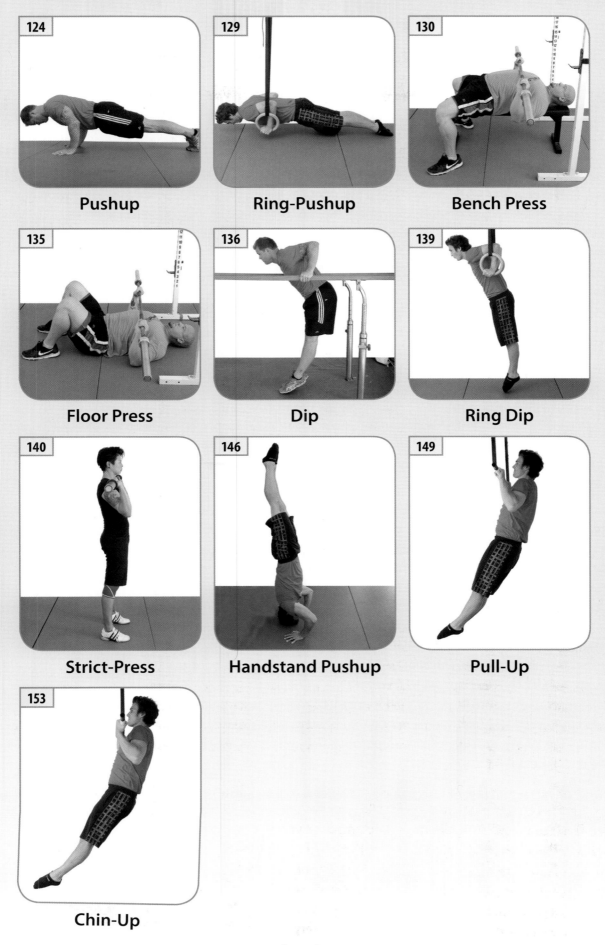

124 Pushup

129 Ring-Pushup

130 Bench Press

135 Floor Press

136 Dip

139 Ring Dip

140 Strict-Press

146 Handstand Pushup

149 Pull-Up

153 Chin-Up

AIR SQUAT

Squatting and walking. If there are two movements you shouldn't take for granted, it's how to squat and how to walk. Make a good decision. Master both movements.

Think about how many times you sit down and stand up. How much you walk. Walk and squat with crappy mechanics every day for years on end and it shouldn't be much of a stunner that your knees and back glow with chronic pain and a doctor starts describing the modern wonders of a joint replacement.

Don't even get me started on how walking and squatting poorly will gut athletic potential.

How a person walks will tell you a lot. The squat, however, is the looking glass. A full-range, butt-to-ankles air squat is an omnipotent diagnostic tool for identifying problems and fixing the broken athlete.

In this section I will break down the squat in detail, and describe how poor squatting mechanics and missing ranges of motion can lead to back, hip, knee, and ankle pain. I will also detail how poor squatting mechanics can transfer over to repetitive, more dynamic movements such as running and jumping. The bottom line is that if you want to optimize performance and escape pain and injury, it's imperative that you learn how to squat correctly.

There are many types of squats: air squat, box squat, back squat, front squat, overhead squat. We'll take a look at each. First let's talk about the critical principles at work with all types of squatting.

Principles of Squatting:

Squat Stance

If you are trying to break 1,200 pounds for the squat, a wide stance is the ticket. It will allow you to keep your torso upright and squat the equivalent of a Volkswagen. But if you're using the squat as an exercise to improve health and athletic performance, you need a stance that expresses a full range-of-motion, reveals problems, and transfers to other athletic movements.

For most people, positioning their feet just outside the shoulders will accomplish that goal. This all-purpose squat stance has universality in sports—think of the ready position of the linebacker, a tennis player, or a fighter's combat stance. From this same position you can tackle more advanced exercises—the front squat, overhead squat, and Olympic lifts—without having to adjust your feet. Remember the Miyamoto Musashi quote that I referenced in the introduction to this book: "Make your fight stance your everyday stance; make your everyday stance your fight stance."

Make your squat stance your everyday stance and make your everyday stance your squat stance.

Here's the deal: Establish a squat stance that best fits your goals as an athlete and allows you to practice good form. Personally, I mostly use an all-purpose stance, but on occasion experiment with a wide stance to throttle the stimulus.

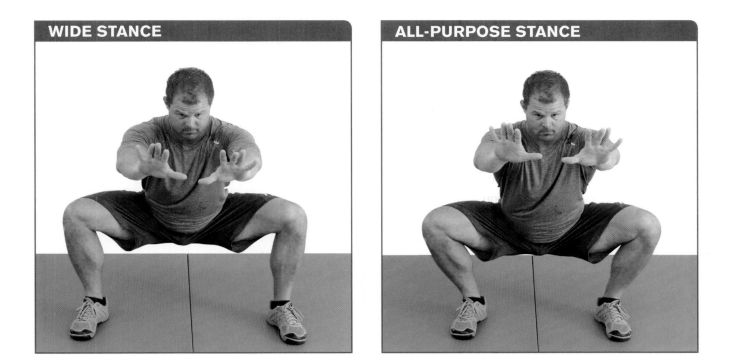

WIDE STANCE — **ALL-PURPOSE STANCE**

Keep Shins Vertical

This tip is worth the price of this book 100 times over. At least.

Keep your shins as vertical as possible when you descend and rise out of the squat. Vertical shins will allow you to channel the power of your hips and hamstrings and consequently unload weight from the knees. If you fail to keep your shins vertical and your knees lurch forward out over your feet, you'll lose power from the posterior chain and increase the shear and twisting forces to the soft tissues within the joint, especially to the cartilage, the patellar tendon, and the ACL. Not good. Keep shins vertical and experience more power.

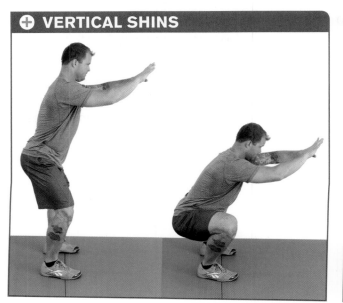

➕ **VERTICAL SHINS**

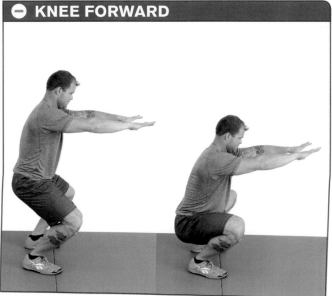

➖ **KNEE FORWARD**

Load Your Hips and Hamstrings

Keeping your shins vertical is one thing. You also must initiate the squat by loading your hips and hamstrings. You do this by tilting your torso forward and driving your hamstrings back. This will load the right muscle groups. It will allow you to hinge at the hips with a flat back and maintain proper torque through your arms and legs. It will fortify your posture so you don't break at the lumbar spine.

For example, a lot of athletes will mistakenly keep their chest up and reach their butt back as a way to keep their shins vertical, which causes an overextension fault (aka anterior pelvic tilt). To avoid this, think about sitting your hamstrings back as you initiate the movement. If you think about reaching your butt back instead, you're more likely to default into an overextended position.

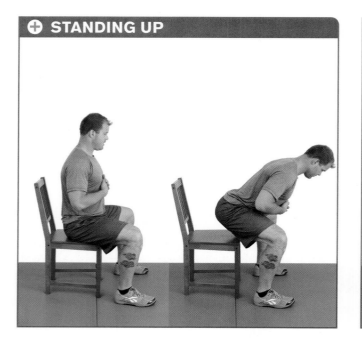

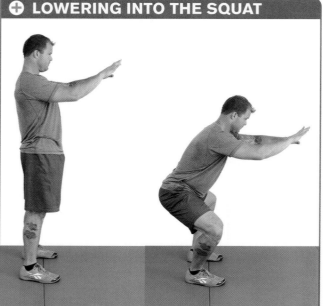

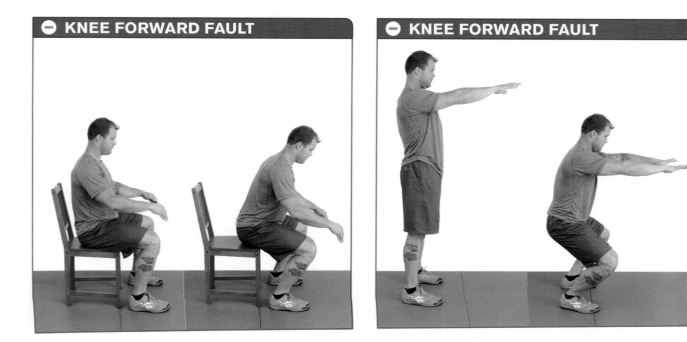

Distribute Weight in the Center of the Foot

To create and maintain maximum torque, imagine screwing your feet into the ground with your weight distributed over the *center* of your feet. Not the balls of your feet, not the heels, the center of your feet, with your mass right in front of your ankles.

People learning how to squat will often mistakenly roll up on the balls of their feet. This stems from either a lack of technique or missing range-of-motion in the quads. Or both. Many coaches like to try and cure the problem by having a beginner shift his weight to his heels. The problem with this fix is that it opens the door to other weight-distribution faults as the athlete develops in the future. Centering your weight on your heels will make it difficult to create the torque necessary for full stability. This habit will likely transfer to other movements as well. Imagine trying to make a big Olympic lift or dunk a basketball with your weight on your heels. It's not going to happen.

Center your weight in front of your ankles and keep your entire foot in contact with the ground.

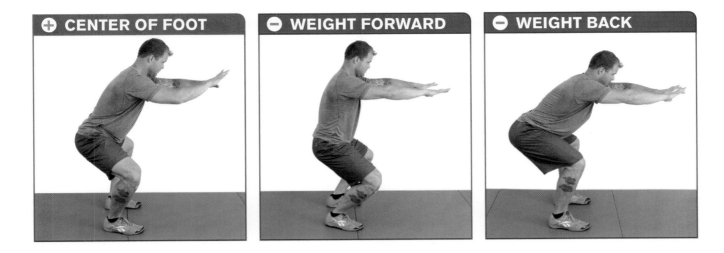

Create a Stable Shoulder

The position of your arms will vary depending on the squat you're doing. Regardless, always set your shoulders in a stable position by creating force from external rotation.

If you're setting up for an air squat, pull your shoulders back while turning your thumbs toward the inside of your body.

If you're setting up for a barbell lift, screw your hands into the bar—your right hand clockwise and your left counter-clockwise—as if you were trying to snap the bar in half. This resulting tension will stabilize your shoulders and turn on the muscles across your upper back, resulting in a braced-neutral spine. This all-powerful ready position becomes more critical the more weight you're dealing with.

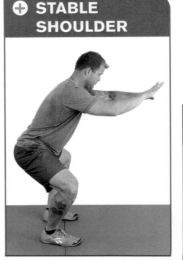

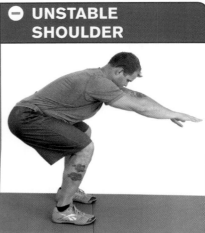

Air Squat Sequence

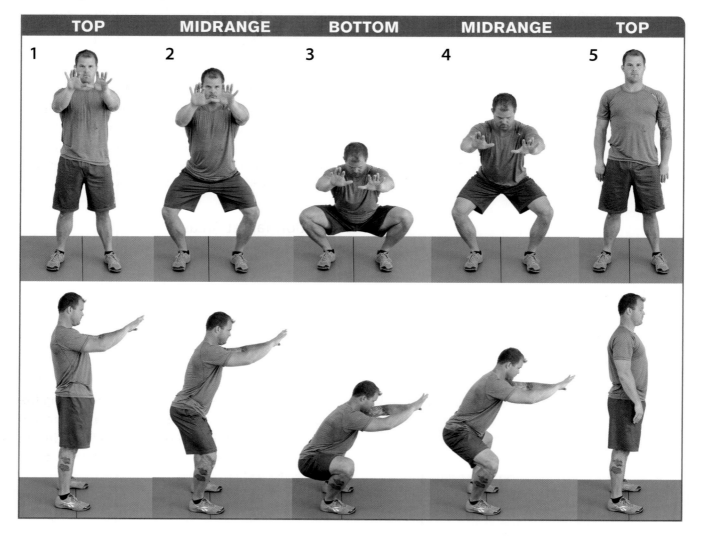

TOP	MIDRANGE	BOTTOM	MIDRANGE	TOP
1	2	3	4	5

1. To set up for the squat, establish your squat stance with your feet straight, somewhere between 5 and 12 degrees. Once accomplished, go through the bracing sequence: Squeeze your butt, pull your ribcage down, and get your belly tight. With your spine braced in a neutral position, screw your feet into the ground as if you were trying to spread the floor. Next, set your shoulders in a stable position and tighten your upper back by raising your arms, pulling your shoulders back, and externally rotating your hands slightly. Look forward to maintain a neutral head position and keep your weight centered over the front of your ankles.

2. Reach your hamstrings back—keeping your shins as vertical as possible—drive your knees out laterally, and start lowering into the bottom position. To help maintain tension and maximize torque, think about pulling yourself into the bottom position instead of dropping into the bottom position.

3. As your hip crease drops below knee depth, continue to drive your knees out laterally, keeping your shins as vertical as possible. As you reach full depth, you should feel very stable. In other words, there should be no slack in the system. Your back should be tight, your knees at the limits of their external rotation range, and your hips at peak tension. Note: You may need to adjust your knees slightly forward to reach full depth. The key is to maintain as much external rotation force as possible by pushing your knees out.

4. Still making a conscious effort to drive your knees out and screw your feet into the ground, pull your shins back to vertical and extend your hips and knees. Rise out of the bottom position in the same way you entered: with your spine neutral, knees out, and shoulders and upper back tight. Put simply, it's the same as descending but in the reverse order.

5. As you stand up, reclaim a stable top position by squeezing your butt. This will set your pelvis in a neutral position and prepare you for the next movement or repetition.

Knee Forward Fault

You squat and your knees move forward out over your feet. Wham! What happened? It's usually a technique problem—motor-control—and you may be fighting against brutally tight muscles in the thighs and hips.

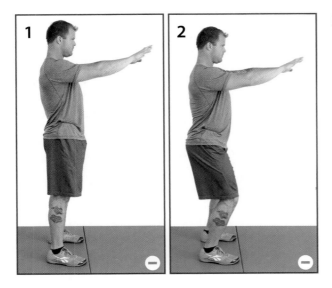

Motor-Control Fix:

▶ Isolate the first 6-inches of the squat.

▶ Focus on creating external rotation torque by screwing your feet into the ground and pressing your knees out.

▶ Initiate the squat by sitting your hamstrings back (load your hips and hamstrings), keeping your shins as vertical as possible while continuing to shove your knees out.

Mobilization Target Areas:

▶ Posterior High Chain (Glutes)

▶ Anterior Chain (Hip and Quads)

Overextension Spinal Fault

Failure to organize your spine in a neutral position with the muscles of your belly tight is like pulling the plug on a cyborg. You will collapse into an overextended position as you initiate the squat. The moment you lose control of your pelvis, stability through the chain is lost. Screwing your feet into the ground and driving your knees outward won't matter. Power will bleed from the system. This fault is also characterized by a gross reversal of the pelvis in the bottom position (see butt wink fault, page 91).

Most people have enough mobility to initiate the first 6-inches of the squat so correcting this fault becomes a learning related task. However, if your anterior hip structures are brutally tight (anterior hip capsule, hip flexor, quads), you are more likely to default into an overextended position to feed slack to your hip system.

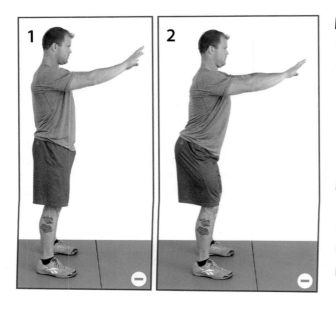

Motor-Control Fix:

▶ Isolate the first 6-inches of the squat.

▶ Create external rotation torque by screwing your feet into the ground and shoving your knees out.

▶ Initiate the squat by sitting your hamstrings back. Keep your shins as vertical as possible while maintaining external rotation torque.

Mobilization Target Areas:

▶ Anterior Chain (Hip and Quads)

▶ Posterior High Chain (Glutes)

▶ Posterior Low Chain (Hamstrings)

▶ Trunk

Valgus Knee Fault

Before you begin a squat, you want to tighten your core and squeeze the muscles of your butt. This creates external rotation force at the hip. Torque. Failure to create this stability will cause your knees to cave in. This is called valgus knee collapse. Remember, if you fail to create torque at the start of a squat, your body will have to create stability somewhere else, which is expressed through this fault.

Turning out your feet past the 12 to 15 degree range increases your vulnerability to this problem. Wide angled feet can also make it difficult to produce torque that will stabilize your knees.

The motor-control fix is simple: Screw your feet into the ground in the top position and focus on driving your knees out as you lower into the bottom position. Past the 6-inch point, however, mobility weaknesses in the ankle, hips, and quads will play a part.

In some cases, spotting torque faults in the air squat can be difficult, especially if someone has full hip and leg range-of-motion. That's why we always challenge these movements with weight, speed, and high-repetitions. Challenge the movements and the faults will become apparent.

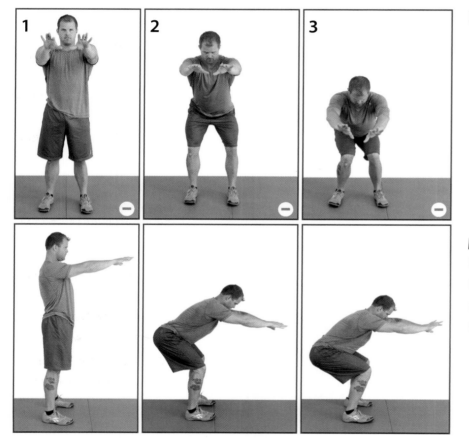

Motor-Control Fix:

► Isolate the first 6-inches of the squat.

► Create external rotation torque by screwing your feet into the ground and shoving your knees out.

► Initiate the squat by sitting your hamstrings back. Keep your shins as vertical as possible while maintaining external rotation torque.

Mobilization Target Areas:

► Anterior Chain (Hips and Quads)

► Anterior Low Chain (Hamstrings)

► Posterior High Chain (Glutes)

► Calf and Heel Cord

Shoulder Fault

If you don't organize your shoulders into a stable, externally rotated position, your upper back becomes soft and rounds and you can't maintain a stable spine. This is usually a setup error, caused by people forgetting to set their shoulders before launching into the movement. Poor mobility in the shoulders can also lead to this fault.

Motor-Control Fix:

► Wind up your shoulders into a stable, externally rotated position.

Mobilization Target Areas:

► Thoracic Spine

► Anterior Shoulders and Chest

► Posterior Shoulders and Lat

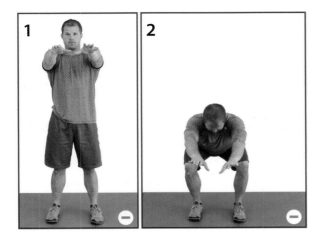

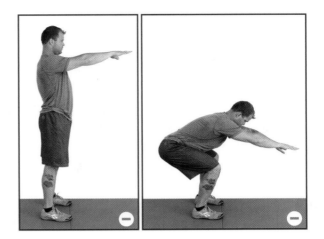

Open Foot Fault

If you glance at the photos, you'll notice that I set my feet up at optimal angles, but as I sink into the squat, my feet spin apart. This fault dumps torque and bleeds force all over the place. Stability throughout the system dribbles away.

Lack of mobility is usually the culprit—either missing range-of-motion in the ankle or hip, or the thigh muscles are just wound up like a top.

This fault can also happen when you put your weight on your heels instead of smack in the center of your feet. Screw your feet into the floor.

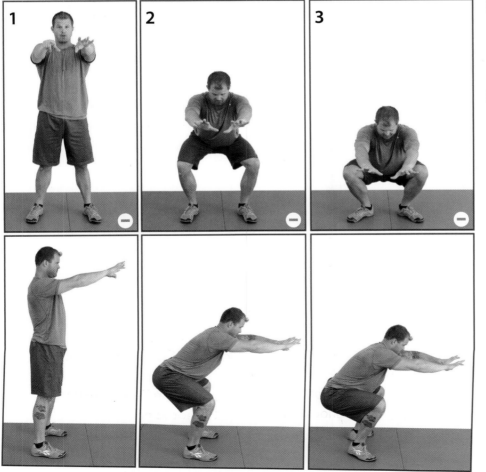

Motor-Control Fix:

▶ Distribute weight evenly between your heel and the ball of your foot.

Mobilization Target Areas:

▶ Ankle and Plantar Surface

▶ Calf and Heel Cord

▶ Anterior Chain (Hips and Quads)

▶ Medial Chain (Adductors)

▶ Posterior High Chain (Glutes)

Range-of-Motion Squat Tests: Ruling Out the Ankle

When you can't get into an ideal position because you're missing key ranges of motion, you have to ask yourself: Where is the problem? Is it my ankle, quad, anterior hip? Chances are it's a system of systems, meaning that it's a combination of tight tissues. This is why we take a systems approach to dealing with these problems by using simple tests to rule out specific areas of the body.

For example, the ankle wall and pistol test are two ways to see whether or not you have full ankle range-of-motion or if you are missing critical corners. What's great about these tests is you don't have to memorize the anatomy or joint measurement of a full range-of-motion. All you have to determine is whether you can you get into a pistol position. Yes or no?

Ankle Wall

The pistol test and ankle wall both tell you if you have full ankle range-of-motion, but more specifically, the ankle wall lets you know where you are coming up short. For example, say you lower into the squat with your feet together, keeping your back flat as you descend. If you're missing ankle range-of-motion you will literally hit a wall, at which point you will either lose your balance, causing you to fall backward, or you will compensate into a rounded position. In either case, the moment you hit the wall, that is the limit of your ankle range-of-motion.

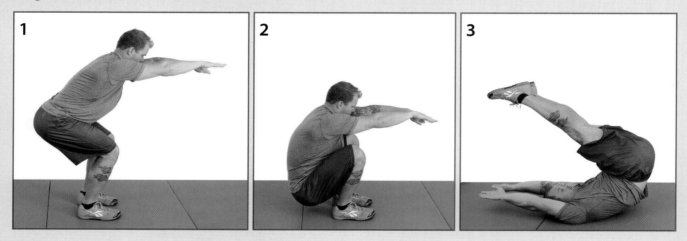

Pistol Test

There is nothing that we do as human beings that requires more ankle range-of-motion than being in the bottom of the single-leg squat position (pistol). If you can lower into the squat with your back flat and extend one of your legs out in front of your body while keeping your grounded foot neutral, you have full dorsiflexion range-of-motion in your ankle.

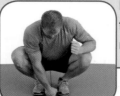

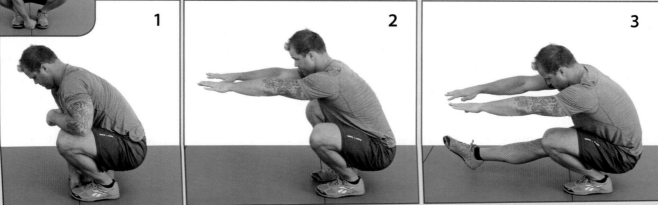

Lumbar Reversal Fault: The Butt Wink

The butt wink fault occurs when your pelvis tucks underneath your body near the bottom position of the squat. If you start a squat by reaching back with your butt and unlocking your abs—overextending the lumbar spine—your femur runs into the top of your hip joint and literally drives your pelvis back like a slow-motion truck accident. The butt wink is the pelvis realigning to a better position. However, the overall system then becomes horribly unstable and poorly braced. This is not a happy place to be, especially with a loaded barbell on your shoulders.

If this is your problem, here's the plan: You need to create and maintain midline stability and torque. If you have tissue restrictions that compromise your movement, reduce the depth of your squat and address your posterior chain and hamstring mobility. Remember, you never want to compromise safe form for depth.

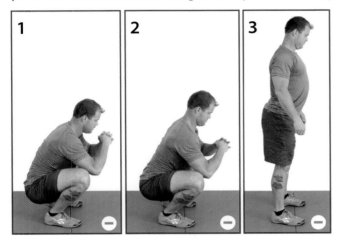

Motor-Control Fix:

▶ Squeeze your butt and stabilize your spine in the top position.

▶ Initiate the squat by driving your hamstrings back, not your butt.

▶ Shove your knees out as far as possible and screw your feet into the ground as you lower into the squat.

Mobilization Target Areas:

▶ Anterior Chain (Hips and Quads)

▶ Posterior High Chain (Glutes)

▶ Posterior Low Chain (Hamstrings)

▶ Calf and Heel Cord

▶ Trunk

Knee Forward Fault: Bottom Position

It's important to mention that a slight forward translation of your knees will happen as you reach full depth. The key is to make a conscious effort to drive your knees out and keep your shins as vertical as possible as long as possible, to avoid loss of position and power.

Ideally, an athlete will fight to maintain a vertical shin for as long as possible and will use additional knee flexion—the knee moving forward—to adjust for increased depth of the squat or to maximize the plumb line uprightness of the torso. As the knee moves forward, the stabilization demands at the hip become untenable and the knee experiences significant shear forces.

When you hear, "Don't squat below 90-degrees, it's bad for your knees," it means that most people can't help but move their knees forward once they drop below the parallel mark. The knees moving forward is a nightmare position. It's exposing the soft tissues of your knees to garden scissors. And it doesn't end there; because the system is now so horribly screwed, the knees tend to remain forward on the ascent out of the squat. Now you're just movement fault road kill and the shearing forces continue their shredding ways.

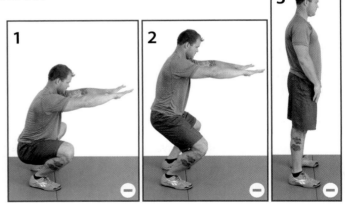

Motor-Control Fix:

▶ Load your hips and hamstrings as you initiate the squat. Keep your shins vertical as long as possible.

▶ If your knees translate forward in the bottom position, pull your knees back, making your shins as vertical as possible, as you rise to the top position. Go up the same way you went down.

Mobilization Target Areas:

▶ Anterior Chain (Hips and Quads)

▶ Medial Chain (Adductors)

▶ Posterior Low Chain (Hamstrings)

▶ Posterior High Chain (Glutes)

Head Fault

Anybody who has played high school football can relate to this cue: "Head up, chest up!" It's another classic cue that coaches use to correct or prevent an athlete from rounding forward into flexion. (Or correcting a good morning squat fault—see good morning squat fault—stripper squat—page 105). Although tilting your head back will help keep your torso upright, it's exchanging one spinal fault for another: Instead of rounding forward into a flexed position, you default into a grossly overextended position. Whether it's a learned pattern, ingrained from bad cueing, or you don't understand the relationship between a neutral head and spine, the solution is simple: don't throw your head back.

Motor-Control Fix:

▶ Don't throw your head back. Maintain a neutral spinal position—see bracing chapter (page 26).

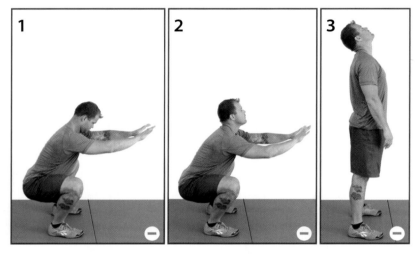

Walking And Stepping Mechanics

Walking Mechanics

Walking is a complex movement. I could spend a lot of time breaking down the joint position and phases of walking, but that is beyond the scope of this book. Nor is it necessary. When I address walking with my ath-

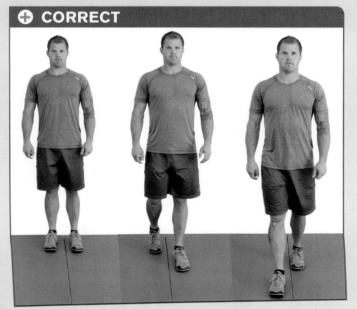

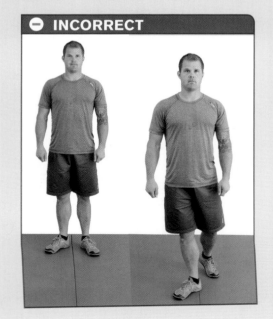

letes for example, I just tell them to keep their feet straight and their spine neutral. It's that simple.

If you turn out your feet out as you walk, your ankles will collapse into an unstable position with every step. This is a mechanism for bunions and a lot of people's foot and knee-related problems. And just think of the number of duty cycles you go through. Again, the key is to get organized before you start moving. Go through the bracing sequence and focus on keeping your feet straight.

Stepping Mechanics

Stepping onto an elevated platform or walking up or down the stairs shares all the same principles as squatting. Think of it as a single-leg upright squat. You want to keep your torso vertical, spine neutral, knees out, and feet arched (neutral). The higher the step, the more you will have to hinge from the hip. Regardless of the height, the key to success is to keep your shin as vertical as possible.

When people have problems walking up and down stairs or stepping onto a box, it's because their knee is translating forward and their ankle is collapsing inward. It's the equivalent of initiating a squat with zero stability. There's no torque at the hip, so they overextend and the downstream structures shift into a wrenched position. The solution is simple: Keep your foot straight, drive your knee out, and maintain a well-organized, stable trunk.

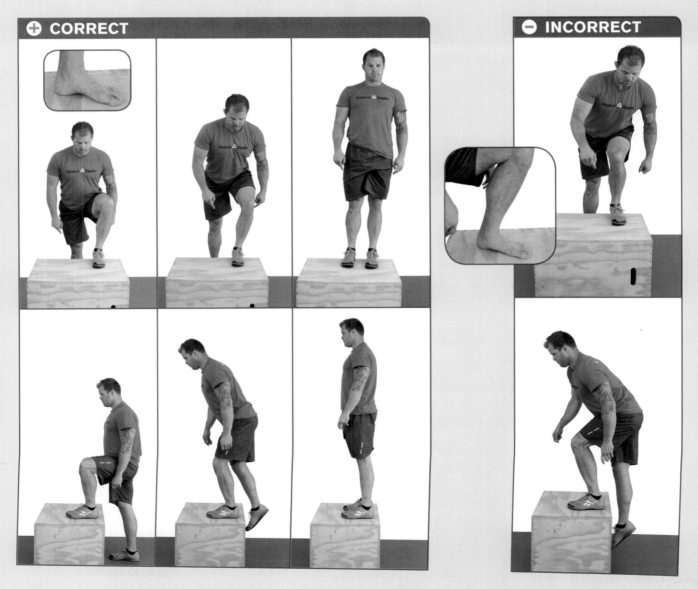

BOX SQUAT

The box squat is a movement that average people perform thousands of times a week. Every time you sit down and get up from a chair, toilet, or couch, you perform a close iteration of this squat.

Although the air squat is the first movement that I teach to novice athletes—it's my way of layering fundamental squat principles—most people don't have the mobility to squat to full depth (even though it's something that every human being should be able to do). If squatting butt to heels is not a viable option, positioning a box at knee-level or slightly higher is a great way to layer good squat mechanics.

Unlike the air squat, the box squat allows people to fix problems that they may or may not be aware of. For example, say you're struggling to load your hips and hamstrings and pull your knees back to get your shins vertical. Having a stable target like a box or a chair to reach for is an easy way to reverse knee forward faults and ingrain functional movement patterns. In addition, you can focus on spinal mechanics and weight distribution in the bottom position without worrying about falling over. It's a simple way to scale or adjust the depth of the squat without compromising form.

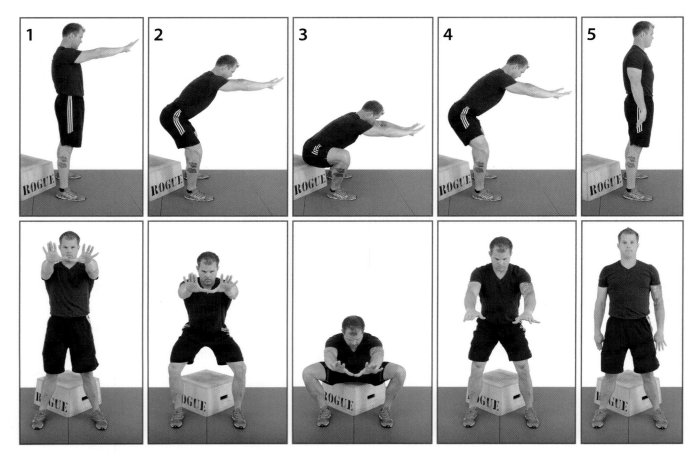

1. Assume your squat stance. Note: position your heels a few inches from the box with a corner angled between your legs. Once accomplished, screw your feet into the ground to create torque, squeeze your butt, stabilize your midline, and set your shoulders in a stable position.

2. Keeping your shins vertical and back flat, sit your hamstrings back and hinge forward at the hips.

3. Lower your butt to the box, maintaining tension in your hips and hamstrings and back as you sit your butt down.

4. Drive out of the bottom position the moment your butt touches down.

5. Reestablish the top position.

Standing Out of the Bottom Position

When you execute the box squat as an exercise, you never completely release tension in your hips and hamstrings. The moment your butt touches down, reverse the sequence by standing back up. However, if you're having trouble in the bottom position, pausing on a box or chair is an excellent way to work on standing up with good mechanics. It gives you a new start position, and allows you to focus on getting your shins vertical, shoving your knees out, and keeping your back flat as you rise out of the bottom position.

This is the key: If you start from the seated position, keep your belly tight and reload your hips and hamstrings by hinging forward at the hips, just as you would when initiating the squat.

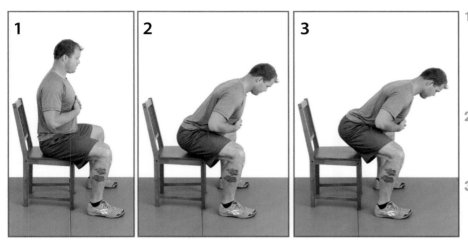

1. Sitting is just a box squat with a long pause in the bottom position. Even if you remain seated for an extended period of time, your back stays flat, shins vertical, and knees out.

2. When you stand up, reclaim tension by loading your hips and hamstrings by hinging forward at the hips.

3. Keeping your back flat, shove your knees out and stand up just as you would when performing a squat.

Knee Forward Chair Fault

When your knees come forward as you get out of a chair it's usually one of two things: either you are not comfortable creating tension in your hips and hamstrings as you stand up, or you haven't created sufficient torque. As with the air squat, driving your knees forward out of the bottom position is primarily a motor-control error.

If I notice that an athlete's knees come forward every time he squats out of the bottom position, I'll have him sit to a box or chair and put my hand in front of his knee. Every time his knee touches my hand, I have him sit back to the box and try again. In addition to illuminating the fault, this simple tactic brings consciousness to the movement, dramatically reducing the probability of committing this error.

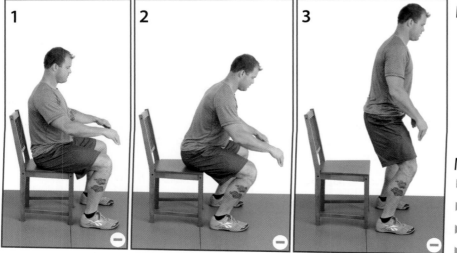

Motor-Control Fix:
▶ Create torque by screwing your feet into the ground and driving your knees out.

▶ Hinge forward with a flat back, load your hips and hamstrings, and get your shins as vertical as possible.

Mobilization Target Areas:
▶ Posterior High Chain (Glutes)

▶ Medial Chain (Adductors)

▶ Anterior Chain (Hips and Quads)

▶ Posterior Low Chain (Hamstrings)

Overextension Fault

As with the knee forward fault, an overextension spinal error is almost always a motor-control issue. As you can see from the photos, my spine flexes in the seated position (same as the butt wink fault) and then as I stand up, I immediately default into an overextended position. Once my pelvis dumps forward, my lumbar spine stabilizes the load of my torso instead of my hips and hamstrings. My shins are vertical so I saved my knees from the load, but I trashed my spine. Not good. To rectify this problem, sit down with a braced spine and keep your belly tight while seated. Remember, you need at least 20 percent tension in your trunk to maintain a neutral posture.

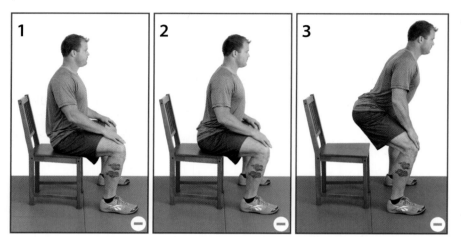

Motor-Control Fix:

- ▶ Address the bracing sequence.

- ▶ Get organized before sitting down and keep your belly tight while in the bottom position (seated).

- ▶ Hinge forward at your hips to load your hamstrings and pull your shins vertical before standing up.

BACK SQUAT

It's one thing to be able to air squat and box squat, it's an entirely different thing to squat with a weight on your back. Spend a day at the zoo shouldering your three-year-old and you'll know what I'm talking about.

Once you understand the universal laws of squatting and you've practiced the movement with the air and box squat, you need to up the ante on your positions and add load. With additional weight on your torso and hips, small errors that may go unnoticed in the air squat and box squat become obvious, making it another way to diagnose poor movement patterns. Not only that, adding a barbell to the equation changes the level of trunk stiffness and torsion force that is applied to the movement, which translates to more complex actions.

This is the idea: If you're air squatting you might be managing 30 to 40 percent torque and tension levels. While this is great for simple tasks, the stabilization demands don't transfer to more dynamic movements. For example, jumping and landing or squatting with a heavy load requires much higher levels of trunk stiffness and torsion force. If you never challenge your setup and your movement with larger loads, generating higher levels of force is difficult.

The back squat involves a lot of complex steps: Take the barbell out of the rack, walk back and assume a squat stance, execute the movement, walk forward, re-rack the weight. It takes skill, practice, and razor sharp focus to perform each step correctly. To ingrain the correct movement patterning and reduce errors, it's important that you go through the same load-order sequence. The idea is to minimize the variability of your movement so that you can preserve the quality of your position with each transitory step. If you take the bar out of the rack seventeen different ways, you're going to start your squat seventeen different ways.

This is not to say that you shouldn't change the bar position or change your squat stance from time to time. Those changes are fine—just be sure to practice the same step-by-step setup every time you lift. If you step back with your left foot first, then do that every single time. That way, when you're tired, under stress, or in competition, you don't make fundamental mistakes because you've ingrained the same motor pattern over and over again. It's instinctual.

To shorten your learning curve, I broke down the back squat into three phases: lift out (taking the barbell out of the rack), walking back, and then squatting. It's worth mentioning that the lift out and walk back are universal steps used in lifts that require you to take a barbell out of the rack—the front squat, overhead squat, strict-press, push-press, push-jerk, split-jerk.

Phase 1: Lift Out_(The 6-Inch Squat)

Anytime you take a barbell out of a rack, you have to set your shoulders and get your belly tight before adding a load to your spine. It's a perfect example of the tunnel concept: If you take the bar out of the rack and your spine is disorganized, or your hips are in a bad position, it's impossible to reclaim a good position.

The first phase, which is essentially a 6-inch vertical squat, sets the tone for the rest of the lift. Most injuries and missed lifts relate back to errors made in this phase, so it's imperative that it's done right. If you don't perform a good lift out, reset the bar and start from scratch. Additionally, make sure to set the rack to a height that allows for a good lift out, which is roughly chest level.

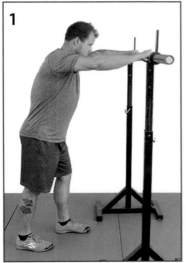

1

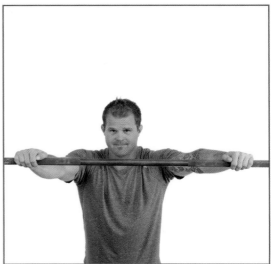

Find a comfortable distance for your grip. Personally, I like to position my hands just outside shoulder-width. As with stance, grip distance is different for everyone and is predicated on mobility and frame size. The key is to form a grip that allows you to create sufficient external rotation force and tension in your upper back and shoulders. Put simply, it's a grip that allows you to keep your wrists straight and your elbows underneath your shoulders.

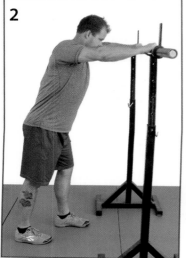

2

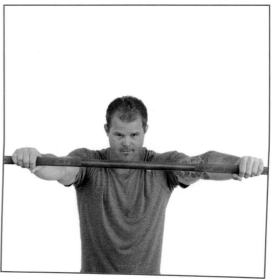

Once you set your hands, create torque in your shoulders. To accomplish this, pull back on the barbell and create an external rotation force by creating torque off the bar. Imagine trying to break or bend the bar with your hands. It's important to mention that you can hook your thumb under or over the bar. Personally, I prefer the thumb under grip because it allows me to generate a stronger torsion force off the bar.

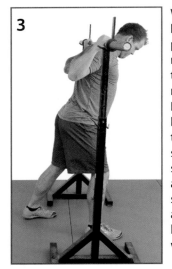

3

With your shoulders set and your upper back tight, step underneath the barbell, positioning the bar somewhere on the mass of your deltoids, otherwise referred to as the spine of your scapula. (To learn more about barbell positioning, see Jesse Burdick Shelf Test on page 101, and high bar back squat on page 102.) Whether the bar is high or low, the goals are the same: create as much torque in your shoulders and tension in your upper back as possible. As you step under the bar, screw your foot into the ground to create a stable hip position. Take your time. The barbell isn't just riding on your back. You want to make it part of your body.

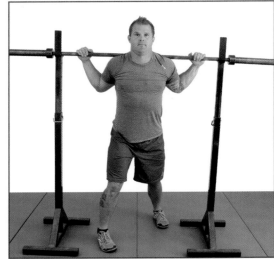

4

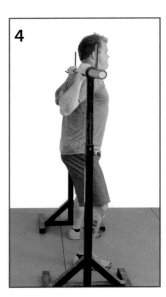

Step underneath the bar with your opposite foot and assume your squat stance. The goal is to create tension in your upper back and get your torso as vertical as possible. To accomplish this, press your neck back into the bar, eyes level at the start, and then twist your arms, bringing your elbows down underneath the bar—pulling your shoulders back and maintaining as much external rotation torque as possible. As you do this, squeeze your butt, get your belly tight, align your ribcage over your pelvis, screw your feet into the ground, and shove your knees out as far as possible.

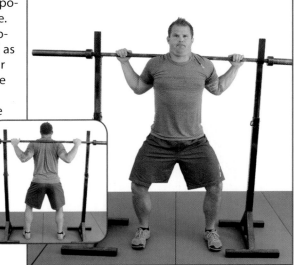

5

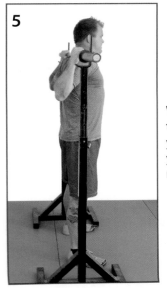

With your spine braced in a neutral position, your shoulders and back tight, and your torso as vertical as possible, extend your knees and lift the weight out of the rack.

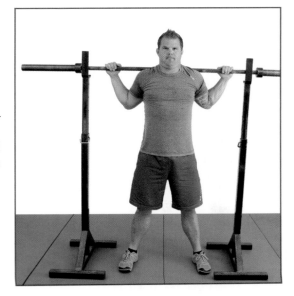

Phase 2: Walk Back

Walking with a significant weight on your back is a tricky endeavor. This is why the lift out is so important; it sets up the efficacy of the walk back. If you lift out with a disorganized spine, walking back is only going to make your bad position worse.

To prevent this, execute a good lift out and walk back in the same pattern every time you back squat. For example, after I lift the weight out of the rack, I always step back with my left foot, step back with my right foot, and then establish my squat stance. The steps are short and deliberate. Don't walk ten feet from the rack, look down at your feet as you establish your stance, or do anything that will compromise trunk and upper back stiffness.

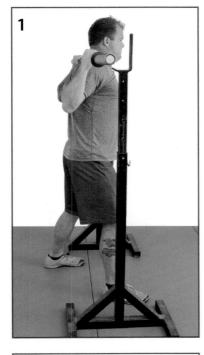

After you've lifted the bar out of the rack, step straight back. The key is to take a short and straight step. Unless you're transitioning into a wider stance, try to keep the same distance as your lift out stance to reduce the variability of your movement. All the same rules apply: Your belly is tight, your spine is neutral, and your back and shoulders are on tension.

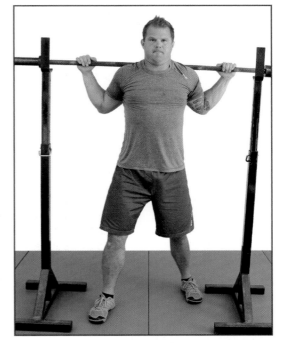

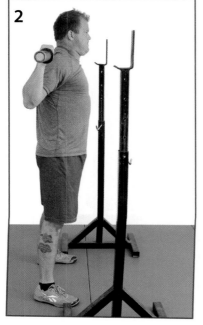

Step back with your opposite foot. Try to position your feet in your squat stance as you step back. The less you have to shift and adjust your stance, the better.

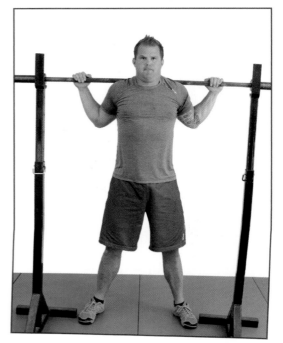

Phase 3: Squat

After you've taken the weight out of the rack, walked back, and established your squat stance, you're ready to perform the third piece of the movement sequence, which is the squat. Aside from managing a heavier load and organizing your arms in a different position, the back squat is performed in the same manner as the air squat.

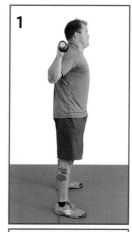

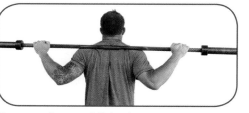

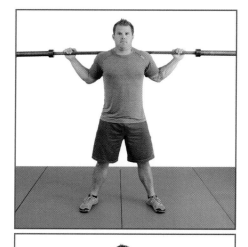

Once you've established your squat stance, squeeze your butt, screw your feet into the ground, and turn your knees out. Your shoulders and upper back should be tight, with wrists straight, head pressed back, and your elbows positioned underneath or slightly behind the bar to support the load. Nothing should have changed from the lift out phase.

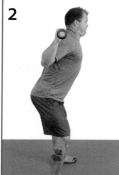

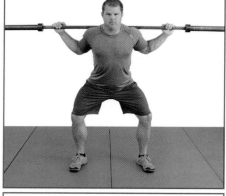

Keeping your back flat and your shins as vertical as possible, reach your hamstrings back.

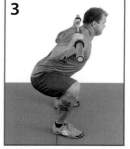

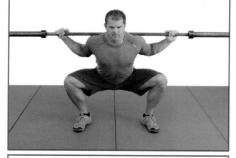

Still driving your knees out, lower into bottom position until your hips pass below your knee crease, or until your thighs are parallel with the floor. To maintain maximum knees-out force, think about pulling yourself into the bottom position.

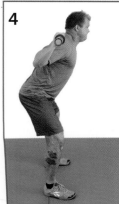

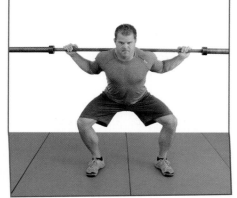

The moment you reach end-range, pull your shins to vertical and stand up.

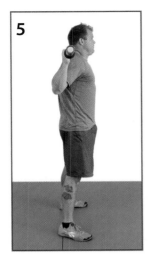

5

As you stand up, squeeze your butt and reestablish the start position.

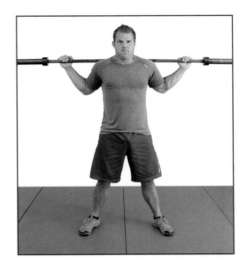

Jesse Burdick's "Back Squat" Shelf Test

There are clearly many possible positions for the bar on your back, but all will be ultimately categorized as low bar or high bar. The low bar back squat (performed in a more athletic stance, not a wide powerlifter stance) allows you to tilt your torso forward and load tension in your posterior chain (hamstrings and hips). The high bar back squat requires a more upright torso and shifts more demand onto your quadriceps. The former is typical of most powerlifters (although the only way to support 1000-plus pounds on your back is with an upright torso), while the latter is common with Olympic lifters. While it's good to learn and practice both variations, you're probably going to gravitate toward one rather than the other, which is fine as long as you can perform both.

The best back squatters in the world will adopt a more "low-ish" position for the bar during their squatting. The key is to find a comfortable and tight position for the barbell on your upper back. To find the sweet spot, perform this simple test:

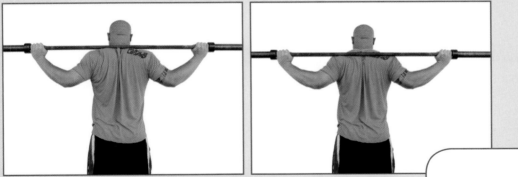

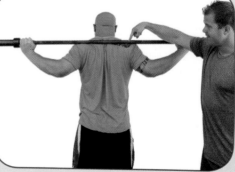

Position a PVC pipe or barbell on your back with your hands spaced far enough apart so that you can get your wrists vertical and your elbows underneath the bar. Then, slide the bar up and down the meat of your upper back (thoracic spine) and shoulders (deltoids, scapula) to find the tightest position. For some that might be a high bar position while for others a low bar position. (For most people, that's just above the scapula and on the deltoids.) You don't want it too high on your neck above your traps (cervical spine) or below the meat of your external rotators (back of your shoulders). Remember, you should have enough range-of-motion to place the bar anywhere. But, when it comes time to have a squat-off dance fight, adopt the best and most effective position for you.

High Bar Back Squat

If you're just learning how to back squat, sticking with either the low bar or high bar variation is what I recommend. However, for the intermediate generalist athlete, there's no reason not to learn how to back squat with the bar in different positions. In fact, if you fall into that category, you should switch your stance, change the positioning of the bar, and change the thickness and weight of the bar often.

Remember: Strength-and-conditioning is a tool for learning and layering complex movement patterns in a controlled environment. With the bar higher on your back, you have to position your torso in a slightly different manner, providing a completely different squat stimulus. Put simply, this gives you a brand new motor pattern to solve. Unlike the low bar back squat, which allows you to load your hips and hamstrings and drop your torso slightly forward, the high bar back squat forces your torso upright, loads more weight onto your quads, and increases range-of-motion demands on your hip and ankles. You're abiding by the same principles, but now you're forced to adapt to a new position—see Mark Bell's Underloading Method.

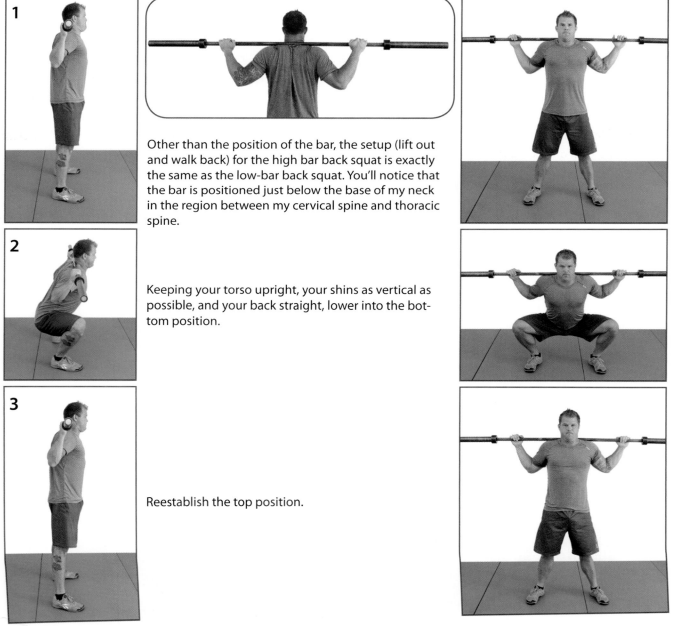

1

Other than the position of the bar, the setup (lift out and walk back) for the high bar back squat is exactly the same as the low-bar back squat. You'll notice that the bar is positioned just below the base of my neck in the region between my cervical spine and thoracic spine.

2

Keeping your torso upright, your shins as vertical as possible, and your back straight, lower into the bottom position.

3

Reestablish the top position.

Mark Bell's Underloading Method

Underloading is a concept that Mark Bell—elite American powerlifter and super coach—uses to train athletes by introducing new positions.

Here's an example: say you're trying to get stronger with the deadlift. Rather than add weight, increase the speed of the lift, or manipulate the set and rep scheme, he will challenge range-of-motion or position. He does this by making you pull from a deficit, changing the bar position, changing your grip, or changing the bar type.

Without adding any additional load, he increases the difficulty of the movement. This is a clever way to help the lifter progress without having to make the weight heavier. It's also a great way to teach people how to apply the rules of movement and the load-order sequence for a movement in a new position. It builds an athlete who can adapt to new positions and quickly understand when they're in a bad position, and what they need to do to adjust.

Grip Fault (Broken at the Wrist)

If you're missing internal rotation in your shoulders or missing extension in your thoracic spine, you lose the ability to pull your shoulders back and brace your spine in a neutral position. As you can see from the photos, this is characterized by rounding forward into a flexed position and breaking at the wrists. If you're not supporting the weight with your shoulders and wrists in a good position, your elbows end up taking the full blunt of the load. Experiencing murderous elbow pain when back squatting? This might be the problem.

Motor-Control Fix:

▶ Find the shelf of your upper back—see Jesse Burdick's Shelf Test, page 101—and make sure your wrists are straight and your elbows are positioned underneath or just behind the bar.

▶ Press your head back into the bar to create a neutral upper back.

▶ If you're missing range-of-motion, adjust your grip by sliding your hands out until you can get your wrists in line with your arm.

Mobilization Target Areas:

▶ Thoracic Spine

▶ Anterior Shoulders and Chest

▶ Posterior Shoulders and Lats

▶ Downstream Arm (Elbow and Wrist)

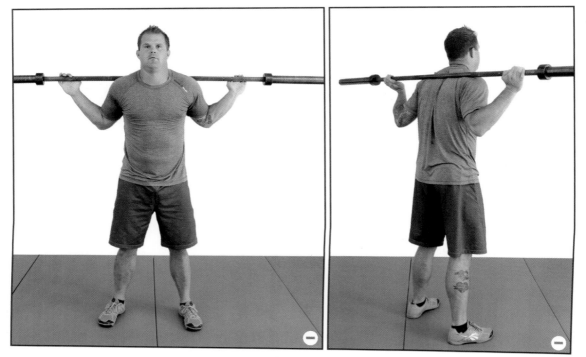

Grip Fault (Elbows High)

Lifting your elbows and pressing the bar into your upper back is another common grip fault that is characterized by poor shoulder and thoracic mobility. As with the previous grip fault, failing to create a stable barbell platform forces you into a forward flexed position, places strain on your elbows, and opens the door to other movement errors down the line. Note: this fault is not limited to athletes with poor mobility. A lot of people mistakenly elevate their elbows in an attempt to create tension in their upper back. This is simply a motor-control error that needs to be addressed in the setup.

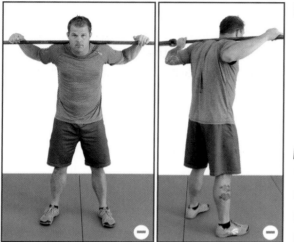

Motor-Control Fix:
▶ Find the shelf of your upper back—see Jesse Burdick's Shelf Test. page 101—and make sure your wrists are straight and your elbows are positioned underneath or just behind the bar.

▶ Press your head back into the bar to create a neutral upper back.

▶ If you're missing range-of-motion, adjust your grip by sliding your hands out until you can get your wrists inline with your arm.

Mobilization Target Areas:
▶ Thoracic Spine

▶ Anterior Shoulders and Chest

▶ Posterior Shoulders and Lats

▶ Downstream Arm (Elbow and Wrist)

Head Fault (Checking Stance)

Looking down to check the orientation of your feet is something that coaches tell beginners to do while warming up. And with good reason: If the positioning of your feet is different—one foot is turned out more than the other—it wreaks havoc with your ability to generate power and creates an uneven force across your spine. What happens? The body simply shuts down. While this is not a big deal in the early stages of development when the weight is light, it ingrains a bad habit that will inevitably cause breaks in spinal position. This is why it's so important to have defined motor patterns—meaning you step back the same way into the same stance every single time—so that you don't have to sacrifice neck position to look down.

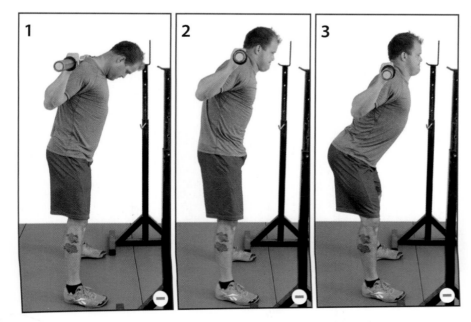

Motor-Control Fix:
▶ When you're first learning how to squat and walk back, try not to exaggerate looking down.

▶ Walk back using the same sequence every single time and practice with a light load until you feel comfortable.

Good Morning Squat Fault (Stripper Fault)

We also call this the stripper fault. It's characterized by shooting your hips up and extending your legs out of the bottom position. It occurs when there is not enough external rotation torque and you don't feel stable in the bottom position, so you raise your hips and hamstrings as a way to support the load.

Without torque, keeping your back and hip connected throughout the movement is impossible. As a result, you hinge at the lumbar spine as if it were a hip joint and use the strength of your back to complete the movement.

Again, if you have good motor-control patterning and the strength to handle the load, your position won't change: You'll go up the same way you went down. If you start to compensate, stop and have your spotter assist the movement or bail out from underneath the bar. (Note: Dumping weight off a failed lift is a complex task that you should learn before handling large loads.) This is easier to see with the deadlift because if you fail there's no change in spinal position. You don't worm around, collapse forward, or look up; you just stop or drop the weight. That's it.

Motor-Control Fix:

▶ This is very common with athletes who squat with their feet turned out, so make sure your feet are straight to allow for maximum torsion force.

▶ Create and maintain torque through range. Think about screwing your feet into the ground, shoving your knees out, and pulling yourself into the bottom position.

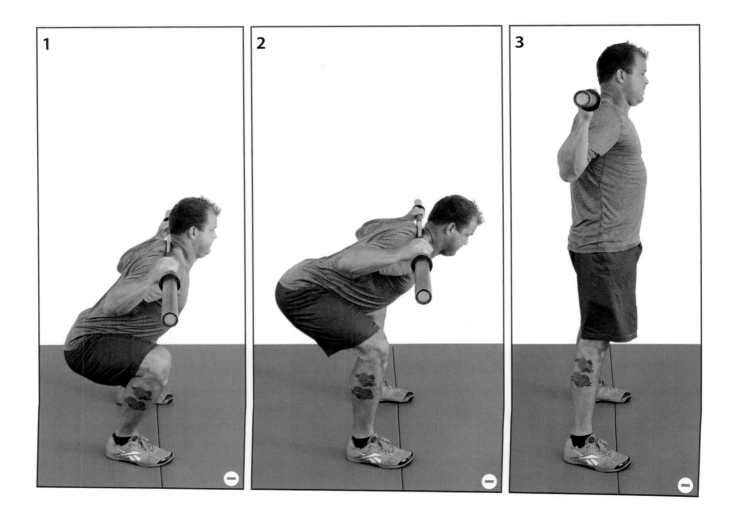

FRONT SQUAT

Imagine picking up a keg of beer and lowering it back down to the ground. Can you do that without ripping apart your knees or back? If you know how to front squat, yes, you can.

Lifting a keg of beer, a couch, a bag of charcoal, your kid: Most lifting-related tasks that we perform on a daily basis require picking something up or lowering something to the ground with the load supported in the front of the body. What's more, the majority of these tasks require the torso to remain upright. The front squat is a great example of a gym movement that transfers to the tasks of daily life.

The front squat will ferret out shortages in shoulder, hip, quad, and ankle range-of-motion—weaknesses an athlete may be able to hide during the air or back squat. In an air or back squat, the athlete can tilt his chest forward and reach his hips farther back, giving the hips, hamstrings, and ankles some breathing room. The upright-torso demands of the front squat will reveal these mobility limitations and, once addressed, present opportunities for snagging more performance.

The front squat is a progression to category 3 movements, specifically the clean and jerk—pulling a weight from the ground to shoulder level in one movement and then pressing the weight overhead.

Front Rack Position

Whether you receive the bar in the clean or take it out of a rack, the priority is the same: Organize your shoulders into a stable position by creating external rotation torque with your arms. Failure to do this results in a rounded upper back. Upper back tension and external rotation torque are what you're after. Grip is the place to start.

The conventional method for establishing an ideal grip is to measure a thumb's distance from your hipbone. As you can see from the photos, raising your arms from this spot can cause your shoulders to internally rotate and the elbows to flare out, leaving you unsecured. A better bet is to align your wrists with your elbows to build a supportive platform.

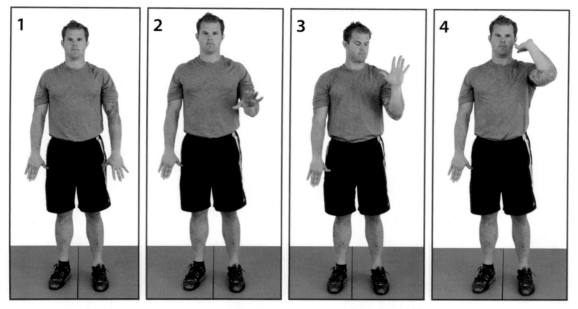

In most cases, when you use the conventional front rack setup method to find your grip, it forces you into a compensated position. As you can see, my grip is too narrow, making it impossible to get my elbows inline with my wrists, which is necessary to support the load and create external rotation torque.

This is how you do it. Turn your palm toward the front of your body, curl your hand to your shoulder, raise your elbow to a 90-degree angle, and then flip your palm toward the sky. (Sometimes it's helpful to have a Superfriend give you an assist by directly manipulating you into this position). You may require a dash of fine-tuning, but this technique will start to get you dialed in on grip width.

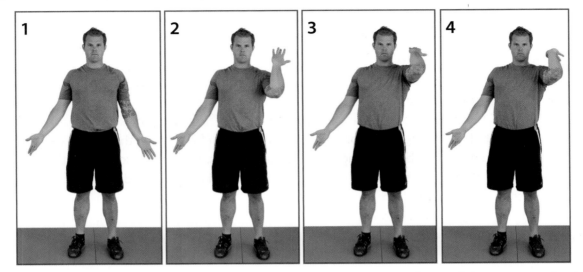

If you flex your arm with your palm forward (externally rotated position), your elbow will deviate out to the side, putting the wrist inline with the elbow. This also sets your shoulders in a stable position, allowing you to maximize torque. As with your squat stance, you may have to tinker around to find the most comfortable and stable position. In most cases, these adjustments are made based on arm length and shoulder mobility. Note: For a more detailed description of the lift out and walk back, refer to the similar phases in the back squat section (see page 96).

Phase 1: Lift Out

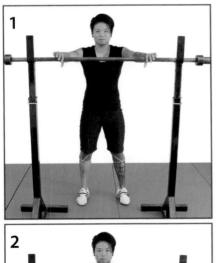

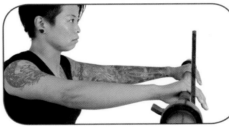

Grip the bar with your hands positioned far enough apart so that you can create a stable shoulder position.

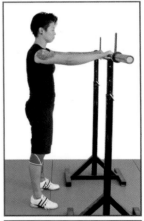

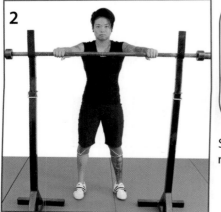

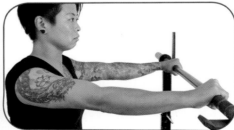

Screw your hands into the bar to light up external rotation torque.

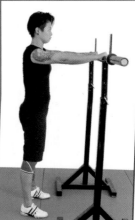

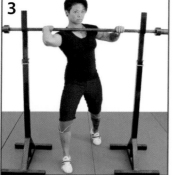

3

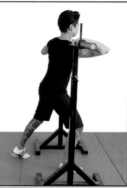

Maintaining as much torque as possible, step directly underneath the bar with one foot. Twist the same-side arm underneath the barbell so that the plane between the shoulder and the arm is parallel to the ground. The idea is to wind up your shoulder to create more tension in your upper back.

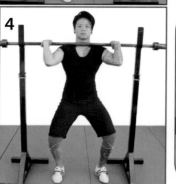

4

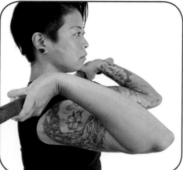

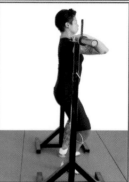

Step in with your opposite foot. Assume a squat stance. As you do this, twist your arm underneath the barbell to establish the front rack position. The bar should be resting on your shoulders and fingers. Note: That doesn't mean you want your shoulders forward to support the weight.

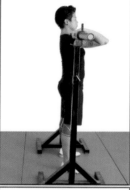

5

Keeping your elbows high to maintain torque, screw your feet into the ground, drive your knees out laterally, and lift the bar straight out of the rack.

Phase 2: Walk Back

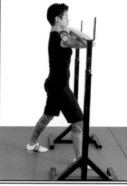

6

Step straight back. Again, step back with the same foot every single time.

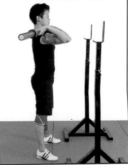

7

Step your opposite foot back and assume your squat stance. Make your steps short and deliberate.

Phase 3: Front Squat

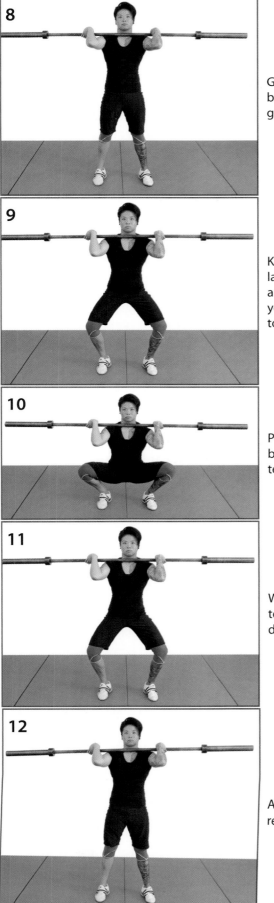

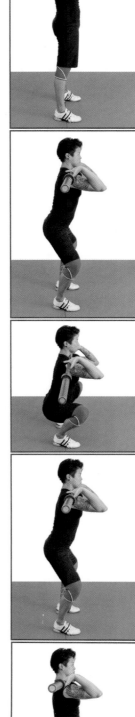

8

Get organized: Squeeze your butt, get your belly tight, and screw your feet into the ground to create tension in your hips.

9

Keeping your elbows up, drive your knees out laterally, draw your hamstrings back slightly, and lower your hips between your feet. Keep your head back and eyes fixed straight ahead to lock in torque and tension.

10

Pressing your knees outward, lower into the bottom of the squat. Keep elbows high and tension on.

11

With an upright torso, drive out of the bottom position. The ascent should mimic the descent.

12

As you stand upright, squeeze your butt and reestablish the top position.

Narrow Grip Fault (Elbows Out)

If your wrists are positioned to the inside of your shoulders in the front rack, it's a blinding giveaway that your shoulders are about as stable as uranium 235. As you can see from the photos, Diane's elbows flare out to the side, unloading tons of force on her wrists. That's when it all crumbles. The shoulders internally rotate and she can no longer create tension in her upper back. If this is what's happening to you, don't be shell-shocked when you have to bail on lifts because your wrists feel like they've been chopped at with a dull axe.

Moral of the story: You can't manage a heavy load or maintain an upright torso unless your wrists are inline with your elbows.

The motor-control fix for this issue is simple: Slide your hands out and address the stable shoulder front rack setup. If the problem can't be solved with motor-control, it's possible that you're missing thoracic extension (upper back flat), internal rotation of your shoulders, and flexion and external rotation of your shoulder.

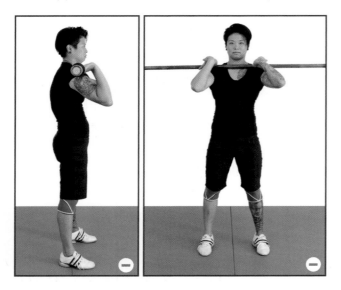

Motor-Control Fix:

▶ Address front rack mechanics and grip position—see stable shoulder front rack setup (page 106).

Mobilization Target Areas:

▶ Thoracic Spine

▶ Anterior Shoulders and Chest

▶ Posterior Shoulders and Lats

▶ Downstream Arm (Elbow and Wrist)

Cross Arm Fault

The cross arm front rack position is a classic bodybuilder setup to the front squat. With your arms crossed in front of your body, you can create a platform for the bar without challenging shoulder range-of-motion. This makes for an easier front rack position. Although this variation still gives you a front squat stimulus, it compromises your shoulder positioning and doesn't transfer to more dynamic lifts. Body-builders typically don't perform Olympic lifting variations, so the fact that it's not a transferable exercise might not matter. However, not being able to create torque off the bar will always present problems. Your shoulders will internally rotate and your upper back will round forward, making it difficult to achieve a neutral position under heavy loads.

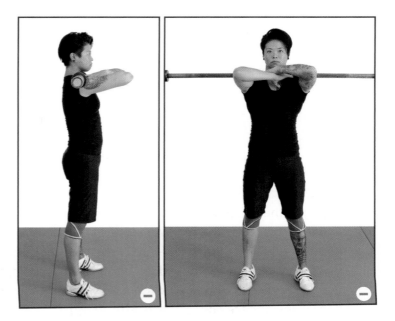

Chest Forward Fault

When your elbows drop and your chest translates forward in the squat, it's an indication that a) you failed to create torque in your hips and shoulders, creating an untenable front rack position, or b) you are missing range-of-motion in one or all the following areas: shoulder (flexion and external rotation), elbow (flexion), wrist (extension), thoracic spine (extension), hip (external rotation), and ankle (dorsiflexion).

Motor-Control Fix:

▶ Address front rack mechanics and grip position—see stable shoulder front rack setup (page 106).

▶ Create and maintain external rotation torque in your shoulders and hips.

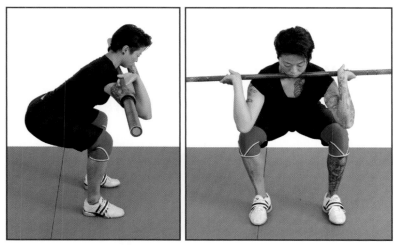

Mobilization Target Areas:

Front Rack

▶ Thoracic Spine

▶ Anterior Shoulders and Chest

▶ Posterior Shoulders and Lat

▶ Downstream Arm (Elbow and Wrist)

Squat

▶ Anterior Chain (Hips and Quads)

▶ Posterior High Chain (Hamstrings)

▶ Calf and Heel Cord

▶ Medial Chain (Adductors)

"Elbows Up!"

Telling athletes to get their elbows up during a front squat or clean is not going to fix the position. It might prevent a missed lift, but it will not prevent faults. The only way to correct the problem is to systematically address the issue: Are they creating enough torque to maintain an upright torso? Can they achieve a good front rack position? Can they squat to full depth with their torso upright? If an athlete misses the lift, meaning he drops the weight, it's probably a combination of a bad rack and missing range-of-motion in his hips and ankles. However, if he has a good rack position, he can come forward a little bit without dropping his weight because he can keep his elbows high and maintain a rigid upper back position.

OVERHEAD SQUAT

When it comes to making the invisible visible, the overhead squat will smoke out the truth. It's the most challenging of the squat iterations. In the front squat you hold the barbell in front of your body. In the overhead squat, you stabilize the bar over your head. Nothing will test your ability to create a stable trunk, generate torque, or reveal your range-of-motion like the overhead squat. In the same fashion that the front squat reveals weaknesses that can be hidden within a back squat, the overhead squat trumps the front squat as a diagnostic tool. Various disguises of motor-control faults or mobility restrictions will be scorched away when you open up the furnace door of the overhead squat.

Let's light this up with an example: Say you're missing a bit of external rotation in the hips and dorsiflexion in the ankles. Doing a front squat, you compensate by tilting your torso slightly forward. Your front rack is good, your spine is rigid, and despite the missing ranges you can execute the front squat. But take this show down the road to the overhead squat and things unravel. Tilt the torso offline in the bottom position of the overhead squat and the shoulders destabilize and unlock, causing the barbell load to sway precariously above like an anvil in a Wile E. Coyote trap.

If you can overhead squat with exceptional technique, it shows that you not only understand the fundamental principles of bracing and torque, but you also have full range-of-motion in your shoulders, hips, and ankles.

This is why the overhead squat with a PVC pipe is such a popular assessment tool. Within two seconds, a good coach can see spot motor-control problems and mobility restrictions.

As with all movements, the key is to become competent with the movement under light loads (like a PVC pipe or empty barbell), and then increase the weight or work output to test your ability to maintain good form under increased demand.

Note: Although the overhead squat retains all the same preliminary phases of the back squat and front squat—lifting out of the rack and walking the load back—before you begin the lift you need to power the load up into the overhead position. To do this you can either push-press or push-jerk the weight. The push-press (dip and drive) is fine for lifting light weight. But for more taxing loads or for workouts with multiple reps, the push-jerk is the preferred method because it costs you less energy.

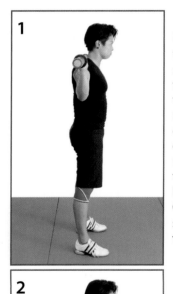
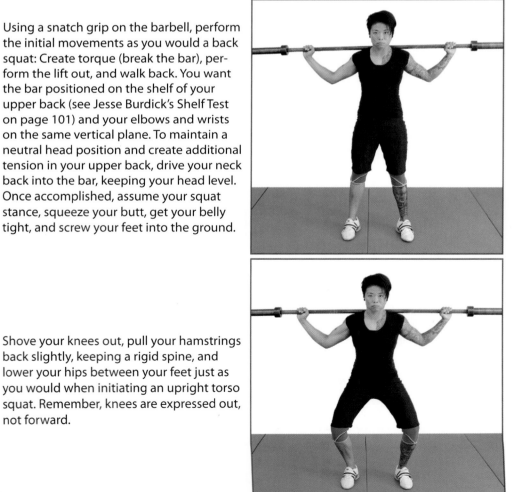

1 Using a snatch grip on the barbell, perform the initial movements as you would a back squat: Create torque (break the bar), perform the lift out, and walk back. You want the bar positioned on the shelf of your upper back (see Jesse Burdick's Shelf Test on page 101) and your elbows and wrists on the same vertical plane. To maintain a neutral head position and create additional tension in your upper back, drive your neck back into the bar, keeping your head level. Once accomplished, assume your squat stance, squeeze your butt, get your belly tight, and screw your feet into the ground.

2 Shove your knees out, pull your hamstrings back slightly, keeping a rigid spine, and lower your hips between your feet just as you would when initiating an upright torso squat. Remember, knees are expressed out, not forward.

3

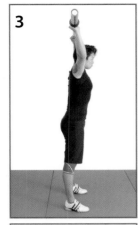

Extend your knees and hips and press the bar overhead. To maintain a stable shoulder position, externally rotate your armpits forward and continue to create torque off the bar. Once the bar is stabilized overhead, readdress the top position sequence (squeeze the butt, screw the feet into the ground, belly tight, etc.). It's important to notice that the bar is positioned in the center of her palms and her wrists are inline with her forearms (they are not bent or flexed).

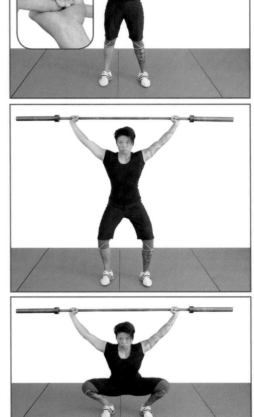

4

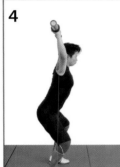

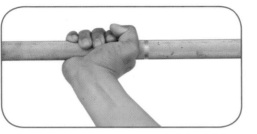

Keeping your shoulders in a stable position, draw your hamstrings back slightly, shove your knees out to the limits of your range, and slowly lower your hips between your feet.

5

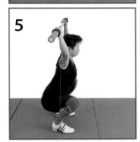

Still making a conscious effort to drive your knees out, lower into the bottom position. If you have to pause in the bottom to stabilize the weight overhead, that's fine. The key is not to bounce out of the bottom, tilt the chest forward, or have the bar move behind or in front of your center of mass.

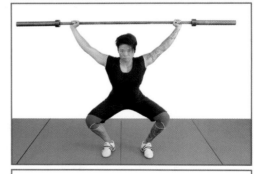

6

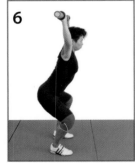

Extend your knees and hips and ascend into the top position.

7

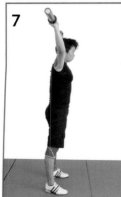

Reestablish the top position. Note: If you're executing another repetition, go through the top position load-order sequence. If you've completed the set, you can lower the weight down to your neck, or guide it out in front of you. The former should only be exercised when you're doing extremely light loads, like the bar. If you're handling anything heavier than that, dump the weights out in front of your body. Don't be that guy that tries to receive 300-pounds on your cervical spine.

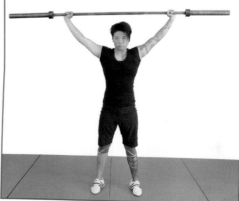

Shoulder Shrug Fault

A lot of people will mistakenly shrug their shoulders to their ears in an attempt to create a stable position. Shrugging your shoulders is another one of the pointless cues that coaches have been telling their athletes to do for years. The only way to stabilize your shoulders in a good position is to create external rotation torque, which is cued with armpits forward. It's that simple. Telling someone to press their shoulders up to their ears will cause them to internally rotate into an unstable position.

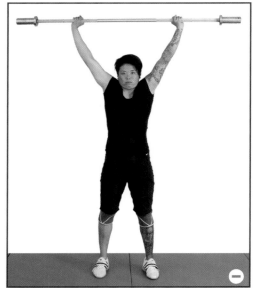

Motor-Control Fix:

▶ Create torque off the bar, keeping your wrists in a neutral position, and externally rotate your armpits forward.

▶ Make sure the bar is aligned directly over your center of mass.

Unstable Shoulder Fault (Bent Elbow)

If you can't lock your arms out overhead, it's an indication that you a) don't understand how to create a stable shoulder position or b) you are missing internal rotation in the shoulder. Bending your elbows internally rotates your arms, which unloads tension in your shoulders, lats, and upper back. While this compensation allows you to get overhead, it puts your shoulders in an unstable position, creating a toxic motor pattern that will leak poison into pulling movements like the pull-up, press, and deadlift. Power is lost by the metric ton and this fault opens the door to elbow injury and pain.

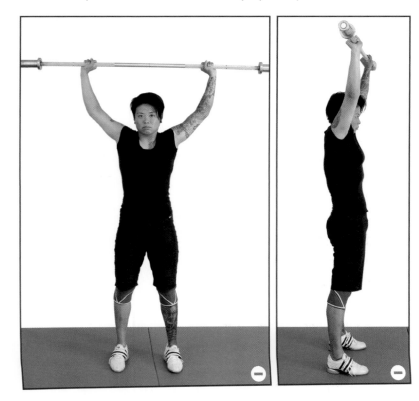

Motor-Control Fix:

▶ Create torque off the bar, keeping your wrist in a neutral position, externally rotate your armpits forward, and lockout your elbows.

Mobilization Target Areas:

▶ Thoracic Spine

▶ Posterior Shoulders and Lats

▶ Anterior Shoulders and Chest

▶ First Rib Mobilization

Grip Fault

Wrist pain is a common complaint associated with the overhead squat. This is due to a faulty grip. As you can see from the photo, when your hands are bent back, your fingers have to support the load, placing severe stress on your wrists. In most cases, athletes will default into this grip position if they are missing shoulder range-of-motion. Unable to pull their shoulders into an ideal position as they press overhead, they will throw their wrists back to balance the bar over the center of their body. In addition to inviting wrist pain, this broken wrist grip makes it difficult to create torque off the bar, compromising power and stability.

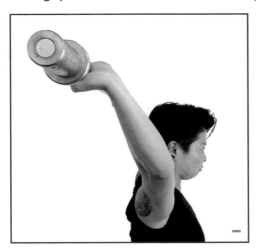

Motor-Control Fix:

▶ Position the bar in the center of your palms and keep your wrists in a neutral position (straight).

▶ Make sure the bar is centered over your hips and shoulders.

Mobilization Target Areas:

▶ Thoracic Spine

▶ Posterior Shoulders and Lats

▶ Anterior Shoulders and Chest

▶ First Rib Mobilization

Chest Forward Fault

If your chest drifts forward—whether you're missing range-of-motion or you failed to set your shoulders in a good position—your shoulders will unlock so that you can maintain balance overhead. This is an untenable position.

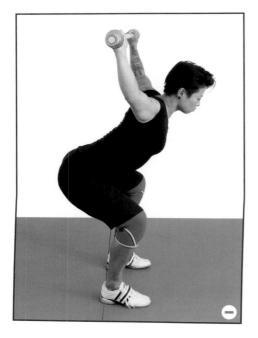

Motor-Control Fix:

▶ Create torque early and maintain that force through range.

▶ Stabilize your shoulders in a good position by locking out your arms, creating torque off the bar, and getting your armpits forward.

Mobilization Target Areas:

▶ Anterior Chain (Hips and Quads)

▶ Posterior High Chain (Glutes)

▶ Medial Chain (Adductors)

▶ Posterior Low Chain (Hamstrings)

▶ Calf and Heel Cord

DEADLIFT

Bend over to pick up a toolbox and you're deadlifting. The deadlift is both common and crucial to the world of work: A fireman hoisting someone onto a stretcher, a soldier in the field bending over to grab an ammo box, or a construction worker picking up an electric saw.

Each time you bend over to pick something up off the ground, you're essentially executing a deadlift. Yet few people understand how to do it correctly. The fact that so many people round their back when they bend over to pick something up may explain why millions suffer from lower back pain.

People who understand how to deadlift with good form—meaning they know how to brace, create torque, and never sacrifice form for range-of-motion—typically have fewer back problems. They have a model for picking something up that is universally applicable: If you know how to set up for a deadlift, you know how to pick something heavy off the ground without compromising your back.

To protect your back and maximize force production, you need to bring consciousness to this fundamental movement pattern so that you can reproduce a good position in all situations. You need to optimize and in-grain the deadlift setup so you have the same movement outcome every single time. Whether you're tired, or stressed out, or both, you have a blueprint that will allow you to produce maximum power with minimum risk.

The deadlift shares the same load-order sequence and universal laws as the squat: Brace, create torque, load your hips and hamstrings, keep your shins vertical, and distribute your weight in the center of your feet. (For an overview of these principles, review the air squat on page 82.) This makes the deadlift a very easy movement to learn and significantly shortens your learning curve. And as with all category 1 movements, the deadlift serves as a diagnostic tool for assessing range-of-motion restrictions and motor-control errors. (You can really see spinal errors and posterior chain restriction with this movement). But before you start down that path, you need to learn how to optimize the setup.

Deadlift Range-of-Motion Test

To get a read on your mobility in regard to good dead-lifting technique, it's important to assess your posterior chain range-of-motion—specifically in your hips, ham-strings, and back.

One of the best ways to do this is to hinge forward at your hips with your back flat and legs straight. If you can touch the barbell without rounding your back or internal-ly rotating your shoulders (essentially a straight leg dead-lift setup with your body forked at a 90-degree angle), you have full range-of-motion and are good to go. If you come up short, you may need to use the top-down setup option 2 (see page 121).

Here's another way to assess posterior range-of-mo-tion: To start, sit on the ground with your legs out in front of you. With your belly tight, you should be able to sit tall with your back and legs straight. If you bend your knees,

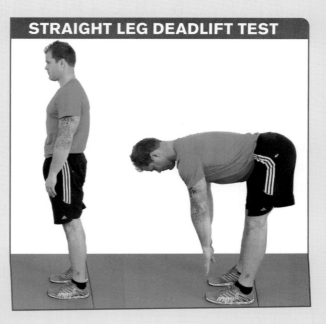

STRAIGHT LEG DEADLIFT TEST

round your back, or break from the upright-seated position, it's a dead giveaway that your posterior chain range-of-motion is wanting or there's a motor-control issue.

This is not to be confused with the classic sit and reach test, where in gym class you sat with your feet flush against a box, clenched your teeth, and reached your hands as far past your toes as possible. Once you acknowledge the laws of bracing, this test becomes comical because it reveals exactly nothing about functional range-of-motion or motor-control. It does, however, tell you how good you are at rounding the back into a horrible, broken position.

Compared to the long sit position test, the straight leg deadlift is the preferred measuring tool. You don't do a lot of movements from a seated position unless you're a kayaker or rower. So adding a weight-bearing element—the torso—makes it more realistic.

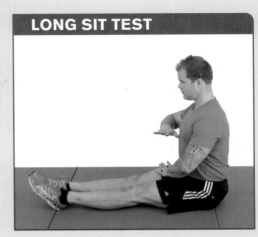

LONG SIT TEST

Top-Down Deadlift Setup

The top-down setup is the easiest and most effective model for lifting something off the ground. By organizing your spine in the top position, you minimize load on your spine and optimize trunk stability prior to forming your grip on the bar, dumbbells, stone, or other heavy object. Again, it's the same bracing sequence as the air squat. One of the mistakes that people make is to bend over, establish their grip, and then try to organize their spine and put their hips in a good position. If you set up for the deadlift by rounding forward, you have to recapture a flat back from the bottom position, which is difficult. This is no different than trying to brace your spine in the bottom of the squat. While you can get your back flat, you will most likely end up in a compromised position because you can't create tension in the upper back or stabilize the spine.

To correctly execute the deadlift, you have to take all the slack out of the system by creating as much tension in your body as possible prior to lifting the weight off the ground. You need to actively seek tension. If you lose tension in the setup, specifically in the hips and hamstrings, you have to adjust with your knees to reload the area. Bottom line: The more tension you can create, the more force you can apply to the movement.

Let's use a simple example to help illustrate this principle. Imagine a car that is stuck in a ditch. To pull it out, you hitch a rope from the ditched car to another car. If there is slack in the rope and the tow car hits the gas, it's either going to rip off a bumper or break the rope. To prevent that from happening, the car in front must eliminate the slack and create tension on the rope, *then* pull. It's the same thing with the deadlift: Create tension by loading the hips and hamstrings and pulling on the barbell (see caption 7). You almost want the bar to float before initiating the lift. If you have a 135-pounds on the bar, you should be thinking about putting a 130-pounds of tension into the bar. If you're lifting 400-pounds, you need to preload at least 200-pounds into the system to avoid breaking the metaphorical rope or tearing apart the metaphorical bumper—as in your lower back.

Top-Down Setup

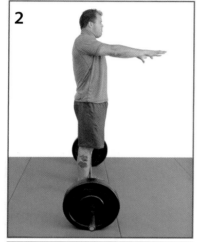

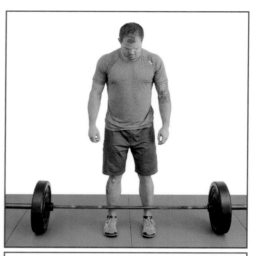

To establish a deadlift stance, walk your shins up to the bar and position your feet directly underneath your hips. The bar should bisect the center of your feet. If you glance at the photos, you'll notice that my feet are pointed straight and positioned underneath my hips, slightly narrower than my squat stance. This is a close iteration of my jumping stance or running stance.

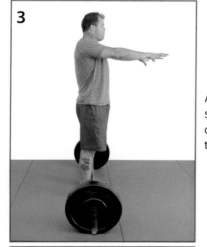

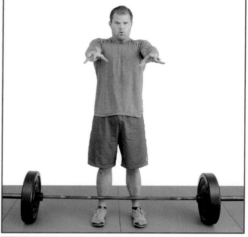

Go through the same load-order sequence as the air squat: Squeeze your butt to set your pelvis into a neutral position, screw your feet into the ground, raise your arms, pull your shoulders back while externally rotating your arms, and take a breath in.

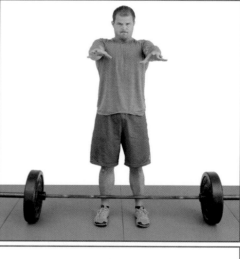

After setting your shoulders into a stable position, pull your ribcage down over your pelvis and get your belly tight.

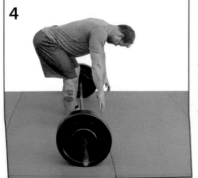

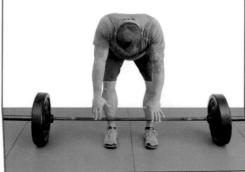

Keeping your back flat, reach your hamstrings back and hinge forward at the hips until you can touch the barbell, or until you reach end-range. Note: If can't reach the bar without compromising spinal position due to a lack of hip and hamstring mobility, use the top-down setup option 2.

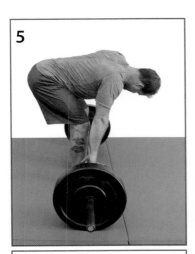

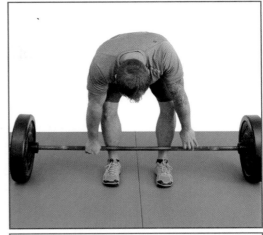

5 Grip the bar one hand at a time, forming your grip just to the outside of your shin with your palm facing your body. This allows you to form a hook grip on the bar—see hook grip, page 120—while maintaining tension in the hips, hamstrings, and upper back. For most people, a thumbs distance from your leg is a good start. The key is that you have enough room to press your knees out. So before you start your lift, get into position, shove your knees out as far as possible, and make sure that your arms are not in the way.

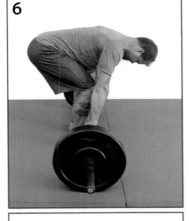

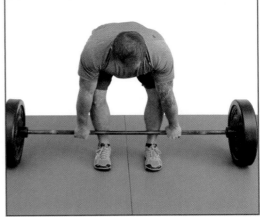

Reload Hips and Hamstrings:

6 Form a hook grip with your other hand in the exact same fashion. Note: I prefer the double over-hand grip (pronated grip) as illustrated in the photos. This allows me to maximize torque and tension in my upper back. While the mix grip is certainly a viable option, it does not allow you to create torque and stabilize your shoulders to the same degree—see mix grip, page 122.

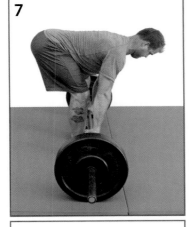

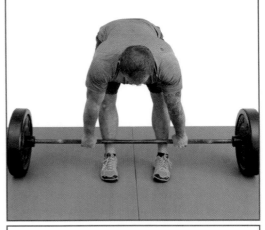

7 As you form your grip, you'll probably notice that there is not as much tension in the system—meaning your back is not as tight and your hips and hamstrings are not loaded to the same degree. To reclaim tension, screw your hands into the bar as if you were trying to break or bend the bar. As you do this, raise your hips and pull your knees back, creating as much tension in your hips, hamstrings, and back as possible. Again, there should be no change in spinal position.

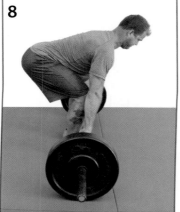

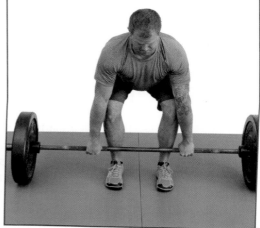

8 After reloading your hips, hamstrings, and back, lower your butt slightly while pulling on the barbell, keeping your shins as vertical as possible. To help with this step, imagine pulling yourself into position. It's also important to notice that the bar is positioned underneath my scapula. If your shoulders are too far over the bar it's usually an indication that your shins are not vertical. You will lose some capacity to generate force.

Lift

9

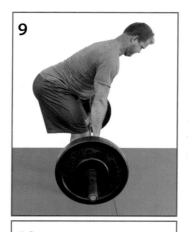

Still screwing your feet into the ground and your hands into the barbell, lift the weight straight off the ground. As you start the pull, the position of your spine should remain unchanged.

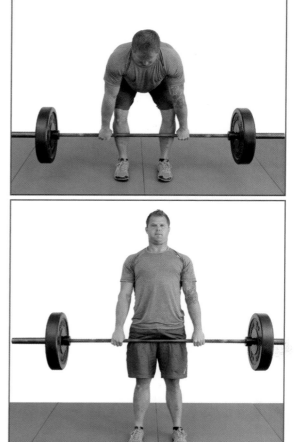

10

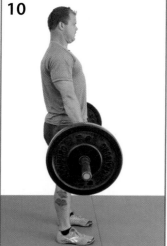

Keeping the barbell as close to your body as possible, stand up with the bar, squeezing your glutes as you extend your hips in the top position. Don't lean back or try to shrug your shoulders. To lower the bar to the ground, simply reverse the order of the movement: keep your back flat, head neutral, load your hips and hamstrings, and maintain as much tension in the system as possible. Or you can just drop the bar from the top position.

Hook Grip

The hook grip is a technique commonly taught to Olympic lifters. As you can see from the photos, instead of clasping your thumb over your fingers, which is a conventional grip, you wrap your thumb around the bar, and then wrap your fingers around your thumb. This lock prevents the bar from rolling out of your hand and puts your wrist in a good position for creating external rotation torque. The reason I like teaching this for the deadlift is because it allows you to handle larger loads and it transfers to other lifts like the clean and snatch.

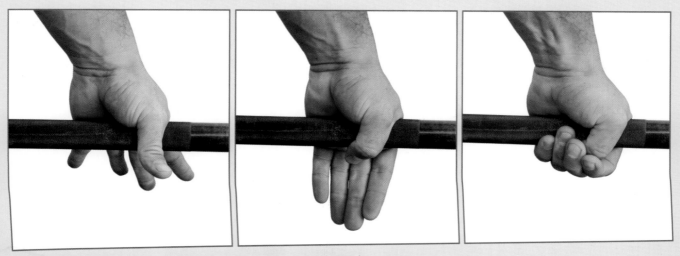

Option 2: Knees Forward Setup

Some people can't quite reach the barbell while keeping their hips loaded and shins vertical using the top-down setup. This is due to tight hamstrings and hips. If that's a problem, use this variation. It's carried out in the same fashion as the previous setup, in that you stabilize your trunk in the top position and hinge forward from your hips while keeping your shins vertical. But the moment you run out of range in your posterior chain—meaning you can't hinge forward or push your hips back any farther without compromising your spinal position—bring your knees forward. This will allow you to adjust for position while still keeping your back flat and your hips and hamstrings loaded. After you establish your grip on the bar, pull your shins back to vertical to reclaim tension. It's the same model: Brace, load your hips and hamstrings, and use your knees to adjust for position.

In some cases, people's ankles (missing dorsiflexion/knee forward range), hamstrings, and hips are so tight they can't set up from the ground without rounding their back position, even when using this setup. In such a situation, scale the setup by setting the bar to a higher position, using blocks, bumper weights, or a rack.

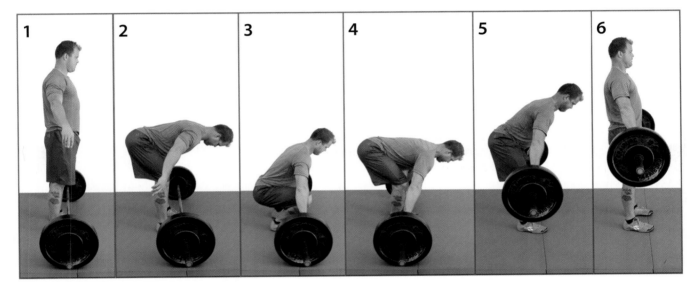

1. Establish your squat stance and stabilize your trunk—see caption 1 in the previous technique.

2. Hinge forward from your hips and drive your hamstrings back.

3. The moment you run out of hamstring and hip range-of-motion, bring your knees forward and establish your deadlift grip. The key is to keep your heels in contact with the ground and your spine rigid.

4. Reload your hips and hamstrings by pulling your knees and hamstrings back. Try to get your shins as vertical as possible.

5. Pull the weight off the ground by extending your hips and knees. Again, there should be no change in spinal position.

6. Keeping the barbell as close to your body as possible, stand up with the bar, squeezing your glutes as you extend your hips in the top position.

Mix Grip

As I mentioned, I generally prefer the double overhand grip because it allows you to maximize external rotation force and builds grip strength. It also transfers to other pull-based exercises (pull-up, clean, snatch, etc.). The mix grip—or what is commonly referred to as the flip grip—doesn't allow for ideal shoulder positioning. As you can see from the photos, my left palm is facing forward and my right palm is facing back. The problem here is I'll never be able to create the same amount of external rotation torque with my left hand as my right, leaving my left arm vulnerable to injury.

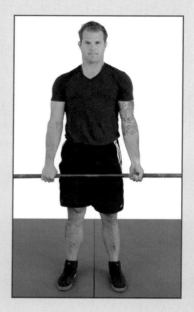

Not only that, it is a dead end grip, meaning that it only applies to the deadlift and doesn't transfer to other movements.

For some people, the mix grip is a more comfortable position and allows them to lift more weight, so it does have a place in your arsenal of techniques. But does that mean it should be used all the time? Not exactly. Here's what I generally recommend: Use the overhand hook grip until your grip starts to fail, which for most people is around 90 percent of a one rep max. Then, implement the flip grip.

Bottom-Up Setup Fault

A lot of people will set up for the deadlift by rounding forward, establishing their grip on the bar, and then trying to set their spine and hips in a good position. Don't get me wrong, I've seen people pick up enormous loads setting up in this manner, but they almost always round forward into a compromised position. Here's why: When you hinge forward from your hips without stabilizing your spine, you rely on the anterior musculature of your pelvis to pull your back into a flat position, shortening the front of your hips. You can pull your back into a neutral position, but you can't lock in or stabilize the position. If you're deadlifting heavy, you will usually round forward. If the weight is light you might be able to maintain a flat back, but because your hips are in a shortened state, standing up into a neutral position is difficult. You will usually overextend to get your torso upright. To put it another way, the bottom-up setup loads your back instead of your hips and hamstrings. So if your lower back hurts after you deadlift, there's a strong chance you're committing this fault.

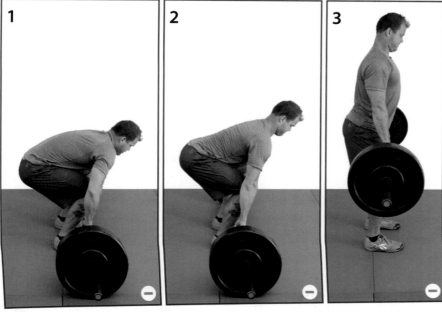

Motor-Control Fix:
▶ Address the top-down setup (both options).

Tension-Hunting Fault

Setting up from the bottom position predisposes people to a rounded back. However, this fault is not limited to the setup. Even if you set up from the top position, if you fail to take all the slack out of the system, you will always default into a bad position. This is what I call tension-hunting. If your hips, hamstrings, and back are not tight, your body will take up the slack, which is expressed with a rounded back. The key to avoiding this fault is to maximize tension in your body by pulling on the bar. Remember, the deadlift is a slow movement. In other words, you never go from 0 to 60; rather, you go from 40 to 60.

Note: Failure to preload the bar will express itself with a definitive click, which is the barbell hitting the bumper weight. Again, the weight should feel like it's floating before you actually lift it from the ground.

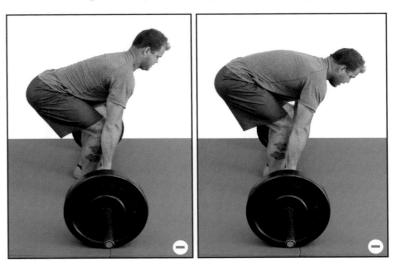

Motor-Control Fix:

▶ After setting your grip, be sure to pull your knees back and raise your hips to load your posterior chain before initiating the pull.

▶ Create sufficient external rotation torque in your shoulders by screwing your hands into the bar.

Powerlifters Rounding Their Back

A lot of powerlifters will pull with a rounded upper back—while keeping the lower back flat—because it shortens the distance they have to pull the weight to the lockout position of the hips. This is where people get confused. The upper back is in fixed flexion, meaning that they round forward and then create tension and torque in that position.

What people have to remember is that rounding the upper back is a conscious decision that professional powerlifters make. And they understand the consequences. A classic case is Donny Thompson, a professional powerlifter and world record holder. He was practicing deficit deadlifts with a rounded back and suffered a disc injury. His reaction was: "I knew better. I was pulling with a rounded back and it got me." At no point will a professional powerlifter ever round their lower back when performing a deadlift. It would be like a bomb going off. However, to get a slight edge, sometimes they will sacrifice the safety of their position if it means being able to lift more weight.

With that said, a beginner or fitness lifter should *never* round their upper back as a means of lifting more weight. Why? Because it increases susceptibility to injury, ingrains a dysfunctional movement pattern into your daily life, and does not translate to other athletic movements like dynamic pulling and jumping.

I like Jesse Burdick's general rule for pulling heavy with a rounded upper back. When you can deadlift 600-pounds, then you can start to entertain thoughts of rounding your thoracic spine. In fact, many of the best Olympic lifting coaches in the world, like Mike Burgener and Glenn Pendlay, won't let their athletes pull heavy deadlift singles for the reason that they don't want to ingrain a pulling pattern with an upper body (upper back and shoulder position) that won't translate to Olympic style weightlifting.

Tension Fault

A properly executed deadlift is expressed with a single movement, meaning that everything goes up at the same time (hips and knees extend simultaneously). If an athlete starts to lift the weight off the floor and his hips come up first and then the torso follows, it's an indication that he didn't take up all the slack in the system. They are tension-hunting. Although he can still maintain a flat back, which is great, he compromises his ability to generate maximum force.

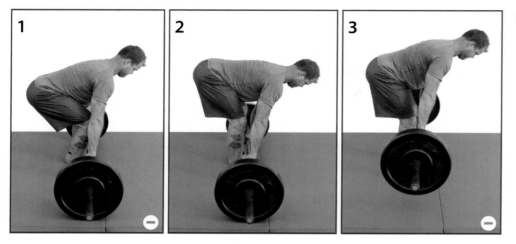

Motor-Control Fix:

▶ Before lifting the weight off the ground, raise your butt and bring your knees back. This will load tension into your posterior chain. With your hip and hamstrings fully engaged, lower your hips and shove your knees out, pulling on the bar as you lower into position.

PUSHUP

Imagine if you will: An adrenaline freak is bombing down a trail of jagged rock on a full-suspension mountain bike. Or a climber is scaling a vertical shelf of blue ice at 18,000 feet. Or a powerlifter is bench pressing a record load surrounded by screaming powerlifting maniacs. Or a 335-pound NFL offensive is tackling with a 4.8 40 speed, pulling, ripping, pushing, and dismantling a blitzing linebacker.

Have one or all of those images in mind. Now what do you think will happen if that athlete doesn't understand how to organize his shoulders into a good position? This is what happens: His shoulders internally rotate and his elbows flare out, sacrificing his ability to create force and opening the door to injury.

Most upper body movements conducive to sport and life are performed at midrange and out in front of your body: feeding, grabbing, carrying, pushing, and pulling. To operate effectively within this domain, you need a model that teaches you how to create a stable shoulder position.

Enter the pushup.

As with the air squat, the pushup is where you can start to layer the principles of bracing and torque. The pushup also serves as a diagnostic tool for assessing motor-control and range-of-motion. But instead of illuminating what's happening at the hips, the pushup tells you what's going on at the shoulder, elbow, and wrist. You go through the same checklist: Does an athlete understand how to brace his spine in a neutral position? Or create external rotational torque by screwing his hands into the ground (set the shoulder in a good position)? Does he have the range-of-motion and motor-control to keep his hands straight and elbows close to his body as he performs the movement? Without having to use any equipment, you can see how well an athlete understands the fundamental principles of bracing and torque, as well as identify restrictions in his mobility.

In addition, the pushup serves as a launch pad to more complex pressing motions—the bench press, dip, and overhead press—and more complex motor patterns as well. If you understand these basic concepts and can apply them to the pushup, you are less likely to default into bad positions when you're training with more complicated movements.

No wonder so many athletes suffer from torn rotator cuffs and dislocated shoulder injuries, and why people experience anterior shoulder pain every time they press. They don't understand the principles that govern good positions as it relates to the shoulder, elbow, and wrist. The pushup teaches and ingrains those fundamental movement patterns and gives coaches and athletes a template for solving problems at the shoulder, elbow, and wrist.

Coaches, athletes, and physical therapists will often relate shoulder issues to a weak rotator cuff or weak shoulders. Although this is a contributing factor, it's not necessarily the root cause. It's about position: If you don't have a model for creating a stable position, generating spontaneous torque and force is difficult. Once you understand how to correctly perform a pushup, it doesn't matter where your hands are, what you are grabbing, pushing, or pulling. Nor does the orientation of your arms matter. You can still create a stable and mechanically powerful position.

Note: The pushup shares a lot of the same principles as the squat and deadlift, but instead of loading your hips and hamstrings, keeping your shins vertical, and distributing your weight over the center of your feet, you load your pecs and triceps, keep your forearms vertical, and distribute your weight over the center of your hands (in front of your wrist). The concept of stance is also transferable. As with your squat and deadlift stance, you should find a comfortable position that transfers to other pressing motions. Positioning your hands shoulder-width apart is a good start. The goal is to establish a position that allows you to perform the movement with good technique. Once you're proficient, start switching up the width of your hands from time to time to create a new stimulus.

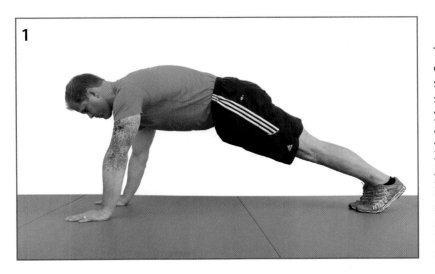

Setup

To correctly set up for the pushup, kneel down and situate your hands at about shoulder-width with your fingers pointing straight ahead. Once accomplished, sprawl your legs back, position your feet together, and squeeze your glutes. Note: Positioning your legs together maximizes glute activation and tension in your trunk. In the photo, you'll notice that I start with my hands out in front of my body. By keeping your weight slightly back, you take load off of your shoulders, making it easier to screw your hands into the floor and create an external rotation torsion force.

Top Position

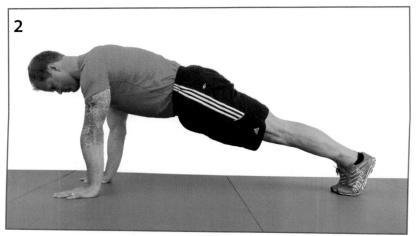

Still actively screwing your hands into the floor, lever forward, positioning your shoulders over your hands. To help maximize torque, think about getting the pits of your elbows forward.

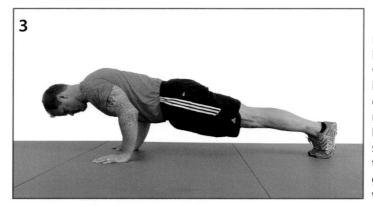

Midrange Phase

Keeping your weight centered over the center of your hands (just in front of your wrists) and your forearm vertical (elbow inline with your wrists), start lowering into the bottom position. This is the equivalent of keeping your shins vertical in the squat in that it maximizes force production and protects your elbows. Remember, you load your triceps and pecs for the same reason you load your hamstrings and glutes in the squat. The pecs help stabilize your shoulder in a good position so that your triceps can do their job, which is to extend the elbow.

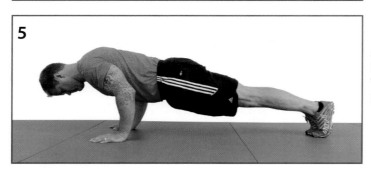

Bottom Position

Lower into the bottom position. Keep your butt squeezed, belly tight, and forearms as vertical as possible.

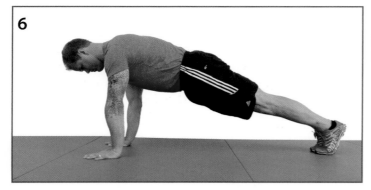

Midrange Phase

As you press out of the bottom position, there should be no change in your spinal or shoulder position. Your back should be flat and your shoulders retracted (pulled back).

Top Position

Still screwing your hands into the ground, extend your arms and reestablish the top position.

Elbows Out Fault

The majority of people can set up for the pushup in a good position, meaning that they can create torque and get their back flat. But just like the squat, the moment they start lowering into the bottom position, errors become easy to spot. For example, a lot of athletes will flare their elbows out and compensate with a shoulder forward position as they lower their chest to the ground. When I see this happen—whether it's in the first few inches or in the bottom position—the first thing that comes to mind is missing internal or external rotation at the shoulder. While a poor setup and weak triceps can contribute to this fault, it's almost always a shoulder range-of-motion issue.

As you can see from the photos, once my elbows fly out to the side, my shoulders get loaded into a bad position. This is why people experience wrist, elbow, and anterior shoulder pain. Whether they are bench pressing a heavy load, stabilizing a weight overhead like with the overhead squat, or performing body-weight movements like pushups or dips, they have no choice but to adopt an elbow-out, shoulder-forward position to execute the movement. It's no surprise that people feel hot, burning pain in the front of their shoulders when they press. They are missing 100 percent or their internal rotation range-of-motion.

Motor-Control Fix:

▶ Address the setup in the top position: squeeze your butt, screw your hands into the ground (elbow pits forward), and keep your forearms vertical as you descend and rise out of the bottom position.

Mobilization Target Areas:

▶ Anterior Shoulders and Lats

▶ Posterior Shoulders and Chest

▶ Downstream Arm (Elbow and Wrist)

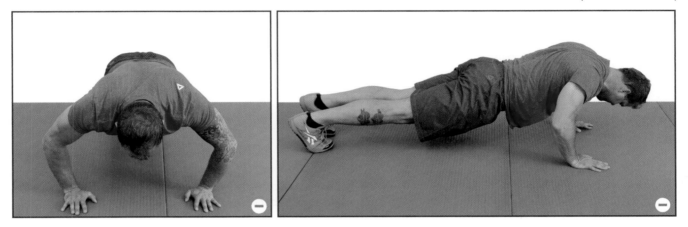

Open Hand Fault

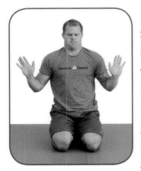

As I explained in the torque chapter and in the squat techniques, if an athlete is missing ankle or hip range-of-motion, he will generally turn his feet out to increase his range-of-motion. The same thing happens in the pushup. If an athlete is missing rotation at his shoulder (internal or external rotation) or flexion at his wrist, he will usually compensate into an open-hand forward shoulder position. As with the open foot, this causes a landslide of mechanical problems up and down the chain, and is what opens the door for a lot of the injuries and pain people experience when they press.

Motor-Control Fix:

▶ Focus on the position of the pushup. Position your hands straight—between 12- and 1-o'clock (right) and 12- and 11-o'clock (left).

▶ Screw your hands into the ground, creating an external rotation torsion force, and try to get the pits of your elbows forward.

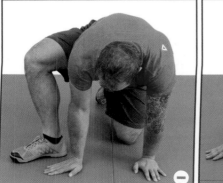
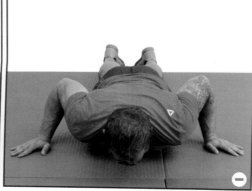

Mobilization Target Areas:

▶ Anterior Shoulders and Lats

▶ Posterior Shoulders and Chest

▶ Downstream Arm (Elbow and Wrist)

Elbow Back Fault

If you've read the introduction to the air squat, you already know that driving your knees forward early in range typically stems from not creating sufficient external rotation torque: You failed to screw your feet into the ground and shove your knees out so your knees track forward to compensate. The pushup exists in

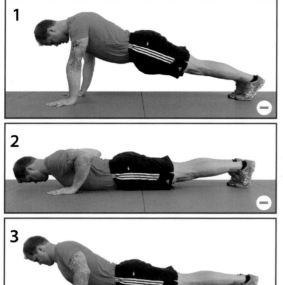

a parallel universe. Failure to screw your hands into the ground results in loading your elbows. What happens? Your back positions breaks, power leaks away, and your elbows hurt.

As a quick recap, loading your chest and triceps is the equivalent of loading your glutes and hamstrings in the squat. Your chest helps keep your shoulders in a good isometric position (just as your glutes keep your hips in a good isometric position). Your triceps are responsible for extending your elbows (just as your hamstrings extend your knees and hips). To accomplish this, screw your hands into the ground and keep your elbows inline with your wrists.

Motor-Control Fix:

▶ Pull your shoulders back and create and maintain torque by screwing your hands into the ground, positioning your elbow pits forward.

▶ Think about keeping your forearms as vertical as possible as you initiate the movement.

Scaling the Pushup

If you are not strong enough to correctly perform a full-range pushup, you can do one of two things: Place your hands on a higher surface (chair, box, or wall) or make the movement easier using Mark Bell's slingshot. Note: If you don't have access to a slingshot (you should), you can loop a Rogue monster band around your elbows. Both methods lower the demand, making the movement easier, while still allowing you to idealize a

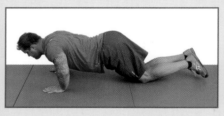

neutral spinal position. What's particularly great about the slingshot, however, is it prevents your elbows from flaring out to the side and supports your weight in the bottom position. So in addition to removing some of the load, it encourages good mechanics. This is the equivalent of doing a pull-up with a Rogue monster band hooked around your feet. You can mimic the movement without compromising form.

Important: A lot of coaches and athletes will mistakenly scale the pushup by dropping their knees to the ground. While this reduces the load and makes the pushup easier, it compromises your ability to squeeze your butt and create tension in your trunk. Doing a pushup from your knees encourages bad mechanics. In or-

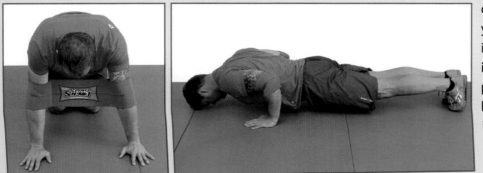

der to create a rigid flat back, you need to set your pelvis in a neutral position by keeping your butt squeezed: If you perform a pushup from your knees, accomplishing this task is impossible.

RING-PUSHUP

Adding rings to an exercise is like injecting the movement with truth serum.

People can perform the pushup in a low torque environment and get away with it. Forget it when it comes to the rings. The moment an athlete climbs on the rings, he has no choice but to generate torque. He has to screw his hands into the rings and keep his elbows over his wrists. This is why athletes sometimes experience pain in the front of their shoulders when performing pushups and the bench press, but don't when doing ring-pushups. The instability of the rings makes it difficult to move with bad mechanics. The athlete needs to provide the stability.

Also, the physics introduced by the rings will show you the light in terms of positioning your hands and the path of your arms—positions and paths that should be applied to the pushup and bench press.

The ring-pushup provides at least two benefits: It challenges an athlete with increased stabilization demands, while also ingraining proper pressing mechanics. Here's why: When athletes perform pushups on the rings, their hands automatically orientate underneath their shoulders. They turn their hands out to create an external rotation force and their forearms remain vertical, allowing their elbows to stay tight to their body.

In other words, people will instinctively create a more stable trunk and adopt an externally rotated shoulder position because it's the easiest way to stay balanced over the rings. If your hands rotate inward (internally rotate), or your elbows deviate back or drift out to the side, your arms will start to shake erratically, making it impossible to stabilize the position.

Note: Don't feel like you have to reserve the ring-pushup for advanced athletes. A lot of novice athletes can benefit by just learning how to stabilize in the top position.

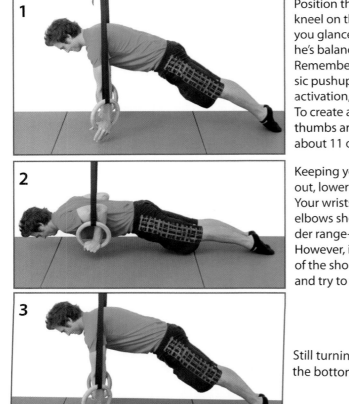

Position the rings so that they hang at roughly shoulder-width. Next, kneel on the ground, form your grip, and then walk your legs back. If you glance at the photo, you'll notice that Carl's feet are together and he's balancing on the front of his toes (not on the balls of his feet). Remember, the ring-pushup requires more trunk control than the classic pushup. By balancing on the front of your toes, you maximize glute activation, which in turn helps create and maintain a stable trunk. To create a stable shoulder, externally rotate your hands so that your thumbs are pointing away from your body. Your left hand should be at about 11 o'clock and your right hand at about 1 o'clock.

Keeping your butt squeezed, your belly tight, and your hands turned out, lower into the bottom position. Note the position of your arms: Your wrists should be in line with your elbows (forearms vertical) and elbows should be in tight to your body. Even if you're missing shoulder range-of-motion, the rings force your arms into an ideal position. However, it's important to note that if you're missing internal rotation of the shoulder, your hands will start to rotate inward. Fight this force and try to reclaim a thumb-out position as you rise out of the bottom.

Still turning your hands out and keeping your back flat, press out of the bottom and reestablish the top position.

BENCH PRESS

Here's a problem with the bench press: Coaches and athletes generally put more stock in how much people lift than how well the movement is performed. It begins with the 300-pound bench press club at the high school gym and the status associated with earning a club T-shirt. The question, "How much do ya bench?" is the defacto joke within the free weight gym culture. While you should know the answer, the question you should be obsessed with if you're sincerely hell-bent on pursuing hot, nasty, high-level athletic performance is this: How good is your bench press form?

Very few athletes understand the variables involved in a proper bench press. It just seems so simple: You lie down on the comfy bench, take the barbell out of the rack, guide it down to your chest, and then extend your elbows. What's the big deal? But like the squat or the deadlift, there are a lot of variables that you have to account for. Setting your shoulders in a good position, bracing while lying on your back, and keeping an ideal bar path takes a lot of practice and technical ability.

A good bench press comes down to using good movement practices. For instance, you should know how to set your shoulders in a stable position and create torque off the bar. You should know how to brace in a globally arched position. You need your wrists in line with your elbows. If one of these steps isn't carried out correctly or you are missing key ranges of motion, you will see horrific movement errors: elbows fly out, shoulders roll forward, the head bobbles into crazy positions, and the back overextends. It's a five-car collision. Because people can press insanely large loads without paying any attention to technique, the bench press is probably responsible for more shoulder injuries than any other movement in the history of the world.

If we can teach people how to bench with good form, we can save millions of shoulders. The bench press doesn't just teach you how to press through midrange, it also gives you a blueprint for creating torque with your shoulders retracted to the back of your socket. The pattern translates to other pulling exercises like the clean and the deadlift. The bench press is also a diagnostic tool: People can disguise their movement and mobility dysfunction in low torque environments like the pushup but can't hide them once the torque demands are increased with load.

Note: As with the squat and standing press iterations, taking the bar out of the rack is a skill in and of itself. To ensure a successful and safe lift out, there several things that need to happen: arch your back, retract your shoulders, create torque off the bar, screw your feet into the ground, take a breath, and get your belly tight. Performing these tasks correctly is predicated on a good bench press setup. If something goes wrong in the lift out phase, completing the movement with good form is difficult. To improve your understanding, I've broken the setup into categories.

Grip

The best way to figure out your grip distance is to establish the top position on the rings with your hands turned out. For most people, this is just outside shoulder-width, which is much narrower than people typically prefer. The fact is you need a grip that will allow you to keep your shoulders blades pulled back, generate sufficient torque off the bar, keep your elbows in a 30-45 degree plane from your body, and maintain a vertical forearm. You also want to keep the bar positioned in the center of your palm, aligned with your wrist. While this may seem intuitive, people will adopt some really crazy grips like centering the bar across the fingers. Not only is this dangerous—imagine a barbell rolling off your hands onto your neck or face—it will also cause a lot of wrist and thumb pain.

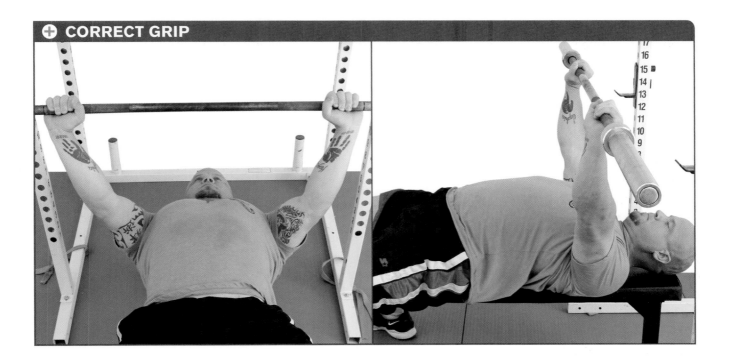

⊕ CORRECT GRIP

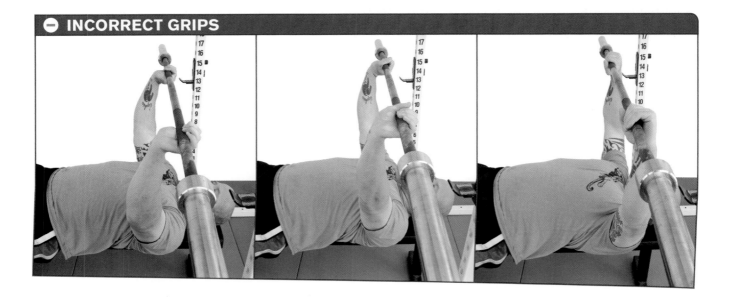

⊖ INCORRECT GRIPS

Stance

Just as poorly organized shoulders compromises the efficiency of the squat, poorly organized hips will affect your ability to bench press. To maintain a rigid trunk, you need a stance that allows you to create sufficient torque. It should look a lot like your squat stance. All the same rules apply: Keep your shins vertical and position your feet as straight as possible, screw your feet into the ground, drive your knees out, and distribute your weight over the center of your feet. People will adopt untenable foot positions that make it impossible to create torque or get into a braced position.

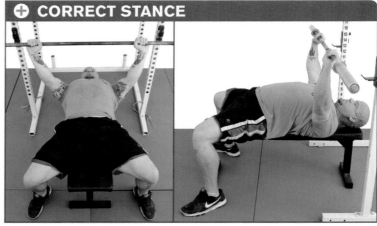

⊕ CORRECT STANCE

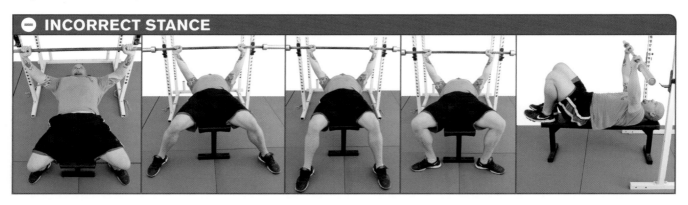

⊖ INCORRECT STANCE

Braced Extension

To correctly perform the movement, you need to create an arch and keep your shoulders pulled back. However, this does not mean you're overextended. The key is to arch back to set your shoulders, brace your abs, and then lower your hips to the bench. If you drop your ribcage or keep your back flat with the bench, keeping your shoulder blades retracted is difficult. This is not easy and takes time to master. Having a tight thoracic spine can also make it difficult to create a good arch.

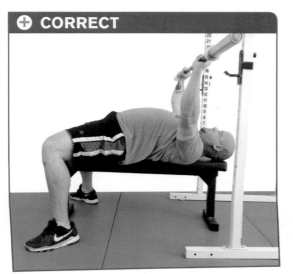

⊕ CORRECT

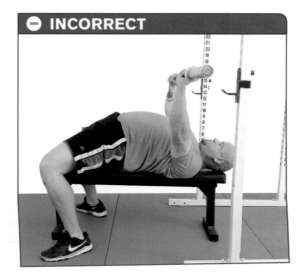

⊖ INCORRECT

Height of the Rack

Although telling you that it's important to set the rack to the right level seems ridiculous, I'll say it anyway: Set the rack to a height that allows for a slight bend in the arm. For an ideal lift out, you should be able to extend your arms and press the weight out of the rack while keeping your shoulder blades pulled back. If the rack is too high, you will have to protract your shoulders, which is a huge setup error.

Bench Press Sequence

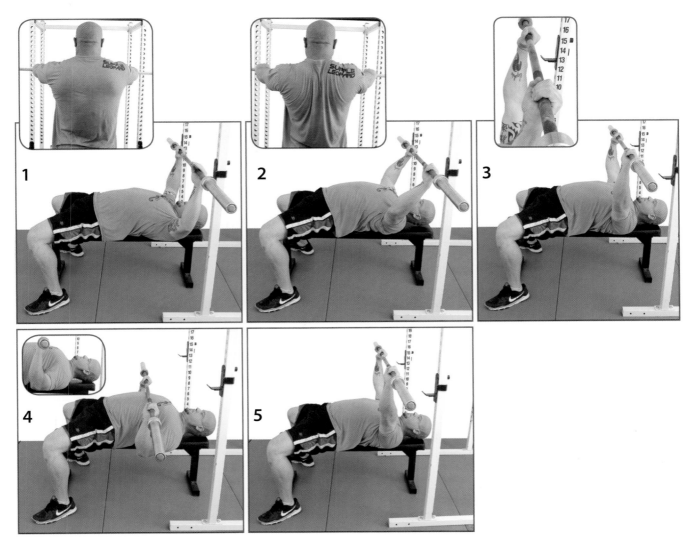

1. To set up for the bench press, lie underneath the bar so that it bisects your collarbone or neck and assume your bench press stance.

2. Before lifting the weight out of the rack, pull your shoulder blades back and create torque off the bar. Imagine trying to break or bend the bar with your hands. This tightens your upper back and sets your shoulders in a stable position. As you do this, screw your feet into the ground, drive your knees out, squeeze your butt, and elevate your hips. You will maintain these actions through every step.

3. Lift the weight out of the rack and align the bar over your shoulders. Notice that the bar is resting in the center of Jesse's palms directly over his wrists.

4. Keeping your shoulder blades pulled back, lower the weight to your chest. Think about loading your triceps and chest by pulling your elbows down and keeping your forearms as vertical as possible.

5. Extend your elbows and reestablish the start position.

Elbows Out Fault

As with the pushup, a lot of athletes will flare their elbows out to the side because they are missing internal rotation in their shoulders or they failed to create and maintain sufficient torque in the setup to the lift. This also happens when people don't keep their shoulders screwed into the back of their socket: If there is slack in your shoulders, your elbows will fly out to the side to take up the tension. If you're missing range-of-motion, you may want to consider implementing the floor press as an alternative exercise.

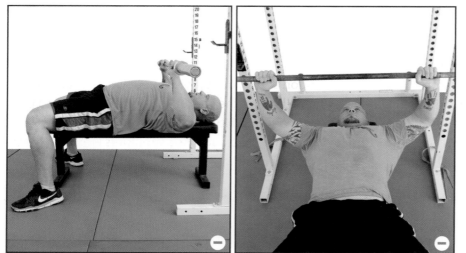

Motor-Control Fix:

► Focus on trying to bend the bar with your hands and pull your shoulder blades back. Maintain high levels of torque during the movement.

► Keep your wrists aligned with your elbows.

Mobilization Target Areas:

► Thoracic Spine

► Anterior Shoulders and Lats

► Posterior Shoulders and Chest

► Downstream Arm (Elbow/Wrist)

Elbows Back Fault

The setup is without question the most complex aspect of the bench press. Once your shoulders are set and the bar is aligned over your shoulders, the bench press is largely a function of just bending and extending your elbows. The goal is to bend your elbows, keeping them in a 30-45 degree plane from your body, while maintaining a vertical forearm. The problem is a lot of people don't feel comfortable lowering the bar to their sternum because it requires a higher degree of mobility, strength, and control. To circumvent their mobility restrictions and lack of triceps strength, they will load their shoulders instead of their triceps and chest. As you can see from the photos, this puts an incredible amount of shear force on your wrists and elbows.

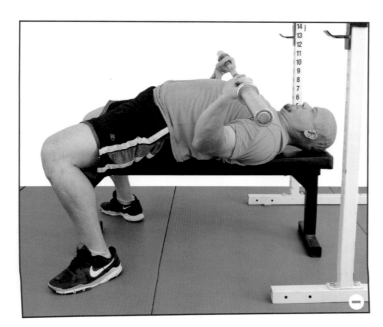

Motor-Control Fix:

► Create and maintain torque by consciously trying to bend the bar.

► Focus on keeping your wrists in line with your elbows while keeping your shoulders back.

► Practice the ideal bar path. You can use the ring-pushup as a tool to practice good bench press form.

Mobilization Target Areas:

► Thoracic Spine

► Anterior Shoulders and Lats

► Posterior Shoulders and Chest

► Downstream Arm (Elbow/Wrist)

FLOOR PRESS

Although the bench press is a fantastic movement, it poses problems for a lot of people. It expresses a high degree of extension and internal rotation of the shoulder—elbows tracking behind your body—and requires triceps strength, something that a lot of people don't have. For example, if you are missing internal rotation range-of-motion in your shoulders or you have underdeveloped triceps, the bench press will exaggerate a lot of faults: your elbows fly out, shoulders roll forward, and you squirm around underneath the bar in search of stability and power. If this is you, know that you are ripe for ingraining a toxic movement pattern. Make a good decision and scale back to the floor press.

The floor press restricts the bench pressing range-of-motion action, but provides you with the same stimulus—meaning that you can still mobilize your shoulders to the back of the socket, load your triceps, and practice a loaded midrange press without having to work around your mobility issues.

To put it in simple terms, the floor press is a valuable tool that protects athlete's shoulders while still teaching them how to press through midrange. This is also a great exercise to throw into a large group of people without worrying about having to correct a lot of faults.

Note: All the same rules apply as the bench press. Your grip, stance, and load-order sequence is exactly the same as the bench press.

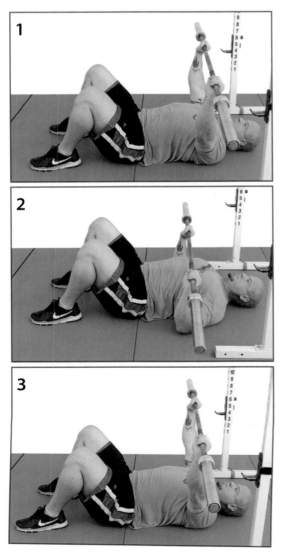

1 The lift out is carried out in the same manner as the bench press. To see the load-order sequence for this step, refer back to the bench press technique.

2 Keeping your forearms vertical, shoulders back, and belly tight, lower your triceps to the floor. The key is to load your chest and triceps by keeping your forearms vertical.

3 The moment your triceps touch down, immediately press the weight back to the start position by extending your elbows.

DIP

The path to developing optimal power output from the shoulders is this: Perform a wide swath of exercises that stabilize the shoulders from a variety of ranges.

The pushup and bench press teach you how to stabilize your shoulders out in front of your body. The strict-press and push-press teaches you how to stabilize loads overhead. And the dip teaches you how to generate stability while your arms are by your side.

Even though the dip is technically a pressing element, it forces the same stabilization demands as carrying heavy objects. The dip transfers to tasks in daily life like carrying a suitcase or getting up out of an armchair.

Although the underlying principles of the dip are the same as midrange and overhead movements—create external rotation torque, pulling your shoulder blades back—it's a new stimulus for the shoulder. If people don't spend time working in these extension ranges, they are more likely to compensate forward into a bad positions when carrying or performing basic tasks with their arms by their side or behind their body.

Plus, being able to perform a full-range quality dip is a prerequisite to more dynamic movements like the muscle-up: If you can't stay in control in the bottom position of the dip, creating spontaneous torque as you transition into a muscle-up is hopeless.

The dip is a complex exercise that requires enormous strength, control, and shoulder range-of-motion. For these reasons, you need to understand how to scale the movement.

To scale the dip, start in the top position and make sure you can stabilize your shoulders in a good position with your arms locked out. If you don't have the strength or range-of-motion to lower into the bottom position, you can use a band or Mark Bell's slingshot to make the movement easier. If you have access to parallel bars, you can walk back and forth with your arms locked out to develop positional strength.

Just because you have the strength to perform the movement doesn't mean you're doing it right. There is a lot that can go wrong. For example, people often struggle to keep their forearms vertical and load their chest and triceps because they are missing shoulder range-of-motion or don't follow the proper load-order sequence. Instead they drive their elbows back, overextend, and keep their chest upright, and then wiggle around in the bottom position in search of a mechanical advantage. This is where a lot of shoulder damage occurs and why people experience pain in their sternum when they dip.

Setup

Don't be half-assed about setting up for the dip. Pay attention to detail. First, you need to make sure your dip station is high enough to straighten your legs. If the apparatus is too short, you will be forced to bend your knees and cross your ankles behind your body. This results in an overextension spinal fault (see page 138).

The width of your grip is also important. The conventional method is to use your forearm (elbow to finger-tips) to measure your grip distance, which doesn't really tell you anything about your start and finish position. The best way to figure out how far apart you need to position your hands is to stand straight with your arms by your sides and then rotate your hands so that your palms are facing away from your body. You want the bars positioned just to the inside of your pinky fingers. Just as in the ring-pushup, you can use the rings to determine proper grip width.

While these are not perfect methods, it will put you in a position where you can maximize torque and shoulder stability. If it works out to be the same length as your forearm and fingers, that's great: You have an easy model for measuring the proper grip distance.

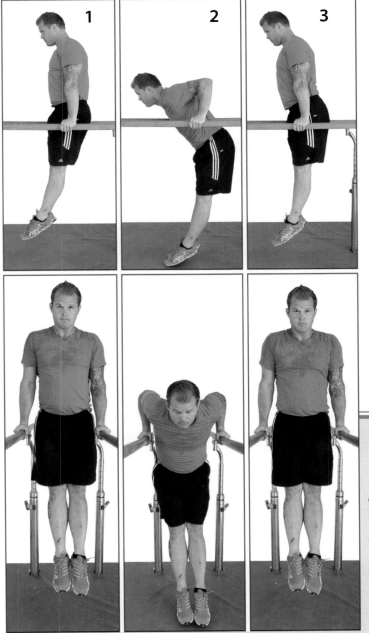

1. The start position for the dip shares a lot of the same cues as the pushup and press: You want to screw your hands into the bars, try to get the pits of your elbows forward, and externally rotate your shoulders into the back of your socket. Ideally, you want your feet together, your toes pointed, and your butt squeezed to maintain that position and support your pelvis in a neutral position. Your feet should be midline or out in front of your body.

2. Keeping your legs straight, feet pointed, butt squeezed, and belly tight, lower into the bottom position by allowing your chest to drop forward. This loads your pecs and triceps. Like the squat, imagine pulling yourself down while screwing your hands into the bars. The key is to focus on keeping your shoulders back (think about squeezing your shoulder blades together as you lever forward), your spine rigid, and your forearms vertical.

3. Still screwing your hands into the bars, extend your elbows and reestablish the top position. There should be no change in torso position.

Stabilizing Your Shoulder

In our gym, there is no such thing as a shoulder stabilization exercise. Every shoulder movement has a stabilization component. This is where coaches and physical therapists miss the mark.

Doing accessory exercises like externally rotating your arm back and forth with a cable machine or light dumbbell is not going to teach you how to pull, push, press, carry, or lift with a stable shoulder. You need to incorporate movements that force you to stabilize your shoulders in a good position. That's why it's so important that you learn how to perform midrange movements like a pushup, overhead movements like the strict-press, and by your side or behind your back movements like the dip.

For example, there are still a lot of coaches out there that dismiss exercises like the press for swimmers, baseball pitchers, and volleyball players—athletes who perform a lot of overhead-type movements—because they believe that overhead exercises are dangerous. This is a valid point if you don't understand what a stable shoulder position looks and feels like. Say an athlete has already put in gazillions of overhead repetitions. If he's doing it with crappy form, the last thing you want him to do is more overhead work with bad technique. What to do?

Answer: Teach him the stable position for the shoulder. Then teach him how to strict-press with good technique. This will not only improve the overall effectiveness of his overhead position, but also allow you to assess his end-range position. He doesn't have to press a lot of weight or perform a ridiculous amount of repetitions. However, as a responsible coach, you need to instill fundamental stabilization principles and highlight mobility and motor-control dysfunction.

Shrug Fault

If you are missing shoulder range-of-motion, pulling your shoulders back into a good position and locking out your elbows is impossible. While the same is true with the pushup and bench press, it's easier to disguise. This is what makes the dip such a great diagnostic tool. With the full weight of your body supported by your shoulders, you can't mask limited shoulder mobility.

If you start in an organized position, but compensate into a bad position as you lower into the bottom position, it's a good indication that you're missing extension and internal rotation in your shoulders or lack the strength to correctly perform the movement.

Your pecs are responsible for stabilizing your shoulders into an externally rotated position. Because the dip requires a high level of stability from your shoulders, your pecs have to work extra hard to keep your shoulders locked into a stable, externally rotated position. If your shoulders roll forward or shrug, your pecs will pull off axis, which pulls the sternum apart—the reason why some people experience intense pain in the sternum when they dip.

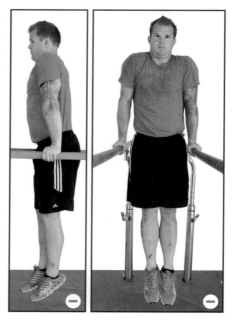

Motor-Control Fix:

▶ Use the pushup as a model to ingrain proper shoulder stabilization mechanics before progressing to the dip.

▶ Isolate the top position: Focus on squeezing your butt with your legs straight and together, screwing your hands into the bars, getting your elbow pits forward, and pulling your shoulders back.

Mobilization Target Areas:

▶ Thoracic Spine

▶ Anterior Shoulders and Lats

▶ Posterior Shoulders and Chest

▶ Downstream Arm (Elbow and Wrist)

Overextension Spinal Fault

Bending your knees and crossing your ankles behind your body is a setup error that can cause overextension fault. The bottom line is you can't engage your glutes and stabilize your pelvis in a neutral position unless your legs are straight and positioned together.

If you glance at the photos, you'll notice that as I press out of the bottom position, I throw my head back and arch into an overextended position. In this example, I've surrendered my spinal position and the stability of my shoulders so that I can generate upward momentum. Arching back, elbows deviating outward, and shoulders compensating forward is my body's way of finding stability so that I can complete the movement. Not good!

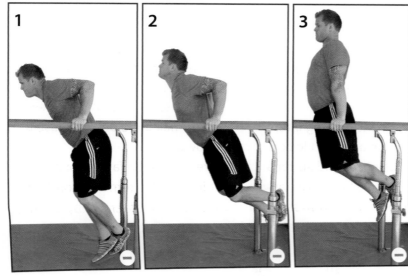

Motor-Control Fix:

▶ Keep your legs straight and pinned together, pointing your toes. Your feet should be positioned underneath or slightly out in front of your body.

▶ Squeeze your glutes and establish a neutral spinal position.

▶ Pull your shoulders back and create torque off the bar.

Overextension Fault

Just because your legs are straight and your shoulders are set in a good position doesn't ensure a quality dip. If you look at the photos you'll notice that my shoulders are pulled back, my feet are together, and my toes are pointed, but I've failed to squeeze my butt and brace my core. As I initiate the dip, my elbows and feet move back, my chest bulges forward, and I instantly lose stability in my shoulders.

Most movements require that you balance your ribcage on top of your pelvis, but in this situation you have to stabilize your pelvis underneath your ribcage, which is challenging if you're just learning the movement. Although the load-order sequence is the same, people will often forget to brace their trunk as they initiate the dip, resulting in this fault.

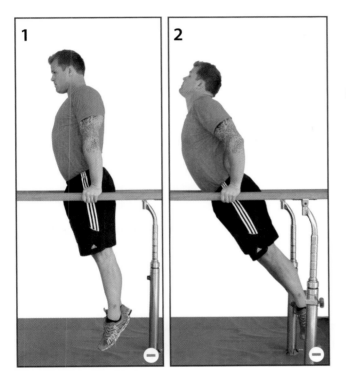

Motor-Control Fix:

▶ Squeeze your glutes to set your pelvis into a neutral position. Keep your glutes engaged and maintain a flat back as you initiate the movement.

▶ Allow your chest to translate forward, focusing on keeping your forearms vertical. This will load your triceps and chest, as well as keep your shoulders locked into a good position.

RING DIP

One of the prime functions of the Movement and Mobility System is to teach and layer movements that transfer learning to other movements. The ring dip is a star example of this. In addition to providing a more challenging stimulus, it preps you for more dynamic movements like the muscle-up.

As with the ring-pushup, the ring dip requires an additional dose of problem solving. Mobility issues are forced out of hiding. You can tell when someone is missing internal rotation in their shoulders because they struggle to achieve an externally rotated position and can't lock out their elbows.

Ring dips also promote good movement practices and automatically correct common faults. For example, a common fault with the classic dip is to pull your elbows back as you lower into the bottom position. This internally rotates your shoulders, sucking you into a compromised position. However, in order to stay balanced over the rings and remain in a stable position, you have to keep your forearms vertical. Put another way, you physically can't press with your elbows behind your wrist.

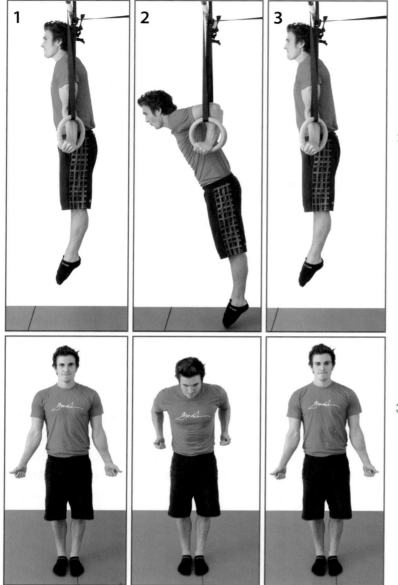

1. To stabilize your shoulders, externally rotate your hands so that your thumbs are pointing away from your body. Now pull your shoulders back. Your left hand should be at about 11 o'clock and your right hand at about 1 o'clock. Position your feet together, point your toes, squeeze your glutes, and then tighten your core.

2. Keeping your butt squeezed, your belly tight, and your hands turned out, lower into the bottom position. If you glance at the photo, you'll notice that Carl levers forward, keeping his feet out in front of his body. This loads his triceps and chest and keeps his shoulders and trunk in a good position. Also note the position of his arms: his wrists are in line with his elbows (his forearms are vertical) and his elbows are in tight to his body. It's important to mention that as you lower your hands you will rotate to about 12 o'clock. If you're missing internal rotation in your shoulders, your hands will continue to rotate inward. Fight this force and try to reclaim a thumb-out position as you rise out of the bottom.

3. Still turning your hands out and keeping your back flat, extend your elbows and reestablish the top position.

STRICT-PRESS

The strict-press is one of the moves that offer a golden opportunity to practice the rules of bracing and torque when your arms are overhead. It's also a magnifying glass for assessing motor-control trouble spots and mobility restriction.

For example, say someone can't get their shoulders into the proper position when they press a barbell overhead. What does that tell you about their motor-control and shoulder range-of-motion? And what do you think will happen when they try to receive a heavy load in the jerk? Or rattle off any overhead movement while burning with met-con fatigue?

If you don't understand the ideal start and finish position or lack the range-of-motion to perform the task, you can't apply these fundamental concepts to more complex overhead actions.

Look for this: Can the athlete keep his back flat with ribcage down and pelvis neutral? Can he get his shoulders into the end-range flexion with his elbows straight? Can he express a stable shoulder position by getting his armpits forward? It's that simple.

This strict-press is also a very useful rehabilitation tool. For example, if you're coaching someone whose coming off a knee injury or rehabbing after ACL surgery, this is one of the first weight-bearing exercises that you can introduce. It still requires a low level of external rotation torque—they have to shove their knees out and screw their feet into the ground—so it will help strengthen the injured joint and surrounding musculature, as well as re-groove functional movement patterns.

Barbell vs. Dumbbell

People will ask me: "Why do you encourage pressing with the barbell … isn't it easier to learn and safer to press with dumbbells?"

Before I answer, it's important to note that the closer you can position the weight to your centerline (general center of mass), the easier it is to press from that position with good form.

If you have limited shoulder range-of-motion or your technique is off, the dumbbell press is a great option because it allows you to keep your shoulders organized in a correct position without compromising form.

So if you have shoulder pain when you raise your arms overhead with a barbell, pressing with dumbbells helps reduce that pain due to improved setup positioning and more rotational options of the arm when the dumbbell is overhead.

There's no arguing the fact that pressing with dumbbells offer distinct advantages. The same goes for kettlebells. In fact, it's something that I encourage all of my athletes to do. However, the dumbbell press will ultimately limit the max load an athlete can put overhead.

Additionally, one of the problems that you will perennially see as athletes move toward more complex lifts like the push-jerk and split-jerk is they don't have a model for creating torque off a fixed object (barbell) and they lack the strength to perform these movements under load. That's why it's so important to get people pressing with a barbell in their developmental stages—because it ingrains fundamental movement patterns that translate to these more complex movements, even as it builds the pressing strength needed to move heavier weight.

However, the barbell does present certain challenges: You have to clear your face as you press the weight overhead; you have to support the load out in front of your body; you have to balance the bar on your chest while keeping your forearms vertical; and you have to generate force from a dead-start position. But like all movements shown in this book, it teaches you a load-order sequence that transfers to other moves and objects.

The objective is to teach movements that express stability in your joints and core through full ranges of motion, as well as allows for a variety of movements. While the barbell is by no means a natural implement, it's the easiest tool for challenging the athlete's competency overhead. There comes a point where lifting heavy dumbbells simply becomes untenable.

Strict-Press Setup

The setup to the press is very similar to establishing the front rack position out of the rack (see front squat, page 106). You still create torque off the bar (breaking the bar and twisting your elbows underneath) one arm at a time, lift the weight out of the rack as if it were a front squat, and walk back. But instead of lifting your elbows to a 90-degree angle and balancing the bar on your fingertips and shoulders, you position the bar on your chest and in the center of your palms.

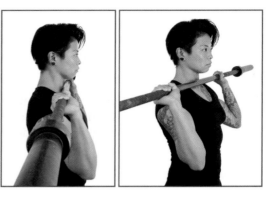

A couple of nuances worth mentioning are the width of your stance and grip. Determining your stance is easy; it's the same as your jumping stance or deadlift stance. Your feet are straight and positioned underneath your hips, roughly shoulder-width apart.

Figuring out your grip is a little trickier. There are a few different methods you can use. You can implement the front rack setup demonstrated on page 106, get into the top position of the ring-pushup (as shown on page 129), or execute the band press test. The keys are this: shoulders screwed into the back of the socket, forearms vertical, wrists aligned with your elbows, and the bar resting in the center of your palms.

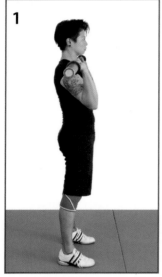

1

To set up for the strict-press, take the weight out of the rack and walk back as you would when performing the front squat—see front rack setup, page 106. To reiterate: The key is to create torque off the bar, wind your shoulders into the back of the socket, and brace your trunk. Your forearms are vertical, with the bar balancing in the center of your palms and chest, and your shoulders are wound tight. The biggest mistake athletes make is to take the weight out of the rack and then try to get tight. This is the equivalent of loading a bar onto your back for the back squat without bracing your midline. Once you establish your stance, screw your feet into the ground and squeeze your glutes.

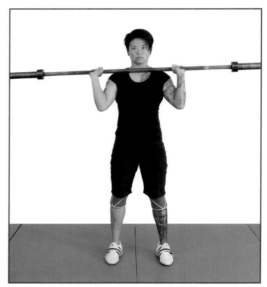

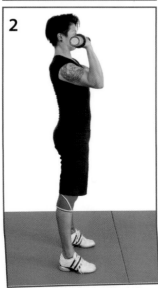

2

Keeping your shoulders pulled back, butt squeezed, and belly tight, pull your head back slightly and press the weight straight overhead. The key is to move your head around the bar, not the bar around your head. Also, focus on keeping your elbows in tight and your armpits forward. Don't shrug your shoulders, flare your elbows out, or lean back. There should be no change in spinal position.

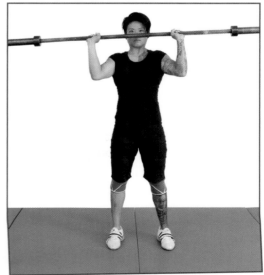

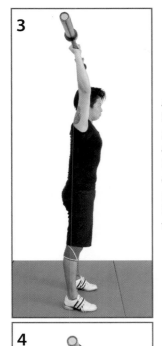

3

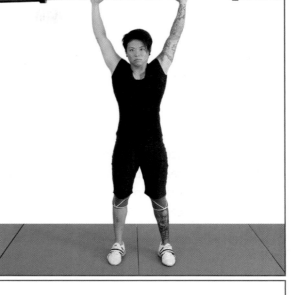

As you lockout your elbows, push your head through your arms into a neutral position. Think about positioning your armpits forward to maximize torque. Notice that the Diane's arm bisects her ears. A lot of athletes will mistakenly push their head through or keep their head back, both of which compromise trunk and shoulder stability.

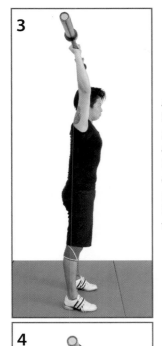

4

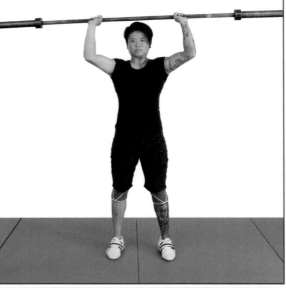

As you lower the bar, pull your head back slightly to maintain a vertical bar path. Again, the way down should look exactly the same as the way up. Keep your elbows tight, shoulders back, and butt squeezed as you lower the bar.

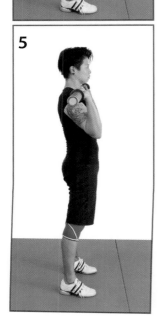

5

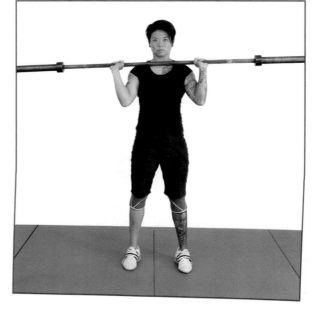

Maintaining the same level of torque, lower the weight back into the start position.

Front Rack Fault

A common mistake is to initiate the press from a front rack position. While you can get away with this when executing the push-press and push-jerk, it doesn't work with the strict-press. With the bar balancing on your fingertips, you can't generate enough force from the start position to lift the weight off your chest. People will do this because they don't have a model for pressing with a vertical forearm or they are missing range-of-motion in their shoulders or their thoracic spine is brutally tight—or all of those things.

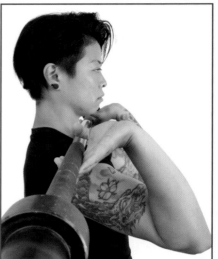

Motor-Control Fix:

▶ Set up for the press out of the rack. Position the bar in the center of your palms and make sure your elbows are aligned with your wrists (and the bar).

▶ Keep your shoulders screwed to the back of the socket by generating torque off the bar.

▶ Perform the band press test—see next page.

Mobilization Target Areas:

▶ Thoracic Spine

▶ Anterior Shoulders and Lats

▶ Posterior Shoulders and Chest

▶ Downstream Arm (Elbow/Wrist)

Arch Fault

The trunk stabilization demands are high in the strict-press. Unlike the push-press and push-jerk, which harness the power of your legs and hips, the strict-press requires you to press using the strength of your shoulders and arms. This dead-start phase is what makes the strict-press such a tricky movement. As the weight gets heavier, people will search for a mechanical advantage by arching back and pressing the weight out in front of their body, like a bench press. While this makes it easier to get the weight off the chest, it destabilizes the primary engines, causing the elbows to fly out and the shoulders to roll forward.

This fault is also common with people that try to move the bar around their face instead of pulling their head back. In most cases, this fault can be addressed by simply lowering the weight, keeping the butt squeezed, and maintaining a vertical bar path by moving the head back. However, if someone has a tight thoracic spine and is missing rotation in their shoulder, they might not be able to set their shoulders into a good position. If that happens, they will always press the weight out in front of their body as illustrated in the photos.

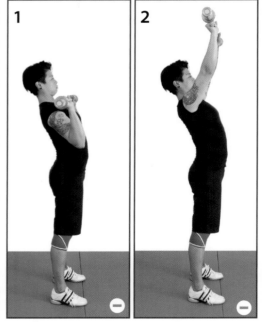

Motor-Control Fix:

▶ Squeeze the glutes and keep the belly tight.

▶ Prioritize the setup out of the rack by screwing your shoulders into the back of the socket.

Mobilization Target Areas:

▶ Thoracic Spine

▶ Anterior Shoulder/Lat

▶ Posterior Shoulder/Chest

▶ Downstream Arm (Elbow/Wrist)

Band Press Test

The band press test is great for a couple of reasons. For starters, it illuminates the importance and efficiency of a stable shoulder. Secondly, it shows people that their lovely push-jerk front rack position doesn't translate to the press.

Here's how it works: Hook a band around your foot and adopt a pressing position that is similar to the front rack. Then, try to extend your arm overhead from that position. What you'll find is that your shoulder immediately translates forward into an unstable position and you struggle to raise your arm overhead. Next, pull your shoulder back into a good position and press. Right away, you will see that it's much easier to lockout your arm. As soon as you bring your shoulder back and get your elbow tight to your body, it's much easier. You're able to harness all the stability of your shoulders and transmit energy effectively to the band.

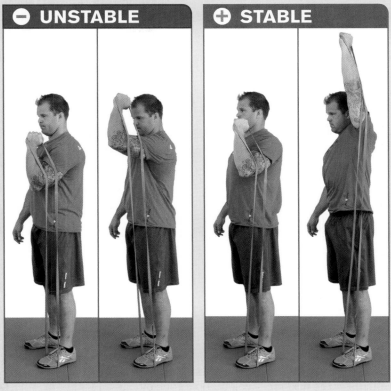

In a nutshell, the press test is a great way to challenge the efficiency of your press and sheds light on what an effective press should feel and look like.

Elbows Out Fault

If your elbows flare out to the side as you extend your arms overhead it's an indication that you're not generating enough torque or failed to set your shoulders in a good position during the setup. However, if you're unable to lockout your arms overhead, which is very common, chances are good that you're missing range-of-motion in your shoulders. This is a detrimental mechanical pattern that will become a real problem when the weight gets heavy or you graduate to more complex lifts like push-pressing and push-jerking.

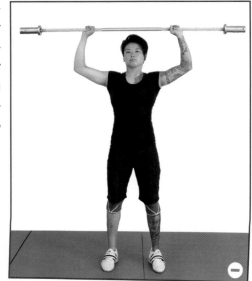

Motor-Control Fix:
▶ Generate sufficient torque in the setup and keep your elbows in as you press overhead.

Mobilization Target Areas:
▶ Thoracic Spine
▶ Anterior Shoulders and Lats
▶ Posterior Shoulders and Chest
▶ Downstream Arm (Elbow/Wrist)

Head Forward Fault

Another common fault is to push your head through your arms as you extend your elbows overhead. Coaches will often cue their athletes to push their head through because athletes will mistakenly pull their head back to clear their face and then leave it there as they lockout their arms overhead, causing a lean back fault. Telling them to push their head through aims to correct this fault by reminding them to move underneath the barbell as it passes their face.

The problem is that a lot of people will overcompensate by pushing the barbell backwards and driving their head forward. In addition to unlocking their shoulders and compromising spinal position, this puts an enormous amount of shear on the cervical segments of the neck. So when people are pressing and their heads penetrate through their arms and the barbell moves behind their body, you have a recipe for a quick neck injury. The correct technique is to bring your head back just enough to clear your face and then move underneath the bar as you press the weight overhead, keeping your torso and head in alignment.

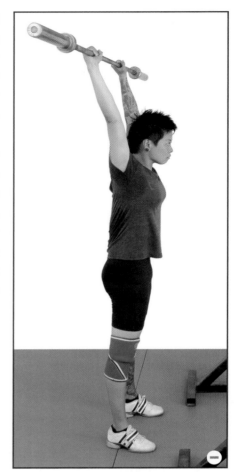

Motor-Control Fix:

▶ Keep your head in line with your torso.

▶ Think about keeping a vertical bar path and moving your head just enough to clear your face.

▶ Practice with lighter weights until you're proficient with the technique.

HANDSTAND PUSHUP
(FREESTANDING)

The handstand pushup is not a natural movement. I mean, aside from gymnastics, break-dancing, and CrossFit, rarely do people do anything inverted.

However, it is still an excellent movement to infuse into your training program. In fact, the handstand pushup is one of the best movements for driving home the relationship between ribcage and pelvis alignment. You have to balance your pelvis and legs on your ribcage, which exposes a lot of holes in people's midline stabilization strategy and shoulder organizational strategy.

Unlike most training movements, the handstand pushup requires that you organize your trunk through your shoulders via your hands, instead of your hips via your feet. For example, when you set up for a squat you create torque (stability) in your hips by screwing your feet into the ground and then balancing your ribcage over your pelvis. But with the handstand pushup, you do the exact opposite, which is very challenging for people. You're basically getting organized in the finish position of a press. From a motor-learning and trunk-stabilization perspective, the handstand pushup is unparalleled.

Again, to improve as an athlete, you have to find different ways to challenge your motor-control. The more training tools an athlete has in his movement arsenal, the better and more stable he will be. Should this belong in the repertoire of all athletes? No. A powerlifter or Olympic lifter is certainly not going to do handstand push-ups. They have plenty of other skill transfer exercises that teach good shoulder positioning and trunk stabilization. But for the average person, it's a fundamental skill that will improve athleticism and, more importantly, it will tell you a lot about your ability to organize your shoulders and trunk in an unfamiliar position.

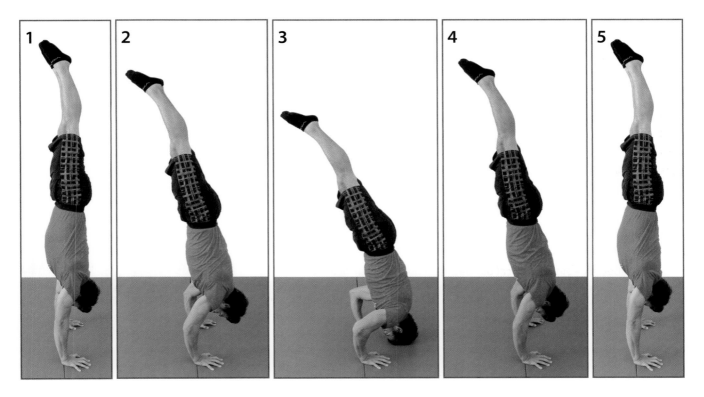

1. To set up for the handstand pushup, go through the bracing sequence and hinge forward from your hips as if you were executing a single-leg deadlift. Using your free leg as a pendulum, place your hands on the ground at your pushup distance, and kick up to a handstand by swinging your legs over your body. Keep your legs straight and create an external rotation force by screwing your hands into the ground as you transition into the handstand. The key is to keep your legs together and your toes pointed to maximize glute activation and stability. Focus on keeping your butt squeezed, belly tight, and armpits forward.

2. Still screwing your hands into the ground, break at your elbows and let your entire body tilt back, keeping your entire body rigid. One of the compromises of doing a handstand upside down is you can't leave your head in a perfect position. If you look at the photo, you'll notice that Carl tilts his head back just enough so that he can see the ground.

3. Lower your body until your head touches the ground.

4. As you press out of the bottom position, think about keeping your body rigid and your elbows in tight to your body.

5. As you lockout your arms, get your head through your arms and underneath your body to level out. At the same time, try to get your armpits forward to maintain external rotation toque.

Handstand Pushup (Supported)

A freestanding handstand or a freestanding handstand pushup—that's the goal. But it takes an extreme amount of strength, stability, and motor-control to pull off. The stepping-stone to such a skill is to use a support like a wall. This is the equivalent of squatting or benching on a Smith machine in that you can move up and down in a straight line. Another option is to have a Superfriend support your feet. This requires higher levels of stability and is great for finding your balance while inverted.

And you don't even need to perform the actual movement; just get into the start position and work on locking out your elbows, getting your armpits forward, and organizing your trunk. It's a great place to teach people about shoulder and trunk stability. Like I said, nothing challenges the ribcage to pelvis relationship like the handstand pushup.

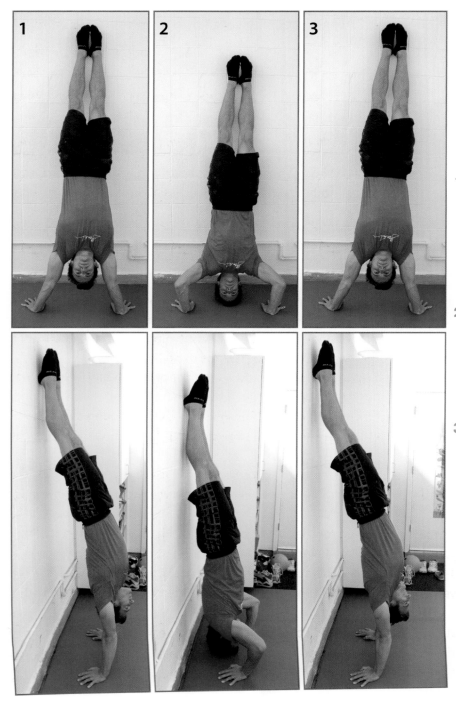

1. Positioning your hands roughly 6-inches from the wall, go through the bracing sequence and then kick up into a handstand. Here are the keys: Keep your hands straight, butt squeezed, legs together, toes pointed, pelvis balanced over your ribcage, and your armpits forward.

2. Screwing your hands into the ground, break at the elbows and lower your head to the ground. As you descend, try to keep your forearms vertical, your elbows in tight to your body, and your back and legs aligned.

3. As you press out of the bottom position and lockout your arms, get your armpits forward.

Scorpion Handstand Pushup Fault

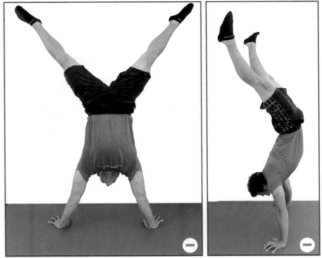

The faults for the handstand pushup are the same as those for the standing press: Ribcage tilt, head up, elbows out, and shoulders forward. And just like the pushup, people will spread their legs, which puts their butt offline, causing a gross overextension lumbar spinal fault. It's a disaster.

Interestingly, this is what most people look like when they try to walk on their hands. I see this all the time and I think to myself: "Congratulations, you're walking on your hands . . . and you're wrecking your motor patterning for all your pressing motions and destroying your back and shoulders." Seriously, there are so many things wrong with this picture I don't know where to begin.

The fact is, you would never press in this position. If we flipped the photo of Carl upside down, put a barbell in his hand and told you to evaluate the position, what would you say? I suspect nothing good.

Here's the deal. You have to get organized at the trunk and work on setting your shoulders into the correct position—armpits forward. Keep your hands straight so that you can maximize torque, keep your feet together, and point your toes to maximize glute activation. If you have to look down to see the ground, try not to exaggerate the movement. Aside from that, the motor-control solution and mobility prescription is the same as the strict-press faults.

- -

PULL-UP

If you view athletic movement through the lens of "how much" and "how fast," the odds of defaulting into a bad position just skyrocket. The pull-up offers a sizzling example. In most cases, little or no attention is paid to how the athlete sacrificed his spine, neck, and shoulder position as if he were drowning at sea. The quality of a pull-up gets reduced to, "Was the athlete able to get his chin over the bar? Yes or no?"

It's not about whether or not a movement was completed, but rather whether or not the movement was completed with good form.

Imagine if I told you that rounding your back when you deadlift heavy is acceptable as long as you complete the lift. That wouldn't make sense, right? It contradicts the underlying theme of this book. Well, it's the same thing with the pull-up.

If you can't perform the movement correctly without compensating into a bad position, it's damaging. You can get away with it for a while, but eventually hanging with bent elbows and overextending your lumbar spine is going to kick your ass.

At our gym, we teach our athlete's the strict pull-up for the same reason we teach the strict-press. It allows us to effectively teach and ingrain good mechanics in a low-risk environment. We can then progress to more dynamic moves like the kipping pull-up with less risk of defaulting into a poor position. The idea is to develop physical competency with the movement from a dead-start at end-range before challenging them with a speed element.

Once we can get athletes to create and maintain a rigid spine and stable shoulders, it becomes an issue of strength. If the athlete can't initiate the movement with good form, we'll simply scale the movement by hooking a band around his feet. In addition to building strength, the band reduces the torque demands and allows him to move through a full range-of-motion.

Hook Grip

Just as the positioning of your feet dictate your ability to generate torque in your hips and maintain a neutral spine, your grip dictates your ability to generate torque in your shoulders and keep your ribcage down when performing a pull-up. For most people, positioning their hands at roughly shoulder-width apart or adopting the same grip distance as their pushup or strict-press is a good start.

The next step is to learn how to grip the bar. If you glance at the photos, you'll notice that Carl implements a unique grip. Instead of adopting a traditional grip of hooking his thumb over the top of the bar, he wraps his thumb over his index or middle finger. In addition, he also positions his pinky fingers over the top of the bar, creating a slight bend in the wrist. This grip is superior because it locks your hand to the bar and allows you to create torque, which sets your shoulders in a stable position.

This modified false grip offers a couple distinct advantages. For starters, it winds his shoulders up into an externally rotated position. In other words, he doesn't have to think about breaking the bar because he's already torqued. When your wrists are positioned directly underneath the bar, you have to work a lot harder to create torque in your shoulders. Secondly, this hook grip dead hang position is also a great diagnostic tool for assessing overhead range-of-motion: If you can keep your torso integrated while hanging with the pull-up hook grip, it's an indication that you have full range-of-motion overhead.

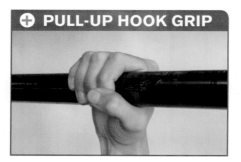

PULL-UP HOOK GRIP

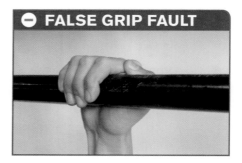

FALSE GRIP FAULT

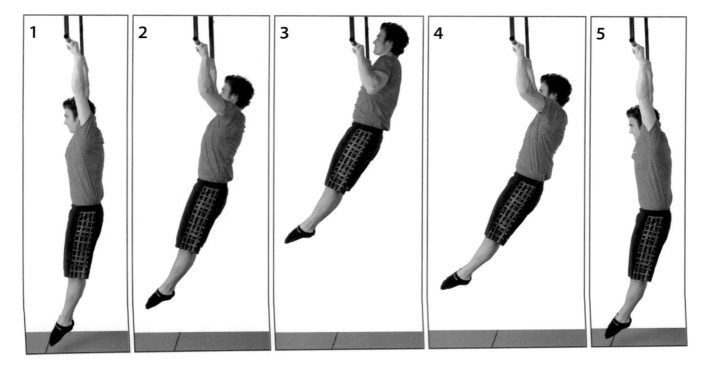

1. Establish a pull-up hook grip. Next, brace your trunk by squeezing your glutes and pulling your ribcage down. Position your legs together with your toes pointed. This allows you to maximize tension in your glutes and core. If you examine the photo, you'll notice that Carl's back is flat, his ribcage is balanced perfectly over his pelvis, and his shoulders are screwed into the back of the socket (armpits forward).

2. Keeping your belly tight and butt squeezed, pull yourself up. To keep your torso and shoulders integrated, imagine pushing your feet forward as you initiate the pull. Don't make the mistake of disengaging your core as your torso deviates back.

3. With your pinky still positioned over the bar, pull your chest to the bar—keeping your head in a neutral position. Note: If you can't raise your chin over the bar with your head neutral, stop. Don't try to throw your head back to complete the movement.

4. As you lower yourself down to the start position, nothing should change: Your back is still flat, butt squeezed, belly tight, pinky over the bar, head neutral, legs together, and feet pointed. As long as you maintain a braced-neutral trunk and your grip stays intact, you don't have to think about breaking the bar—you will remain in a state of high torque.

5. Finish the movement the same way you started, in a good position.

Upper-Back Flinch Fault

As mentioned, very few people are strong enough or have the motor-control to initiate a strict pull-up. To gain a mechanical advantage, athletes often tilt their ribcage back, unlocking their shoulders, and overextend their lumbar spine. This is also common with people that are missing internal rotation in their shoulders or are not comfortable with the hook grip. Rather than create torque, they keep their shoulders soft, which feeds slack downstream to the torso, making it easier to initiate the pull.

If your back, shoulders, and trunk are not on tension entering the movement, your body will hunt for stability. This is characterized by tilting your ribcage, your elbows flaring out, your shoulders rolling forward, and your head cranking back. All the same faults that you see with the strict-press. Coincidence? I think not. You're towing the car out of the ditch with slack in the rope.

Motor-Control Fix:

► Address grip mechanics: make sure your pinky is positioned over the bar.

► Squeeze your butt, pull your ribcage over your pelvis, position your legs together, and point your toes.

Mobilization Target Areas:

► Thoracic Spine

► Posterior Shoulders and Lats

► Anterior Shoulders and Chest

► Downstream Arm (Elbow/Wrist)

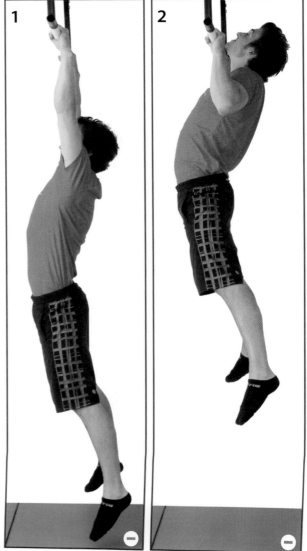

Cross Leg Fault

Just like the dip, a lot of people mistakenly set up for the pull-up by hooking their feet behind their body and bending their legs. This prevents your legs from flying apart, which happens when you're not strong enough to perform a strict pull-up, and allows you to pump your knees up to your chest to generate upward momentum.

This also happens if you set up on a bar that is too low to the ground. Regardless of why you do it, this fault makes it impossible to engage your glutes and set your ribcage over your pelvis, putting you into an overextended position. If you start from an overextended position, there is no way that you can create torque and stability in your shoulders. So in addition to moving with a disorganized spine, your shoulders move up to your ears and your lats turn off. Put simply, you're hanging from an unstable shoulder joint.

Motor-Control Fix:

▶ Address grip mechanics: make sure your pinky is positioned over the bar.

▶ Straighten out your legs, position your feet together, and point your toes. Squeeze your butt and balance your ribcage over your pelvis.

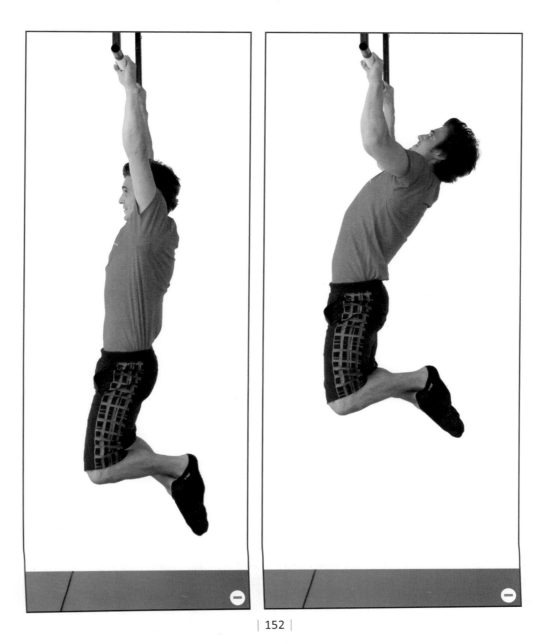

CHIN-UP

The goal is to be able to create torque from any hand position and express a full range-of-motion with every movement. In fact, performing pull-ups with your hands in different positions is a nice way to test your understanding of the movement. However, you don't want to adopt a position that undermines your technique. For that reason, I recommend you start by learning the conventional palm-forward pull-up. It teaches you how to create torque, puts your shoulders into a stable position, and makes it easier to maintain a braced-neutral spine. Once you're competent with a full range-of-motion overhead, test your position by implementing the chin-up.

If you're unable to lock your arms out and keep your ribcage down with a chin-up grip, there's a good chance that you're missing range-of-motion overhead.

Putting your arms in a position of full external rotation provides more stability because you don't have to actively hunt for tension. The problem is that externally rotating your hands makes it difficult to create torque at end-range. Not only that, if you can't get into an end-range start position, your elbows bend and your ribcage tilts, which is less than ideal. So in addition to pulling from a compensated position, you're not expressing a full range-of-motion (no wonder they're easier).

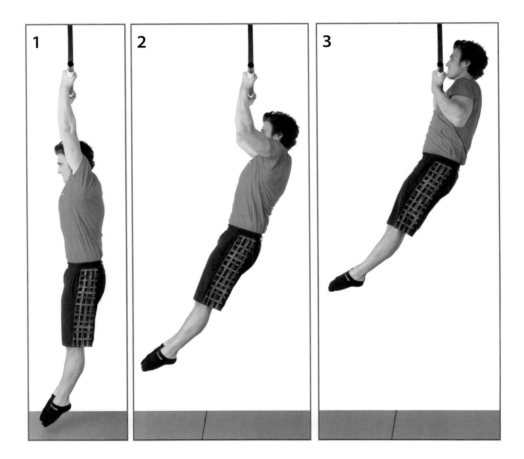

1. The setup for the chin-up is the same as the pull-up: Squeeze your butt, position your legs together and out in front of your body, point your toes, pull your ribcage down, and keep your head neutral. Notice how Carl's shoulders are in a fully externally rotated position. While this sets his shoulders in a good position, he will have to work extra hard to keep his ribcage down and his spine neutral as he initiates the pull.

2. Keeping your elbows tight, ribcage down, head neutral, and butt squeezed, pull yourself toward the bar. Think about keeping your legs out in front of your body as you lever back.

3. Pull your chin over the bar. Keep your head neutral and avoid reaching for the bar with your chin.

CATEGORY 2 MOVEMENTS

Position of High Stability (PHS)	▶	remove connection	▶	Position of High Stability (PHS)

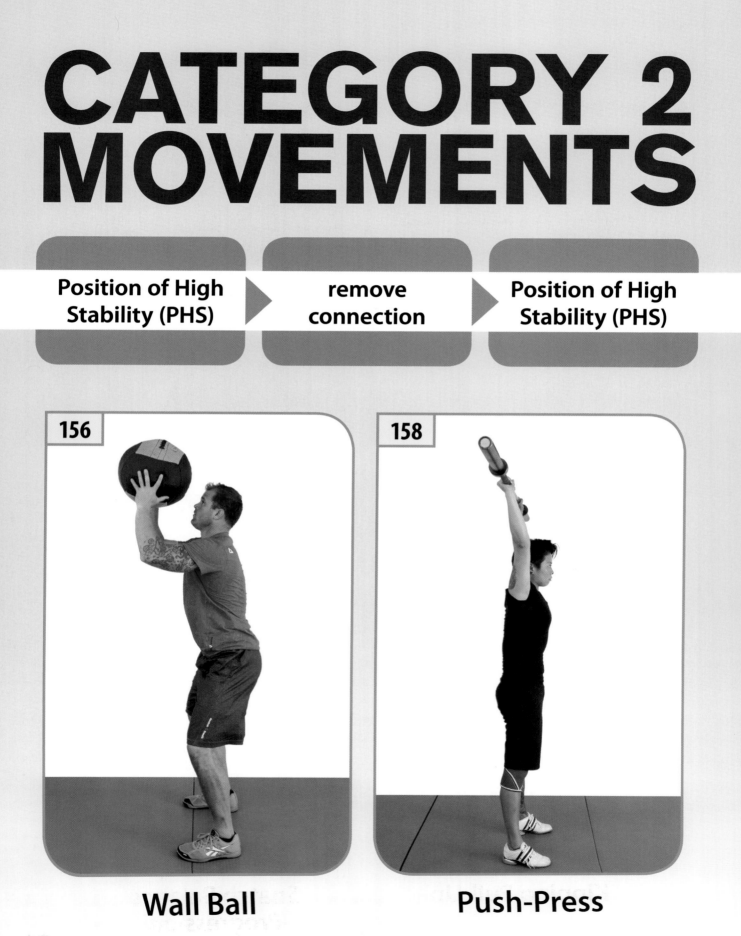

156

Wall Ball

158

Push-Press

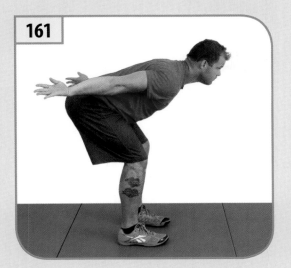

161

Jumping and Landing

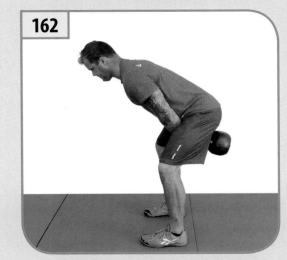

162

Kettlebell Swing

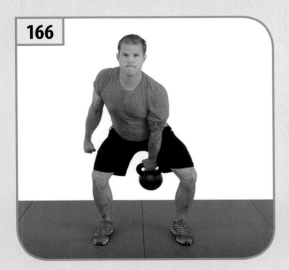

166

One-Arm Swing

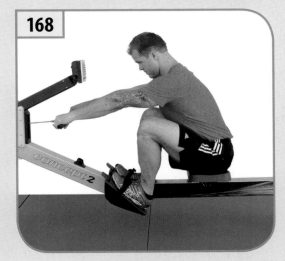

168

Rowing

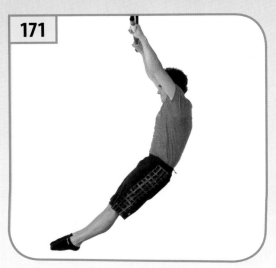

171

Kipping Pull-Up

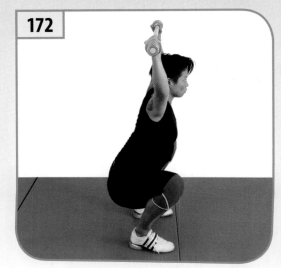

172

Snatch Balance Progression

WALL BALL

As a quick recap, category 2 movements are similar to category 1 movements in that you start and finish in a position that allows you to cultivate trunk stiffness and torque. But instead of staying connected to the movement—meaning that you maintain torque and tension through the movement's entire range-of-motion—you add a speed element and momentarily remove the connection.

The wall ball is one of the first category 2 movements that I introduce to novice athletes or someone who is coming off an injury. It's a simple squat that adds a dynamic stimulus—throwing and receiving a medicine ball—while challenging an athlete's ability to maintain a vertical torso. It's a great way to assess an athlete's motor-control patterns and deficiencies.

Here's an example: Say you're training a novice athlete. He's now competent with fundamental movement principles and category 1 movements. You've also challenged him under load with an upright torso. The next step is to introduce category 2 movements such as the wall ball. What you will find is that the moment he's asked to spontaneously create torque off of an object that is not a barbell, everything falls apart. He starts overextending his lumbar spine, rounding his upper back, and driving his knees forward. And the only thing you asked him to do was squat with a medicine ball, throw it to a target, and receive it in a stable position.

Now, should the wall ball be part of every elite level athlete's training program? Not necessarily.

This is the idea: By adding a speed element, you expose weaknesses in the athlete's profile in an environment where the chances of getting injured are very low. (You can also add a metabolic demand to the equation, making it even harder for him to disguise his poor movement patterns and mobility restrictions.) This is extremely useful for a coach because now you have a simple model for teaching an athlete how to transmit force from his hips to his shoulders. You can teach him how to spontaneously create torque in the bottom position of the squat, as a progression to the Olympic lifts: If he can't receive an 8-pound ball in a good position what do you think will happen with a 95-pound barbell? This is what makes the wall ball such a rich and useful movement.

Note: The common faults associated with the wall ball include: forward inclination of the torso, internal rotation of the shoulders, overextension of the lower back, valgus knee collapse, etc. Revisit the air squat and front squat for motor-control and mobility solutions.

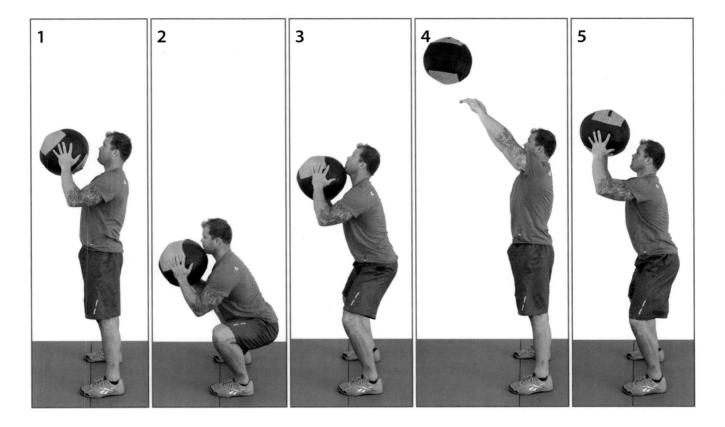

1. To set up for the wall ball, assume your squat stance with the medicine ball positioned at head level, screwing your hands into the ball to create a stable shoulder position. Stand far enough away from your target so that you can receive the ball in the start position. In other words, you don't want the ball to fall in front or behind you, but right at your chest.

2. Keeping your torso upright, lower yourself into the bottom position just as you would when performing a front squat—see front squat, page 106. Keep your head neutral and focus on keeping your back flat. Don't try craning your neck so that you can see your target.

3. As you increase your elevation, focus your gaze on your target. Again, you don't need to throw your head back to do this. If you set up correctly, you'll be standing far enough away so that you can see your target without craning your neck.

4. As you stand tall, extend your arms and throw the ball to the target. The key is to extend your arms equally. In other words, don't try to throw the ball like you're shooting a free throw. A lot of people will overcompensate with their dominant arm, which compromises your ability to receive the ball in a good position. Be sure to squeeze your glutes as you stand tall and reestablish a strong upright position before receiving the ball.

5. Receive the ball out in front of your body in the exact same position you started. The idea is to receive the ball overhead and move down with the ball, screwing your hands into the ball to set your shoulders in a good position as you descend.

PUSH-PRESS

You set up for the push-press like you would a strict-press. But instead of pressing the weight off your chest from a dead-start, you bend and extend your knees to accelerate the weight overhead. The "dip and drive" addition of power allows you to handle larger loads. It also teaches you how to transmit force from your hips to your shoulders, a pattern that transfers to more complex movements, like the clean and jerk.

In the push-press you don't have to generate as much torque in the start position because you're using the power of your legs and hips to press the weight off of your chest. So if you have mobility issues that make the strict-press rack position untenable, the push-press rack position will give you some breathing room and still allow you to go overhead.

Think of the push-press as a weighted vertical jump. In fact, the push-press is a great way to layer and teach proper upright torso jumping and landing mechanics: If you understand how to dip and drive by shoving your knees out and keeping your back flat, you have a model for jumping and landing with a vertical posture that doesn't trash your back or knees.

To help with your understanding, think of the dip and drive as the jump, and lowering the weight as the landing. Most people have not been taught how to jump and land with good form.

Imagine jumping up for a rebound, spiking a volleyball, or performing a strength-and-conditioning circuit that calls for high-repetition box jumps and push-presses, like CrossFit's Fight Gone Bad workout. What happens when you don't have a model for shoving your knees out or keeping a flat back? You drive your knees forward and overextend. No wonder so many people suffer from insidious knee pain—commonly referred to as jumper's knee (patellar tendonitis)—after engaging in such activities.

Note: The most common faults associated with the push-press include: driving your knees forward, overextending your lumbar spine, pressing the barbell out in front or behind your body, flaring your elbows out, and internally rotating your shoulders. To address the knee forward and overextension faults related to the dip and drive, revisit the air squat and front squat. To address the pressing faults, flip back to the pushup and strict-press.

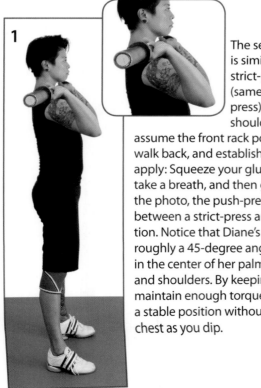

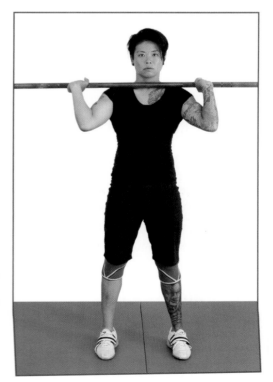

The setup for the push-press is similar to the setup for the strict-press: establish your grip (same grip distance as the strict-press), break the bar to set your shoulders in a good position, assume the front rack position, lift the weight out, walk back, and establish your stance. Same rules apply: Squeeze your glutes, get your belly tight, take a breath, and then go. As you can see from the photo, the push-press rack position is halfway between a strict-press and front squat rack position. Notice that Diane's elbows are positioned at roughly a 45-degree angle. The bar is positioned in the center of her palms, supported by her chest and shoulders. By keeping your elbows up, you can maintain enough torque to keep your shoulders in a stable position without the bar sliding down your chest as you dip.

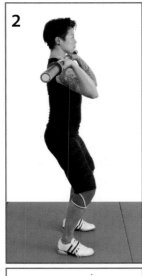

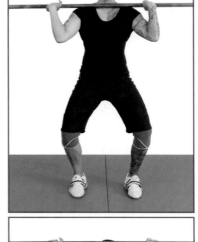

2

Keeping your torso upright, drive your knees out laterally—screwing your feet into the ground—and lower your hips between your feet.

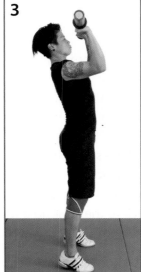

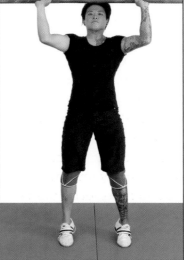

3

In one explosive movement, extend your knees and hips, move your head back slightly (just enough to clear your face while still maintaining a vertical bar path), and press the weight overhead. The goal is to keep your posture as vertical as possible and keep your weight centered over your feet. If you roll up onto your toes, you will fall forward, and if you're on your heels, you'll roll backwards. As the bar accelerates upwards, maintain torque by keeping your elbows in and shoulders back.

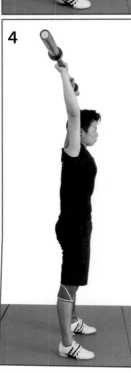

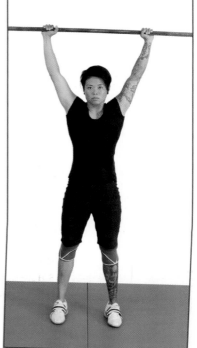

4

As you lock your arms out overhead, pull your torso and head underneath the bar. Continue to squeeze your glutes, maintain tension in your core, and generate torque in your hips and shoulders.

5

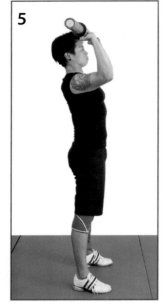

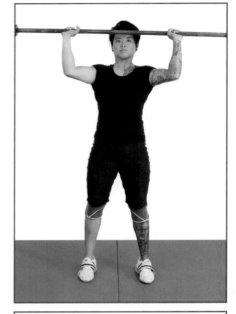

To correctly lower the weight, pull your head and torso back slightly, keeping your butt squeezed to support your back, and lower the weight down. It's imperative that you continue to generate torque by keeping your elbows in and shoulders back.

6

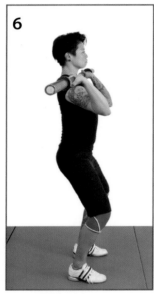

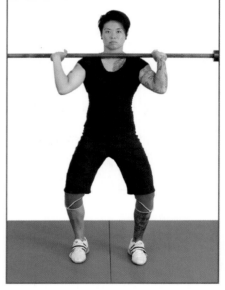

Receive the weight onto your chest by dipping into a quarter squat. To be more specific, shove your knees out, drop your hips between your feet, and reestablish the push-press rack position. It's extremely important that you consciously cultivate torque into the receiving position because it sets you up for the next rep. If you dump torque by letting your elbows flare out or your shoulders roll forward as you lower the weight onto your chest, you will start the next rep in a bad position. This is why it's important to perform high-repetition elements because it teaches you how to create and maintain torque. For example, say you're doing a workout that calls for 15 push-presses. You take the weight out perfectly, press one time, but fail to maintain torque on the way down. Now the next 14 repetitions will be done from a bad position.

7

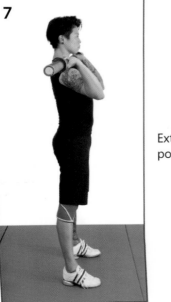

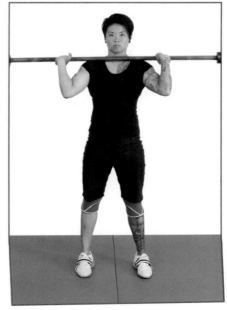

Extend your hips and knees and reestablish the top position.

JUMPING AND LANDING

Jumping straight up and down, or even bounding forward from a square, stationary stance, is essentially an unloaded dynamic squat. You hinge forward from your hips, loading your posterior chain, create torque through your hips by creating external rotation torque, and keep your shins as vertical as possible. You also see the same faults.

People will drive their knees forward. If their feet are angled out, you will see ankles collapse, valgus knee faults, overextension at the lumbar spine, etc. The only difference with jumping and landing is the consequences are much higher, especially if you're coming down from an elevated platform or combining a ton of jumping and landing sequences together in a single workout.

Consider a sport like basketball or volleyball where athletes put in countless jumping and landing cycles. Now imagine what happens if they develop a knee forward or open foot or knee in movement pattern. They're doomed. The insidious load on their knees is insane and the mechanism for how they get jumper's knee. (Note: jumper's knee is caused by an irritation of the patellar tendon, the tendon that connects the kneecap to the shinbone, due to forward and valgus translation of the knee during jumping and squatting movements.) This is also how people invite ACL tears.

Mobilizing and smashing the upstream and downstream tissues will certainly alleviate a lot of the irritation caused by jumper's knee and help you get into a better position. But the only way to fix this issue is to address the technique.

With jumping and landing from a stationary stance, it's easy: Adhere to the movement principles and focus on keeping your shins vertical, feet straight, and knees out. And remember, squatting, pulling, and push-pressing movements are all great ways of building good jumping and landing movement patterns.

Note: If you are executing an upright torso jump—rebounding a basketball, for example—remember that you have to drive your knees out and create higher levels of torque to minimize compression forces on your knees.

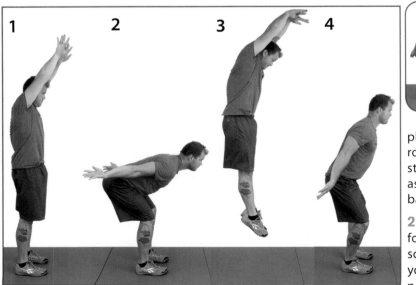

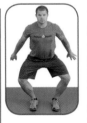

1. If you're trying to jump as high as possible from a stationary stance, position your feet underneath your hips—keeping your feet straight. Then go through the bracing sequence and raise your arms just overhead. Notice in the photograph how my arms are internally rotated. This will leave my shoulders in a stable position, helping me keep my back flat as I tilt my torso forward and swing my arms back.

2. To load up for the jump, tilt your torso forward, loading your hips and hamstrings, screw your feet into the ground, and drive your knees out. Keep your shins as vertical as possible.

3. Swing your arms overhead while simultaneously extending your hips and knees. If you glance at the photo, you'll notice that my legs are together and my feet are pointed. This allows me to activate my glutes and keep my spine organized while airborne. Pointing your toes also sets you up for landing on the ball of the foot, which is ideal.

4. As your feet touch down, create an external rotation force by driving your knees out and screwing your feet into the ground. Let your torso translate forward as you drive your hips and hamstrings back.

KETTLEBELL SWING

When it comes to learning complicated movements efficiently, the key is to make them uncomplicated. We do this by breaking them down into precise, manageable steps. Then we emphatically encourage like-your-life-depends-on-it focus in performing each step. This is the path to a tight learning curve. It's the foundation required for optimal performance. It's also how you reduce the risk of injury.

Consider the back squat. Instead of teaching the back squat as one movement, we break it up into three distinct phases: the lift out, the walk back, and the squat. This not only simplifies the movement and brings consciousness to each step, but it also serves as a diagnostic test. Right away, you can see if an athlete understands how to brace and create torque in the early stages of their setup. If he fails to create torque off the bar and doesn't set his pelvis in a neutral position during the lift out, you can work to correct that fault before he loads his spine. This is extremely useful tool for the coach because you can start to correct faults before your athlete initiates a full-range movement.

The kettlebell swing is another example. In order to perform the actual swing, which is the focus of the movement, you first have to lift the kettlebell off the ground. This phase is no different than performing a deadlift: brace, hinge forward at the hips with a flat back, create torque in the shoulders, and then stand up. It's telling that people will fail to make this connection and immediately begin from a bad position by bending over with a rounded back, drive their knees forward, and lift the weight up with unstable shoulders. No wonder so many people struggle with the kettlebell swing. It's not that they lack the motor-control or range-of-motion to correctly perform the movement, they just set up in a bad position.

This is why layering category 2 movements is so important: It allows you to see what an athlete's default motor patterns are when there is a dynamic stimulus. If you want to highlight why an athlete has jumper's knee, have him perform a kettlebell swing as a diagnostic test. In two seconds, you will see him drive his knees forward instead of pulling his hamstrings back, a fault that may have gone unnoticed in category 1 but gets lit up in category 2.

Russian Swing vs. American Swing

There are two different kettlebell swings commonly used in strength-and-conditioning circles that are worth mentioning. There's the American swing and the Russian swing. The former requires that you swing the kettlebell overhead, while the latter requires you to swing the kettlebell to chest or head level. Both iterations are extremely helpful in terms of assessing motor-control and mobility, but serve slightly different purposes.

The American swing obviously requires more shoulder, trunk, and hip control so it illuminates more faults than the Russian counterpart due to the increased range-of-motion demands. But you can't handle as much weight. And if you don't have full range-of-motion overhead, the American swing will exaggerate bracing and torque faults (overextension in the top position, internal rotation in the shoulders). If you don't have a full range-of-motion, performing the American swing just to reach some arbitrary range is not a particularly brainy move.

Top-Down Setup

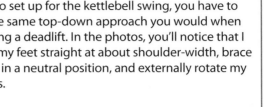

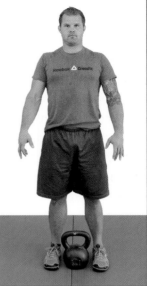

1

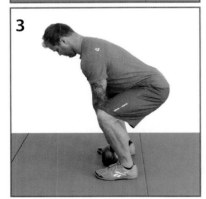

In order to set up for the kettlebell swing, you have to follow the same top-down approach you would when performing a deadlift. In the photos, you'll notice that I position my feet straight at about shoulder-width, brace my trunk in a neutral position, and externally rotate my shoulders.

2

Keeping your shoulders pulled back, shins vertical, and head neutral, drive your hamstrings back and bend over with a flat back.

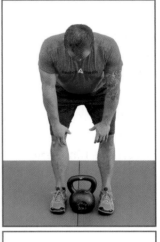

3

As you reach end-range, bend your knees and lower your hips—making sure to keep your belly tight, shins as vertical as possible, and back flat—so that you can assume your grip on the kettlebell. To set your shoulders in a strong position, create an external rotation force by screwing your hands into the handle. It's important to note that if you can't keep your shoulders pulled back because you're missing internal rotation, you can grip the outside of the kettlebell. (Keep reading to see this variation.)

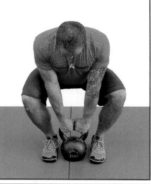

4

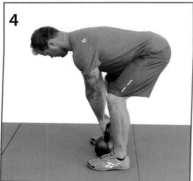

In order to maintain a good position, you need to take out all the slack in your body and put tension back into the system. To accomplish this, continue to drive your knees out, raise your hips, and get your shins as vertical as possible.

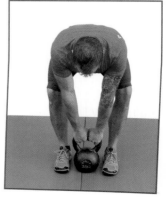

The Swing

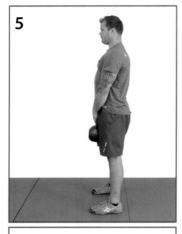

5 Deadlift the kettlebell into the standing position. As you extend your hips and lockout your knees, squeeze your butt in the top position, keep your shoulders pulled back, and screw your feet into the ground.

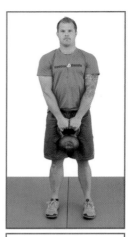

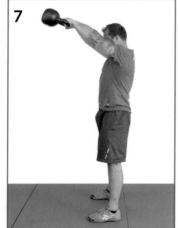

6 To initiate the swing, drive your knees out, sit your hamstrings back, and hinge forward at the hips. Note: It's the same movement sequence as the first 6-inches of a low bar back squat. As you do this, hike the kettlebell between your legs. The key is to keep your head in a neutral position, your shins vertical, and your shoulders pulled back.

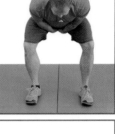

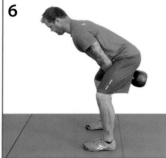

Keeping your weight distributed over the center of your feet, extend your hips and knees simultaneously, squeezing your glutes as you reach full hip extension. The idea is to drive your hips into your forearms and use this explosive hip extension to power the swing. Your arms should not deviate away from your body until your hips reach full extension.

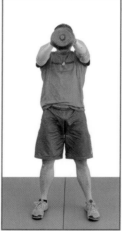

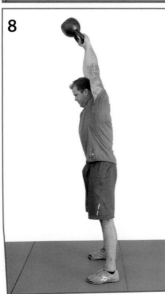

8 Harnessing the power generated by your hips, raise your arms overhead. It's important to mention that there is a moment of weightlessness, so take advantage of this by squeezing your glutes and organizing your position. From here, receive the weight the same way you initiated the swing, by pulling your hamstrings back—keeping your shins vertical and head neutral—and maintaining a rigid spine.

Torque Fault

If you fail to create torque off the kettlebell handle, your shoulders will always compensate into an internally rotated position. This is easily fixed by addressing the top-down setup. However, if you're missing internal rotation in your shoulders, establishing a stable position with a narrow grip is difficult to manage. If that happens,

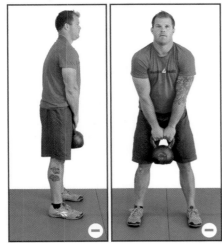

scale your grip by grabbing the outside of the kettlebell handle. This will give your shoulders some breathing room so that you can get into a good position. But remember, this is not normal. You shouldn't have to circumvent your poor mobility by scaling movements. Get to work on improving shoulder range-of-motion like it's your job.

Motor-Control Fix:
▶ Use the top-down deadlift setup to pick the kettlebell off the ground.
▶ Screw your hands into the handle and pull your shoulder blades back.

Mobilization Target Areas:
▶ Posterior Shoulders and Lats
▶ Anterior Shoulders and Chest

Scaling Your Grip

If you can't get your shoulders into a good position because you're missing internal rotation, you can buy yourself some breathing room by grabbing the outside of the kettlebell handle.

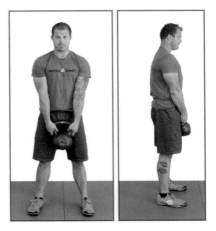

Head Fault

Here's a common scenario: An athlete sets up perfectly for the kettlebell swing, but as he loads his hips and hamstrings to initiate the movement (or receive the weight from the top position), he sacrifices his neutral spinal position by throwing his head back. In most cases, this fault occurs because the athlete is fighting against the down swing, which pulls his torso forward. Throwing his head back is a way to counterbalance that force and avoid falling forward—see hip hinge fault.

Think about it like this: The kettlebell swing shares the same movement pattern as the first 6-inches of a low bar back squat. The key is to keep your head neutral and focus your gaze on the ground about six feet out in front of you. If you're looking straight ahead, you're more likely to commit this fault.

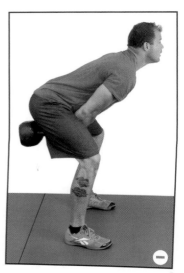

Motor-Control Fix:
▶ Keep your head neutral and focus your gaze about six feet out in front of your body.

Hip Fault

Another common fault is to follow the weight between your legs as if you were hiking a football. This happens when an athlete fails to create torque or brace, or if he has a weak lower back. As you can see from the photos, I demonstrate a grossly exaggerated illustration of this fault. However, it does happen, especially after the last rep. Instead of controlling the weight down, an athlete will count his last rep at the top position and release all tension in his shoulders and hips and let the momentum of the weight pull him forward. This little gem is a great way to finish a workout with a tweaked lower back. Remember, injuries often occur in the beginning or at the end of an exercise. Make the right decision. Start and finish the movement in a good position.

Motor-Control Fix:

▶ Don't chase the kettlebell with your torso, look down, or release tension after completing your last repetition. Control the weight down to the ground as you would with a heavy deadlift.

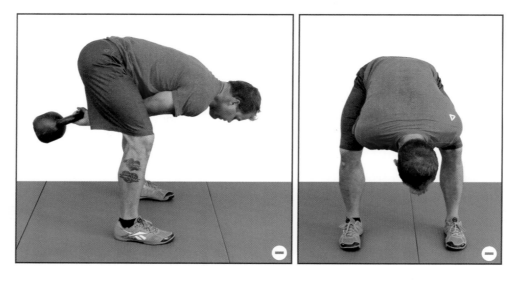

ONE-ARM SWING

In my opinion, the kettlebell is better suited to the one-arm swings than the classic kettlebell swing. It's a surprisingly challenging movement because there's a rotational element that makes stabilizing your shoulders and trunk difficult. For example, on the downswing, with the kettlebell swinging between your legs, the momentum of the weight pulls your shoulder into an internally rotated position. You have to resist that force to keep your shoulder back.

The one-arm swing also highlights an athlete's strategy for stabilizing the non-swinging hand. I know this is a mantra that I have been chatting about throughout this book, but I'll say it again anyway: If you don't create a stable position by bracing your spine and creating torque in your primary engines, your body will find stability somewhere else. You have to organize your opposite hand by making a fist or splaying your fingers, and wind your shoulder into the back of the socket. This idea carries over to all single-arm, unilateral movements like one-arm dumbbell pressing, dumbbell snatches, and the Turkish getup.

The bottom line is this: It's much harder to create stability in a single shoulder, especially when there's a dynamic element, than in two shoulders. You can't create torque off the implement so it really highlights your understanding of fundamental movement patterns.

Note: The setup is exactly the same as the double-arm swing in that you use a top-down setup approach.

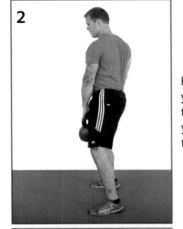

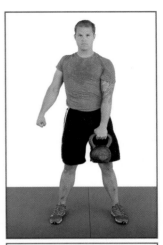

1

Follow the top-down setup as demonstrated in the previous technique. But instead of gripping the kettlebell with both hands, grab the center or far end of the handle. Be sure to set your shoulder back and wind up your opposite arm to keep tension in the system.

2

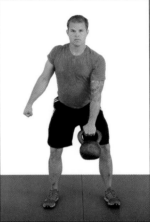

Keeping your shoulder back and your torso upright, rotate your body toward your free arm and maneuver the kettlebell toward your centerline. If you're holding the kettlebell with your left hand, turn toward your right side. If you're holding the kettlebell with your right hand, turn toward your left side.

3

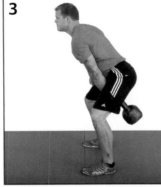

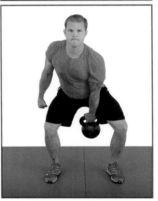

As you maneuver the kettlebell toward your centerline, pull your hamstrings back—keeping your back flat, head neutral, and shins vertical—and hike the kettlebell between your legs. Note: Some coaches will tell you to internally rotate your hand in this step. Personally, I focus on keeping my knuckles forward because it allows me to clear my leg while still maintaining a stable shoulder position. If you internally rotate your hand, it's harder to keep your shoulder back.

4

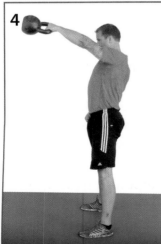

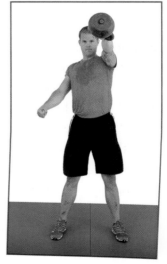

In one explosive movement, extend your hips and knees. As with the classic double-arm swing, think about driving your hips into your arm so that you can effectively transmit force from your hips to your shoulder.

Unstable Shoulder Fault (Hook Hand Fault)

As I just mentioned, if you don't organize your free arm, it will contort into some strange positions. Oftentimes, this is characterized by a hook hand and grossly internally rotated shoulder. In addition to looking really weird, it creates an open circuit fault, which travels through the kinetic chain and makes it difficult to create and maintain stability.

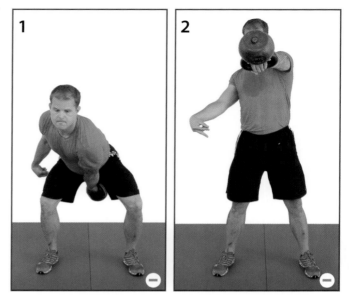

ROWING

If you know how to deadlift with good form, rowing is simple. They share the same load-order sequence and start position. So if I tell you to row 1,000 meters, I want you to automatically think 60-80 deadlifts. This not only makes it easier to sequence the right movement patterns, but also brings consciousness to each stroke.

Unlike the deadlift, however, rowing is a low-resistance, high-repetition exercise. In addition to adding speed, timing, and a metabolic stimulus, you have to reconstitute the same start and finish position over and over again. This is what makes rowing a minefield.

Introduce speed and people start falling apart. Although the consequences for rowing in a bad position are not as immediate as deadlifting with bad form, there's a cumulative effect. For example, say you fail to drive your knees out, causing your ankles to collapse every time you pull and return the handle to the start position. If you're rowing at thirty strokes a minute for 20 minutes, that's six hundred collapsed ankle compressions. You may get away with it for a while without consequence, but injuries result over the long haul. It also grooves in poor movement patterns.

Here are the key takeaways of rowing. First, rowing highlights an athlete's ankle, posterior chain, and hip flexion range-of-motion. Two, you can identify load-sequencing errors. It's easy to see if someone is loading his lower back and rounding forward instead of keeping his spine rigid and assigning tension into his hips and hamstrings. Three, it helps strengthen an athlete's understanding of this principle—namely, if the positioning of his head, shoulders, or spine is off, it's impossible to perform the movement with good form. Finally, it tests an athlete's coordination and ability to repetitively generate force from the same position.

Note: A lot can be said about the technical aspect of rowing, especially the timing, but breaking into the minutia of things like stroke rate moves beyond the scope of this chapter. My intention is to drive home the relationship of bracing, torque, and movement transferability as it relates to functional movements.

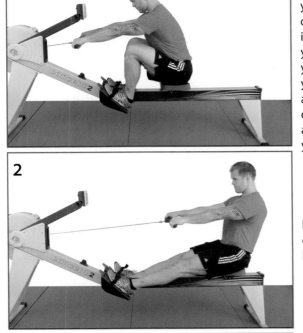

Setting up: First, adjust the footboards so that the straps wrap around the base of your toes. Second, tighten the straps around your feet, grab the oar handle with both of your hands, straighten out your legs and slide your seat back on the monorail. (Note: The idea is to take some of the compression forces off your pelvis so that you can flatten your back.) With your legs straight, sit tall, flatten your back, and then pull your shoulder blades together and screw your hands into the handle. To maximize torque, hook your thumbs around the handle. Keeping your back flat, head neutral, and shoulders back, drive your knees out and slide your hips and seat forward, allowing your torso to deviate forward slightly. As with the deadlift, you want your shins vertical, shoulders back, and hips loaded.

Keeping your arms straight while still creating torque off the handle, extend your knees, lean back slightly, and drive your hips back. To help maintain a neutral head position, focus your gaze on the chain.

As you extend your knees, pull the oar handle to your sternum. If you examine the photo, you'll notice that my forearms are nearly horizontal and my shoulders are pulled back. If you were to flip the photo 90-degrees in a counterclockwise direction, it would look a lot like the bottom of the dip. Much of the same rules apply. You want to keep your shoulders back, head neutral, and wrists aligned with your elbows.

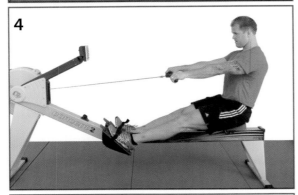

After a momentary pause, straighten your arms. Although this is technically referred to as the recovery phase, you still want to create torque off the handle and keep your shoulder blades pulled back.

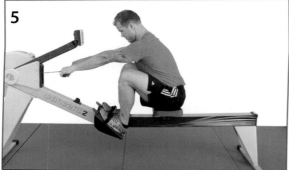

As your hands track over your knees, drive your knees out, hinge forward at your hips, allowing your torso to tilt forward, and slide your hips toward your heels. You should arrive in the same position that you started.

Head, Spine, and Shoulder Fault

Once you surrender head position, your back will round and your shoulders will go soft. If that happens, force transmits to your back instead of your hips and your shoulders internally rotate, affecting the power of your pull. Other factors that can contribute to this fault include missing shoulder range-of-motion and a tight thoracic spine.

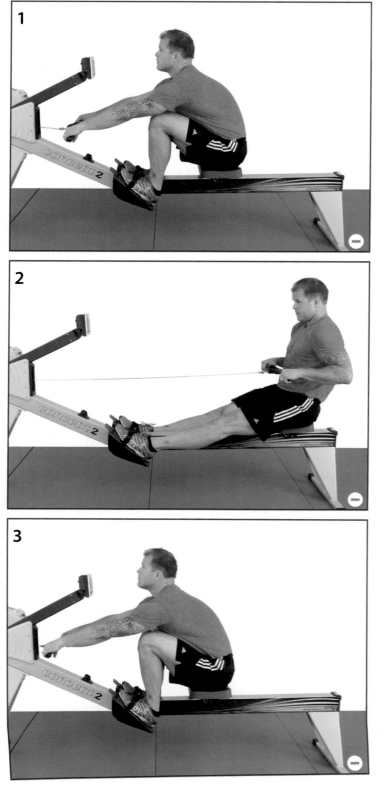

Motor-Control Fix:

▶ Pull your shoulder blades together and screw your hands into the oar handle to generate torque.

▶ To maintain a neutral head position, focus your gaze on the chain.

▶ Keep your back as flat as possible and your shins vertical.

Mobilization Target Areas:

▶ Anterior Shoulders and Chest

▶ Posterior Shoulders and Lats

▶ Thoracic Spine

Sequencing Faults

The start position and initial pull phase of the row is similar to the deadlift in that you simultaneously extend your knees and hips. However, due to the speed and timing element of rowing, a lot of athletes struggle with this sequence. Rather than move their body as a single unit, they will either drive their hips back, leaving their torso forward, and pull with their back, or they will lean back, leaving their knees bent, and pull with their arms.

This also happens during the recovery phase—when they return the oar handle to the start position—but in the opposite order. They will leave their hips back and lean their chest forward, or they will bend their knees before they straighten their arms, forcing them to move the oar handle over their legs. Regardless of the order or phase at which these faults occur, it disrupts rhythm, compromises force, and can cause a ton of problems up and down the athletic chain.

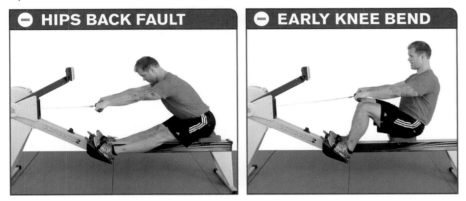

⊖ HIPS BACK FAULT **⊖ EARLY KNEE BEND**

Motor-Control Fix:
▶ Move your body as a single unit and focus on extending your knees and hips at the same time.

KIPPING PULL-UP

The kipping pull-up is a gymnastic-based technique that combines a back and forth horizontal swing with a pull. This swing is powered by a leg kick and hip drive. The idea is to harness momentum along a horizontal plane to make raising your chin over the bar easier to do. A lot of strength-and-conditioning pundits criticize the kipping pull-up as being unsafe. And they're right, but only if it's done incorrectly. The simple fact is kipping pull-ups allow you to execute more repetitions in a shorter span of time, but if performed improperly they will wreak havoc on your shoulders, elbows, and lower back.

So how do you kip without inviting injury?

First, you need to have full range-of-motion in your shoulders, meaning that you can hang from the bar with your elbows straight, armpits forward, and spine braced in a neutral position.

Second, you need to start with the strict pull-up and address the basics before you start spastically swinging from the bar. Once you have a fundamental understanding of how to form your grip and organize your body in a good position, you can start to layer the kip not only as an exercise, but also as a way of assessing shoulder mobility and motor-control. Say you see an athlete's elbows bend and shoulders roll forward while swinging from the bar. That's a good sign that he a) doesn't understand how to set up and swing, or b) he's missing end-range shoulder flexion, internal rotation, or thoracic extension.

Another reason why the kip is such a useful movement is that it fits into our model of movement transfer exercises. If you glance at the photos, you'll notice that the back swing exaggerates a movement pattern that is expressed in a lot of sport activities, specifically throwing motions. For example, a tennis player's serve, a volleyball player's spike, and a baseball player's pitch all mirror the action of a kipping pull-up. In addition, the dynamic opening and closing of the hips used in the kip is similar to Olympic lifting techniques, like the clean and snatch. The hip action of the kip is also a building block to other gymnastic movements like the muscle-up.

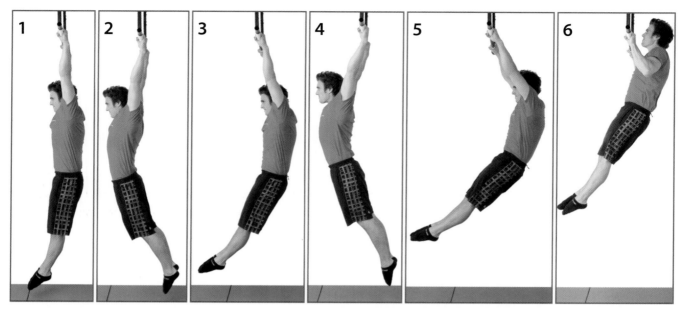

1. Jump up to the bar and establish a pull-up hook grip (see the strict pull-up). With your elbows straight and your armpits forward, squeeze your glutes, pull your ribcage down, and get your belly tight. Position your legs together and point your toes.

2. Keeping your butt squeezed, armpits forward, and legs together, kick your legs back and pull your head and chest underneath the bar. Note: Squeezing your glutes prevents you from overextending your lower back. If you examine the photo, you'll notice that Carl is in a globally arched position. Although his back is in extension, his spine is protected and he's not in a compromised position.

3. With your armpits forward and your elbows locked out, swing your legs forward and push away from the bar.

4. Pull your hips back and push your shoulders forward.

5. Still squeezing your glutes and keeping your belly tight, swing your feet forward and push your body away from the bar.

6. As you swing back, pull your chin over the bar—keeping your elbows in tight and your spine neutral. Again, the idea is to harness the energy of your back swing to help raise your chin over the bar. To seamlessly transition back into your next rep, push yourself away from the bar and then as you extend your arms, pull yourself under the bar as demonstrated in steps 2 and 4. As with all category 1 and category 2 movements, the way down should look exactly like the way up.

SNATCH BALANCE PROGRESSION

The snatch balance is an Olympic lifting exercise that isolates the catch phase of the snatch. Specifically, it's a movement that requires you to transition from the top position of the back squat with your snatch grip and quickly drop underneath the bar into the full overhead squat position. The purpose of this exercise is to get athletes comfortable receiving weight in the bottom of the overhead squat, which is the most challenging and intimidating phase of the snatch. You have to simultaneously organize your hips and shoulders into a good position while maintaining a rigid spine and upright torso.

It's important to note that there are three versions of the snatch balance technique, the first of which falls into a different category within the movement hierarchy. Because these techniques follow a specific progression and are typically layered as such, I thought it best to present all three in sequential order. By lumping these movements together, I hope to illustrate the small differences between each variation, as well as illuminate why going from a category 1 movement (pressing snatch balance) to a category 2 movement (heaving snatch balance, and snatch balance) is so difficult.

Note: The snatch balance progression can be done using a PVC pipe. This makes it applicable to athletes of all ages and ability levels. If you're interested in seeing the common faults associated with the snatch balance, revisit the overhead squat, on page 111.

Pressing Snatch Balance

The first progression in this series is the pressing snatch balance. To correctly execute this technique, assume your overhead squat stance, and without moving the bar, press yourself into the bottom of the overhead squat. As you can see from the photos, Diane does not press the bar over her head. Rather, she presses her body underneath the bar. This is without question the most difficult category 1 movement because it synchronizes two techniques, the press and the overhead squat.

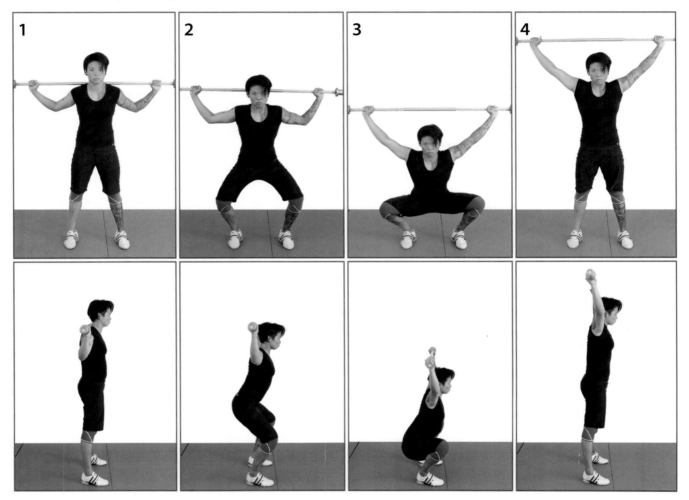

1. If you're using a barbell, assume your snatch grip and take the bar out of the rack just as you would when performing a back squat.

2. Here you do several things at once. With your torso upright and spine neutral, sit your hamstrings back and sink your hips between your feet. At the same time, apply just enough upward force to the bar so that it stays in the exact same position. To help with this step, imagine pressing yourself underneath the bar, as if it were an unmovable object.

3. Keeping the bar in the same position, press yourself down into the bottom position. Your elbows should lockout overhead as your hips drop below knee level. The key is to maintain torque in your hips and shoulders by shoving your knees out, pulling your shoulder blades back, and positioning your armpits forward.

4. Overhead squat the weight into the standing position.

Heaving Snatch Balance

The heaving snatch balance is similar to the pressing snatch balance, in that you drop underneath the bar into an overhead squat without changing your stance (foot position). But instead of pressing yourself underneath the bar from a dead-start, you add a dip and a drive, the exact same technique used when performing a push-press or push-jerk. The idea is this: Harness the energy from your hips to bump the weight off of your back, and then drop underneath the bar into a full squat with your arms locked out. Your focus here is speed, unlike the pressing snatch balance, which you perform slowly.

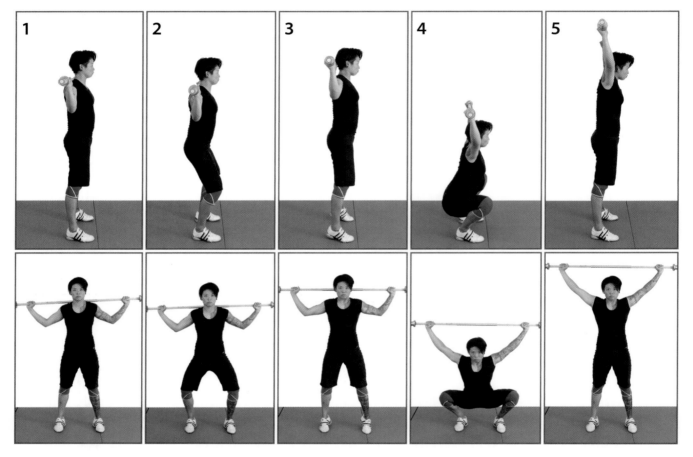

1. If you're setting up for the snatch using a barbell, establish your snatch grip and then take the bar out of the rack just as you would when performing a back squat (see page 96).

2. Driving your knees out and keeping your torso as vertical as possible, sit your hips between your feet.

3. In one explosive motion, simultaneously extend your knees and hips. The idea is to harness the energy generated from your dip and drive to accelerate the weight off of your upper back, just enough to drop underneath the bar.

4. As the bar travels upward, drop into the overhead squat position. The goal is to arrive in the bottom position with your knees out, elbows straight, and armpits forward.

5. Overhead squat the weight into the standing position.

Snatch Balance

The snatch balance adds one more piece to the previous two variations. Unlike the pressing and heaving snatch balance iterations, which start and end in an overhead squat stance, the snatch balance requires that you change the positioning of your feet as you drop underneath the weight. So instead of remaining in your overhead squat stance, you assume your pulling stance (deadlift, clean, and snatch stance). Another way to think of it is that you start in your jumping stance (deadlift) and finish in your landing stance (squat). This uncovers another set of faults because you will notice that people will default into an open foot position as they drop into the full squat to compensate for their lack of mobility or their inability to create spontaneous torque. Put simply, it's a quick and dirty way to highlight an athlete's range-of-motion and understanding of torque and bracing.

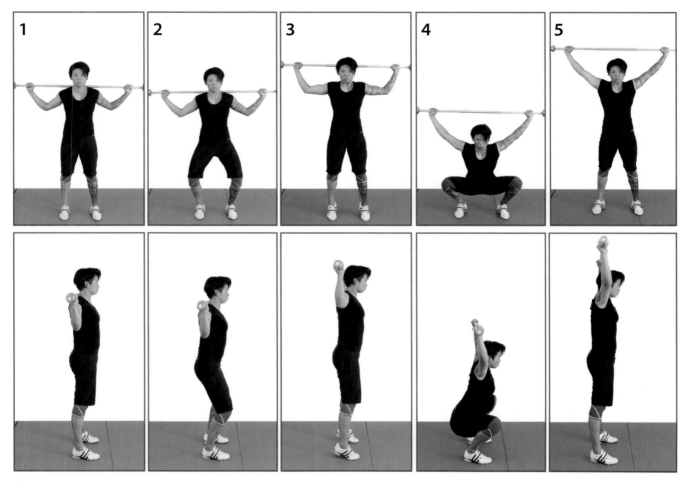

1. Secure your snatch grip on the bar and position it on your upper back as if you were performing a back squat. Then, position your feet in your pulling (snatch, clean, deadlift) stance.

2. Keeping your torso as vertical as possible, drive your knees out and lower your hips between your feet.

3. Extend your knees and hips simultaneously as if you were performing a vertical jump. The idea is to transmit power from your hips to your shoulders and bump the bar off the back of your shoulders.

4. Here you do several things at once. As the bar accelerates upward, drop into the bottom of the overhead squat, pressing your body underneath the bar. At the same time, slide your feet out into your landing stance (squat stance), immediately screwing your feet into the ground, and receive the bar overhead with your arms locked out. Keep your feet straight, your knees out, and armpits forward.

5. Stand up as if you were executing an overhead squat.

CATEGORY 3 MOVEMENTS

| Position of Transition | ▶ | remove connection | ▶ | Position of High Stability (PHS) |

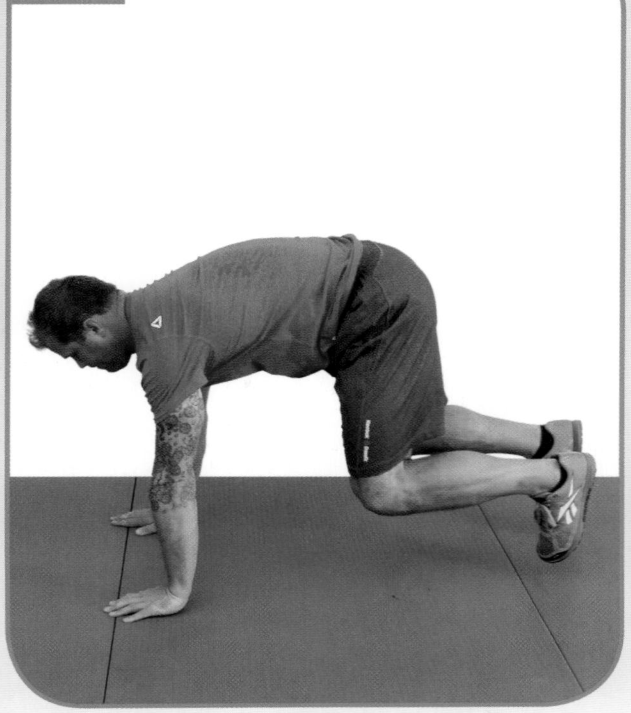

Burpee

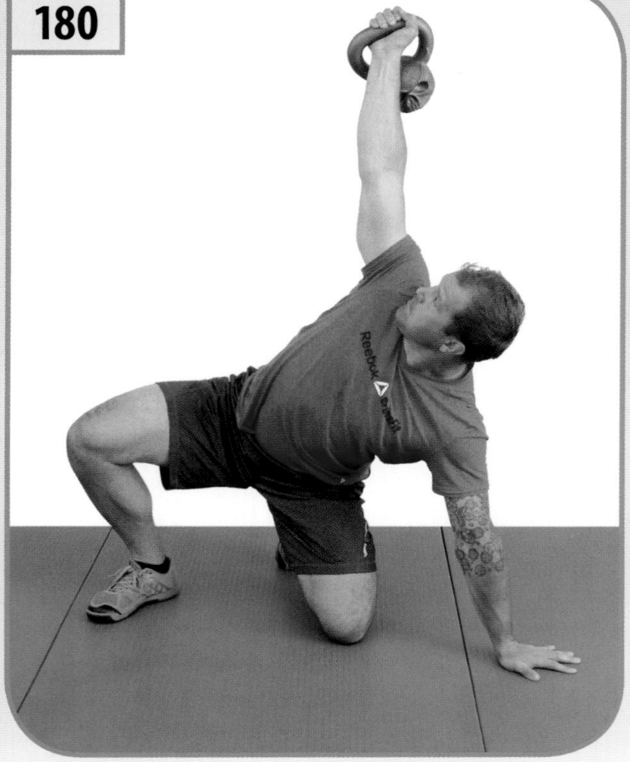

Turkish Getup

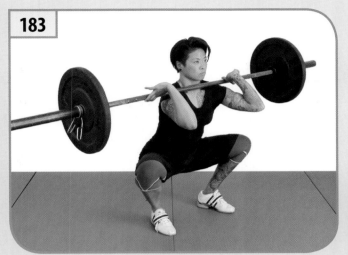

183

Clean

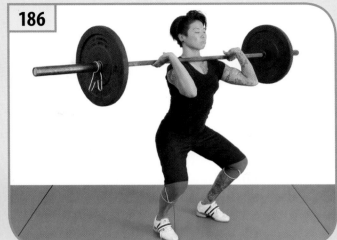

186

Power Clean

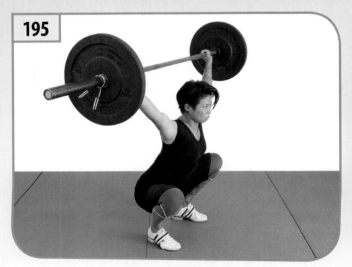

187

Hang Clean

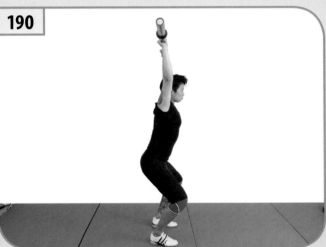

190

Push-Jerk

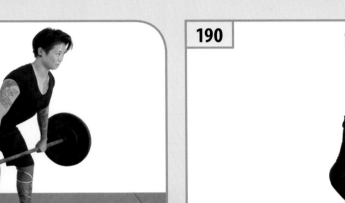

195

Snatch

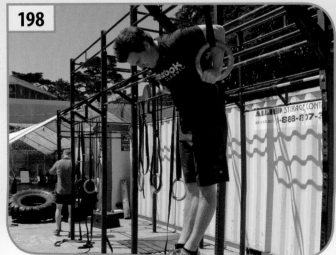

198

Muscle-Up

BURPEE

The burpee is basically a pushup, squat, and vertical jump layered into one seamless movement.

This makes it easy to identify where the problems are because you already know what the start and finish positions look like. And by now you should be able to identify the common faults. All you are doing is reconstituting the same basic positions and reinforcing the same movement patterns over and over again. The difference is you're adding transitions.

Can you drop into a dynamic plank while keeping your trunk stabilized and shoulders in a good position? Perform a pushup with forearms vertical? Transition into the bottom of the squat with straight feet, create spontaneous torque, and then jump with an upright torso?

What's interesting is people will show proficiency with the pushup, squat, and jumping and landing techniques, but the moment you ask them to spontaneously arrive in these positions, everything falls apart.

Think about it like this: You essentially enter and exit three different tunnels. If you start the pushup in a bad position, you will transition into the squat in a bad position, and then by the time you jump, you're a broken mess. The faults from each movement compound the faults of the subsequent movement. Make it a fast, high-repetition workout testing stamina and the injury risk rises as the form degrades.

You have to be able to reproduce the same stable positions with accuracy and speed in every single repetition. It's not a matter of how much work you can get done, but rather how many quality repetitions you can complete. So if the burpee is something that you do often (you should), you need to organize the workout so that you approach the exercise with care.

I'll use a CrossFit group class as an example. Say you're coaching a group of athletes through a workout that calls for 25 consecutive burpees. Rather than have them rip through 25 burpees in a row as fast as possible—which will inevitably result in some burpees that bring to mind dying animals—reconstruct the workout that awards athletes for their movement quality, not who finishes with the fastest time.

For example, pair them up into groups of two, and have one perform a set number of burpees in a row while their partner silently counts a point for every fault they commit. The goal is to get the lowest score possible. It's that simple.

By simply changing the game of the workout, you change the athlete's mindset. Now he's thinking about the quality of his movement and reproducing the same good position over and over again, which is what it's all about!

Another point worth mentioning is the universality of the burpee. Following the theme of using strength-and-conditioning movements that transfer to sport and life, the burpee is something that we tend to see a lot in martial arts and fighting sports (think of an MMA fighter or wrestler defending a takedown by sprawling his legs back and jumping back up to his fighting stance). We also see it in sports like surfing and collision sports like football.

Scaling the Burpee

Consider a soldier lying on the ground with an eighty-pound pack. What's the most efficient way to stand up? It turns out that it's not that different from a burpee. Get into the bottom of the pushup, get your forearms as vertical as possible, press up into a globally arched position, and then bring one leg up at a time and stand up. You can also lunge into the standing position. The goal is to get your foot flat on the ground, your shin vertical, and stand up with your spine in a well-organized, stable position. We use this same model in the gym for folks that can't transition from the pushup to the bottom of the squat with good form.

Think of the scaled burpee as the formal expression of getting up off the ground from your stomach.

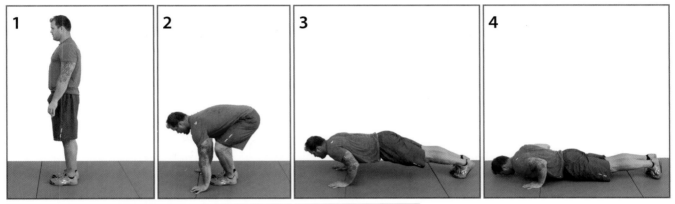

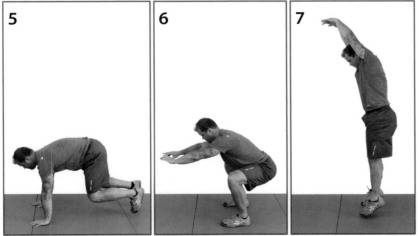

1. Start in your jumping stance and go through the bracing sequence.

2. Reach your hamstrings back, shove your knees out—keeping your shins as vertical as possible—hinge forward at the hips, and place your palms on the ground with your hands facing straight forward. The key is to keep your low back flat and sprawl or slide your feet back as your hands touch down.

3. Jump your feet back and establish the top of the pushup. Remember to screw your hands into the ground, squeeze your butt, and keep your belly tight.

4. As you lower your chest to the ground, keep your elbows in tight to your body and your shoulders aligned over your wrists.

5. In one explosive motion, extend your elbows, drive your hips up as you reach full extension, and pull your knees toward your chest.

6. As you pull your legs underneath your body, try to replace your hands with your feet. The idea is to land in the bottom of the squat with your feet straight, shins vertical, and back flat.

7. Drive out of the bottom position of the squat and perform a vertical jump. Notice that my legs are together, my shoulders are back (armpits forward), and my toes are pointed. From here, I will land in my stance and transition right back into another burpee. To see how to land, revisit the jumping and landing technique.

Burpee Fail

Because the burpee combines so many movements into one seamless, coordinated action, there are a ton of faults that occur. For example, people will bend over with a rounded back, flop on the ground in a broken mess, jump up into the dreaded dog poop position, burn their knees standing up, and then donkey kick their legs back as they jump.

It's as if you combined all the deadlift, pushup, squat, and jumping faults into one movement. Like I said before, it's a disaster. If you see anything that looks like the sequence here (and you probably will), clearly the athlete doesn't understand the concepts presented in this book. The best approach, therefore, is to isolate each movement until competency is reached.

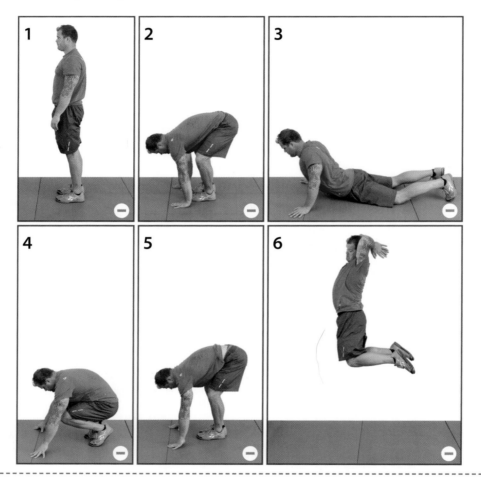

TURKISH GETUP

Martial artists—specifically Brazilian Jiu-Jitsu practitioners—refer to the Turkish getup as the "technical getup." It allows them to get up to their feet using the least amount of energy possible, while giving them options in terms of other movements they can employ.

So that's the critical everyday life application for the Turkish getup. It teaches people how to get up off the ground in the most efficient way possible. Imagine the value this has for an elderly person needing to get to his feet.

The Turkish getup is also an invaluable diagnostic tool. When I have an athlete who is rehabbing from a shoulder injury, or if I simply want to test his understanding of a stable shoulder, one of the first category 3 exercises that I will introduce is the Turkish getup. It forces him to lock his shoulder in a stable position without the benefit of generating torque off a fixed object like a barbell or the ground and to move through a full range-of-motion. And unlike other category 3 movements, it's performed slowly, making it a safe and useful tool for driving home these concepts of stability.

At any point during the movement, you can stop the athlete and make corrections to shoulder position. Not just with the arm overhead, but with the supporting arm as well. The arm holding the dumbbell is expressed with armpit forward, and the arm supporting your body is expressed with shoulder back—screwing your hand into the ground. So it's a nice two-for-one shoulder diagnostic. In addition, you can start to see how loss of shoulder position translates to other problems in the athletic chain: If their shoulder is unlocked, chances are good that you'll see their ankles collapse, knees track inward, lumbar spine overextend, etc.

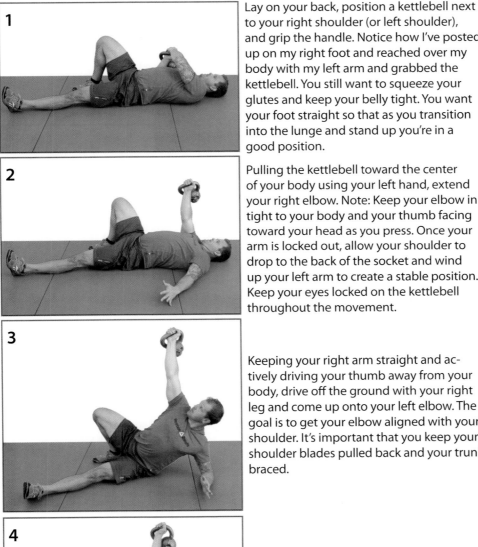

1

Lay on your back, position a kettlebell next to your right shoulder (or left shoulder), and grip the handle. Notice how I've posted up on my right foot and reached over my body with my left arm and grabbed the kettlebell. You still want to squeeze your glutes and keep your belly tight. You want your foot straight so that as you transition into the lunge and stand up you're in a good position.

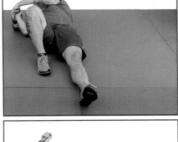

2

Pulling the kettlebell toward the center of your body using your left hand, extend your right elbow. Note: Keep your elbow in tight to your body and your thumb facing toward your head as you press. Once your arm is locked out, allow your shoulder to drop to the back of the socket and wind up your left arm to create a stable position. Keep your eyes locked on the kettlebell throughout the movement.

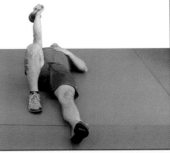

3

Keeping your right arm straight and actively driving your thumb away from your body, drive off the ground with your right leg and come up onto your left elbow. The goal is to get your elbow aligned with your shoulder. It's important that you keep your shoulder blades pulled back and your trunk braced.

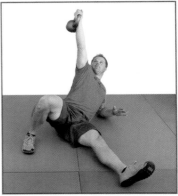

4

Sit up and plant your left hand on the ground. You want your hand aligned with your left shoulder. As you transition into the overhead position think about getting your armpit forward.

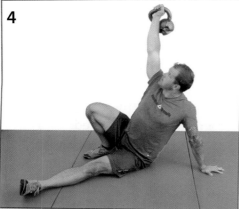

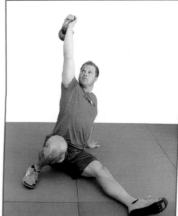

5

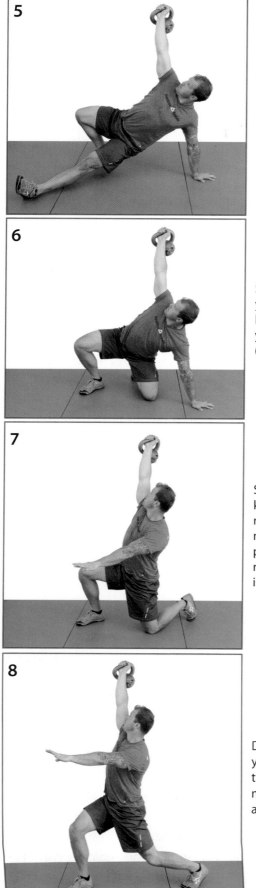

Still squeezing your glutes, push off the ground using your right foot and extend your hips.

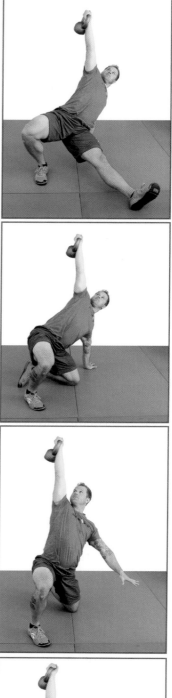

6

Supporting the weight of your body with your left arm and right leg, pull your left leg underneath your hips and the plant your knee underneath your center of mass (aligned with the kettlebell).

7

Still keeping your eyes locked on the kettlebell, shift your weight toward your right side and get your torso vertical. The moment your left hand leaves the ground, pull your shoulder back and externally rotate your arm. Make sure your left leg is internally rotated.

8

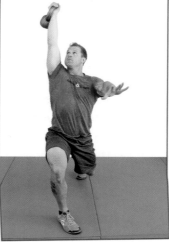

Drive your right knee out, push off of your right leg, and stand tall—keeping the weight positioned over your center of mass. Use your opposite arm for balance and maintain stability in that shoulder.

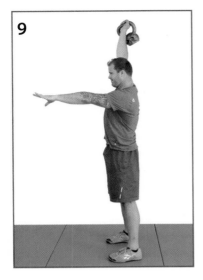

As you stand tall, step your left foot forward, squeeze your glutes, and establish the finish position.

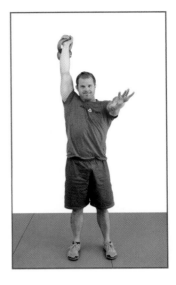

CLEAN

The clean tells you a lot about an athlete. Can he pull dynamically off the floor with speed while maintaining a neutral spine? Can he reproduce the same load-order sequence with every rep? Can he practice stabilization through the trunk, hips, and shoulders while transitioning from one position to another?

With all of this additional complexity, it's true that the possibility of making a technique error increases. But it's also an opportunity to improve performance and highlight potential weaknesses in your athletic profile. This is the mindset that you need to cultivate as you start to introduce, layer, and train category 3 movements.

It's like this: You can deadlift and front squat. That's fantastic. Now show me you can pull with speed and create torque off a fixed object while it's in motion. Show me you have the motor-control and mobility to drop into the bottom of the front squat with speed and accuracy.

If you want to pick something up off the ground and receive it onto your shoulders, you need a model for learning and teaching that skill. The clean is the formal blueprint for layering this movement pattern.

Bottom-Up Setup

Unlike setting up for the deadlift, which works from the top-down, you set up for the clean and snatch from the bottom-up. (To see the top-down setup, revisit the deadlift in the category 1 section, page 116). There are some similarities in the load-order sequence: With the back flat and shoulders pulled back, load your hips and hamstrings and use your knees to adjust for position. But instead of bending over and forming your grip with your hips and hamstrings on tension, you drop into the bottom of the squat and set up from there.

Here's why: First, the bottom-up setup is used for Olympic lifts as it allows you to optimize thoracic extension. By lowering into the bottom of the squat, you can effectively pull your shoulder blades back—using the bar as an anchor—and maximize tension in your upper back. Why is this important? Simple: You're setting yourself up to receive the load in a good front rack position.

You have to consider your finish position as you formulate your setup strategy. It's not just about entering the tunnel in a good position, but also exiting the tunnel in a good position. By setting up in the same position that you finish (bottom of the squat), you improve the stability of your receiving position.

Secondly, the bottom-up approach allows you to prioritize an upright torso position, which is critical in both the pull (lifting the weight from the ground to hip and chest level) and catching phase (dropping into the bottom of the squat while receiving the weight in the front rack).

Most importantly, the bottom-up setup also gives you a template that will yield the same reproducible results every single time you approach the movement.

Note: A lot of people don't have the mobility to implement the bottom-up setup. If that happens, the top-down approach is the best option, and still quite functional—just ask some of the best weightlifters in America. But it's less than ideal because your upper back and shoulder position aren't in the most mechanically ideal position. Figure out what's holding you back and address the issue.

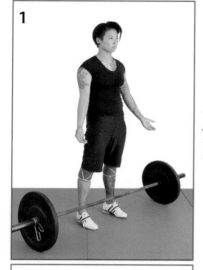

1 Assume your clean stance (same as your jumping and deadlift stance), retract your shoulders, and go through the bracing sequence.

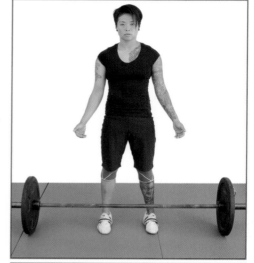

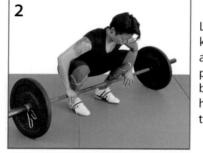

2 Lower into the bottom of the squat—keeping your back flat, shoulders upright and tight—and establish a hook grip (see page 120). Note: Your clean grip should be the same as your front rack grip. To see how to set up for the front rack, flip back to the front squat on page 106.

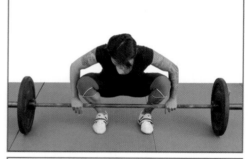

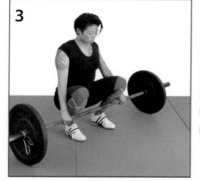

3 Driving your knees out, drop your butt, pull your torso vertical, retract your shoulders, and screw your hands into the bar. This maximizes tension in your upper back and sets your shoulders into a stable position.

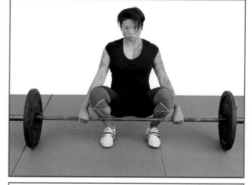

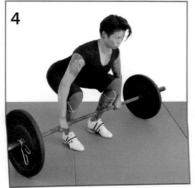

4 Still creating tension off the bar, take a breath and get your belly tight. Then, load your hips and hamstrings by raising your hips.

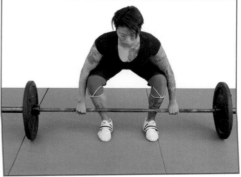

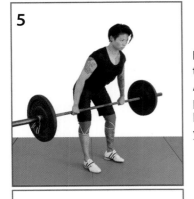

Keeping your back flat, knees out, and shoulders tight, extend your hips and knees simultaneously. Again, there should be no change in your spinal position as you pull the bar off the ground. If your butt comes up first, there's a click on the bar, or your knees come in—those are all errors.

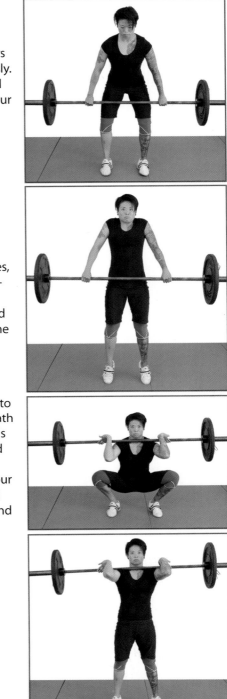

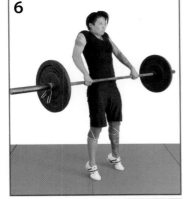

As the bar passes your knees, scoop your hips forward, keeping the bar as close to your body as possible. As you reach triple extension (ankles, knees, and hips in extension), shrug your shoulders. Notice that Diane's arms are straight and that a hundred percent of the energy generated from her legs and hips is being transferred to the bar.

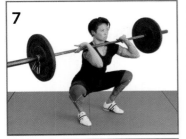

As the bar travels upward, slide your feet out into your landing stance and pull yourself underneath the weight. A common fault is to kick your heels back and stomp your feet—commonly referred to as a donkey kick. Although stomping your feet fires your posterior chain and optimizes your lading position, you want to avoid the dreaded donkey kick. The idea is to slide your feet out and screw your feet into the ground as you land.

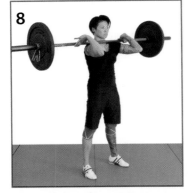

Front squat the weight up to the top position.

A Bad Mix

The top-down approach is without question the best setup for the deadlift, but it doesn't necessarily transfer as well to Olympic lifting. In fact, Glen Pendalay—world-renowned Olympic lifting coach—doesn't allow his Olympic lifters to deadlift heavy singles because he believes that the loss of upper back extension and deadlift "shoulders" wrecks their movement patterns for Olympic lifting.

Although this is a sport specific approach, it fits with our 'practice makes permanent' philosophy. If you pull from a bent over position, you have to get your torso vertical as you pull the bar past your thighs, resulting in a forward hip thrust kettlebell-like action. This transfers your hip energy forward, instead of upward. What happens is athletes either miss the lift or have to jump forward in order to receive the weight.

POWER CLEAN

If you're an NFL lineman you need to know how to go from a 4 point stance to a vertical torso with organized shoulders and ready to hit. You have to do this near light speed. Learning how to power clean helps train this motor pattern.

The power clean is a scaled down iteration of the clean. Instead of receiving the weight in the bottom of the squat, you receive the weight in a quarter squat or top position. A lot of people don't have the mobility to clean, so the power and hang variants are a great way to dial in good motor patterns.

That said, there's no excuse to avoid the full clean and snatch. If you can't drop into a clean or snatch, you need to figure out what is holding you back and address the problem.

The goal is to develop motor-control through a full range-of-motion. If you're consistently hiding the deficits of your motor-control and mobility through shortened ranges, you'll end up compensating into bad positions when you're forced into end-range positions. You end up failing at the margins of your experience. To put it simply, you need develop the motor-control at end-ranges.

Don't hide your weaknesses. Park your ego, get hungry, and go after them.

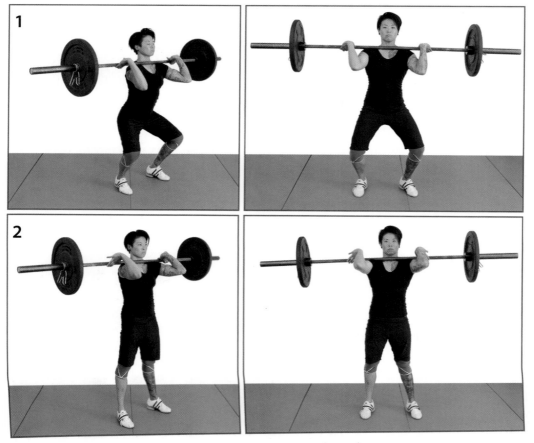

HANG CLEAN

Complex movements like the clean and snatch must be layered accordingly. If you plan on taking the Olympic lifts seriously, you need to isolate and practice each phase of the lift. For example, the hang variants—starting from the standing position—allow you to focus on the second phase of the pull (triple extension), the catch phase of the lift (front rack), and the landing.

This is great for a few reasons: 1) By breaking the movement down to a defined phase you shorten the learning curve; 2) it allows you to highlight areas that are giving you trouble; and 3) you can get around mobility issues (can't set up or receive weight in the bottom position) while still working on other aspects of the movement.

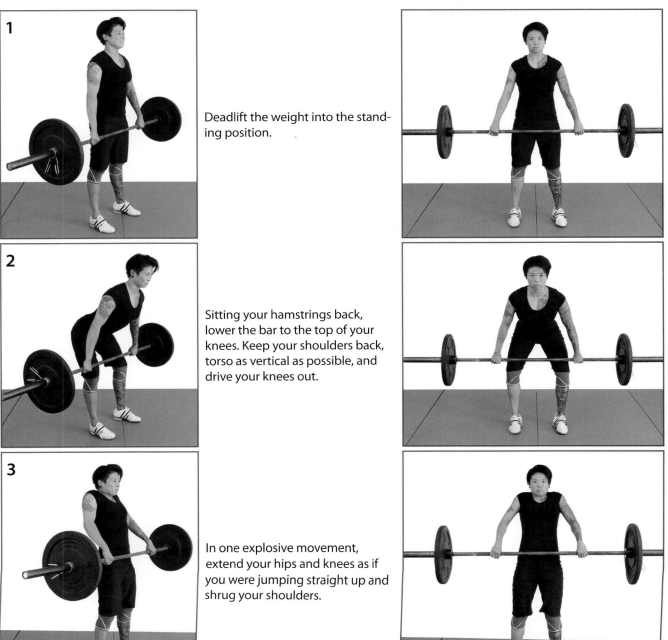

1 Deadlift the weight into the standing position.

2 Sitting your hamstrings back, lower the bar to the top of your knees. Keep your shoulders back, torso as vertical as possible, and drive your knees out.

3 In one explosive movement, extend your hips and knees as if you were jumping straight up and shrug your shoulders.

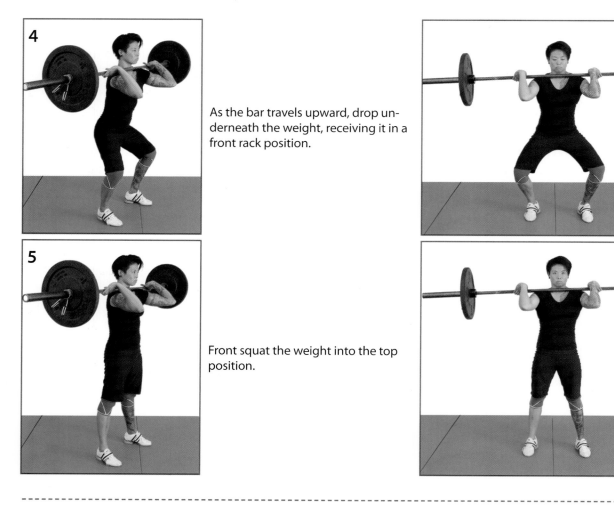

As the bar travels upward, drop underneath the weight, receiving it in a front rack position.

Front squat the weight into the top position.

Tension-Hunting Fault

If you fail to shove your knees out or you're missing flexion and external rotation range-of-motion, your butt will shoot up as you initiate the pull, causing an overextension spinal fault. This is your body's way of putting tension in the system. Take up the slack by driving your knees out in the bottom.

Motor-Control Fix:
▶ Drive your knees out in the bottom position and load your hips and hamstrings before you initiate the pull.

Mobilization Target Areas:
▶ Anterior Hips and Quads
▶ Posterior High Chain (Glutes)
▶ Posterior Low Chain (Hamstrings)
▶ Calf and Heel Cord

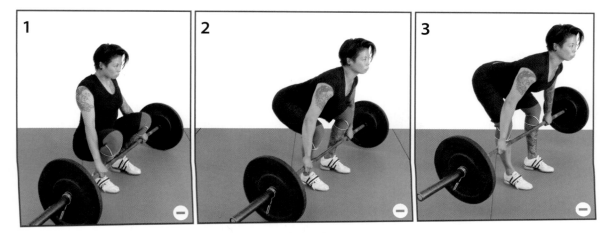

Early Pull Fault

Once the bar moves past your knees, the goal is to get your torso as vertical as possible so that you can open your hips into full extension. This is what allows you to transmit upward energy from your hips to the bar. If you're bent over (implemented the top-down setup) or you're missing extension ranges of motion in your anterior chain (hip flexors, quads), reaching full hip extension is difficult. What happens? You end up pulling with your arms instead of harnessing the power of your hips.

To correct this fault, implement the hang clean variant—deadlift the weight to the standing position, lower to your thigh, and then pull—or just work on extending your hips without transitioning into the receiving position (clean pull). If it's tight hips or quads that are holding you back, pony up and get to work on those stiffened tissue.

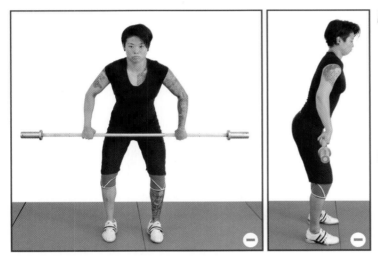

Motor-Control Fix:
▶ Isolate the phase of the pull that is giving you the most trouble by implementing a clean pull or hang clean variant.

▶ Think about getting your elbows high after locking out your hips and shrugging your shoulders.

Mobilization Target Areas:
▶ Anterior Hips and Quads

Next Rep Transition

If you're stringing together multiple repetitions, you need to be conscious of your shoulder position as you lower the weight to the ground. Think about keeping your shoulders back, screwing your hands into the bar, and lowering into your start position. This will allow you to seamlessly transition into your next rep without defaulting into a poor position.

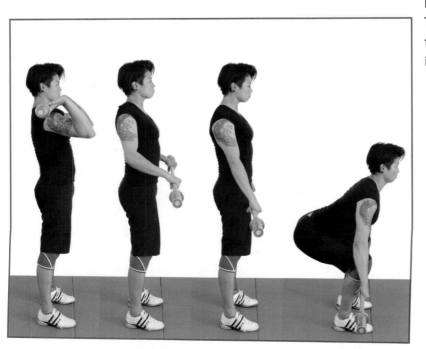

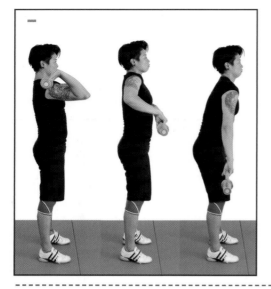

Soft Shoulders Fault

A lot of people mistakenly unlock their shoulders as they lower the bar to the ground. As you can see from the photos, this compromises the integrity of your spine and puts your shoulders in a bad position.

Motor-Control Fix:

▶ Keep your shoulders back and screw your hands into the bar as you lower it to your thighs.

▶ Think about keeping your back flat and driving your knees out as if you were initiating a hang clean.

JERK

We have a saying around our gym: Your shoulders are abnormal unless you can jerk.

While it's important to learn the basic, stable overhead positions, it's not enough to say you have full range-of-motion overhead, or that you can press and push-press. To fully express the stability and effectiveness of your overhead position, you need to be able to lockout your arms, as well as spontaneously generate a stable shoulder position (armpits forward) with speed and accuracy. Put another way, you need to be able to jerk.

If you can do that—lengthen and stabilize both of your shoulders simultaneously—it shows that you understand the stabilization concepts repeated throughout this book and have a model that translates to dynamic overhead actions like swimming, throwing, blocking, etc. And like all category 3 movements, the jerk highlights torque dumps and force bleeds, as well as spotlights shoulder mobility issues that may go unnoticed when implementing the basic overhead pressing elements.

It's important to mention that if you're just learning how to jerk, it's helpful to get the bar from a rack. This allows you to optimize the setup and isolate the movement. (To see how to take the bar out of the rack, check out the front squat on page 107.) However, if you plan on Olympic weightlifting, you have to learn how to transition from a clean to a jerk. To accomplish this, reset your feet back into your pulling stance and adjust your front rack position by lowering your elbows. You want your elbows to be at about a 45-degree angle (about halfway between a front squat rack position and a strict-press rack position).

As with the push-press, you use a dip and drive (bend and extend your knees) to accelerate the weight upward. But instead of staying in your jumping stance, you drop underneath the weight, catching it in either a squat (landing) or split squat position. Regardless of the variation you implement, the goal is to receive the weight in a strong, stable position at the apex bar height. For the average athlete, pausing for a second in the lockout position is a valuable stimulus and allows the coach to evaluate the quality of their position.

Push-Jerk

The push-jerk variation allows you to evaluate vertical jumping and landing mechanics with a dynamic overhead stimulus. The key to correctly performing the push-jerk is to keep your torso upright, drive your knees out as you dip and catch, and position your feet straight as you go from a jumping to a landing stance. The faults to look out for include lumbar spine overextension, knees forward, bent elbow and internally rotated shoulder, and the dreaded donkey kick.

Note: The push-jerk is often implemented in low-weight, high-repetition workouts because it allows for a quick recovery and setup. For most people, the split-jerk allows them to press more weight.

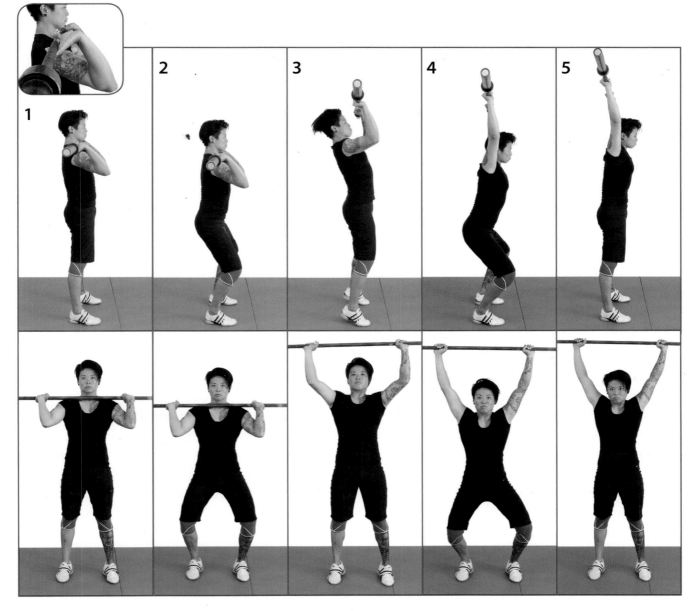

1. Whether you take the bar out of the rack or clean the weight to your shoulders, the setup is the same: Butt is squeezed, belly is tight, feet are straight, and shoulders are back. If you glance at the photo, you'll notice that Diane is in her pulling stance or jumping stance and has the bar balanced on her fingertips and deltoids. Her elbows are halfway between a strict-press and front rack position, about a 45-degree angle. Note: Your jerk grip width should be close to your front squat rack position.

2. Keeping your torso as upright as possible, sit your hamstrings back slightly, drive your knees out, and lower your hips between your feet. The dip should look no different than the first 6-inches of a front squat.

3. In one explosive motion, simultaneously extend your knees and hips into triple extension. As the barbell jumps off your shoulders, pull your head back slightly, just far enough to clear your face and maintain a vertical bar path.

4. As the bar accelerates upward, slide your feet out into your landing stance—screwing your feet into the ground and shoving your knees out—and press yourself under the bar. Catch the weight with your elbows straight, shoulders back, and armpits forward.

5. Overhead squat the weight into the top position.

Split-Jerk

It's a lot easier to maintain an upright torso and stabilize your shoulders in the split stance. This is why you can likely move more weight with the split variation of the jerk. (Unless you happen to be a very competent Chinese Olympic lifter.)

That's wonderful, but the real magic with the split-jerk is that it gives you a model for creating a stable hip position when one leg is in extension—behind you—and the other leg is in flexion. Which is what it looks like when you cut, run, or lunge.

There are a few key points to keep in mind when performing the split-jerk. The first is to create a stable foot position. To accomplish this, land with both of your feet slightly internally rotated—meaning you turn your front foot toward the inside of your body with your weight centered just in front of your ankle, and internally rotate your rear leg with your weight centered over the ball of your foot. The front-foot position allows you to create external rotation without your knee tracking too far out and the rear foot puts your hip into a stable position, allowing you to support an upright torso with a neutral pelvis position.

Second, always draw your feet together at the finish of the lift by moving your front leg first. Don't rush this. Slide your lead foot back and then step your rear foot into a squat stance. Master the habit of this sequence in the same way you walk out the bar when performing a squat.

Third, unless you're a competitive Olympic weightlifter, alternate your stance. Become a switch-hitter of sorts. Sometimes jerk with your left leg forward and other times jerk with your right leg forward. You will have a side that is stronger than the other, which is natural. But just as a good fighter practices from both a southpaw and orthodox stance and a good skateboarder will switch from standard to goofy, a well-rounded athlete should practice jerking from both stances.

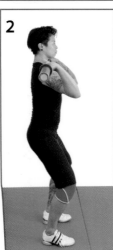
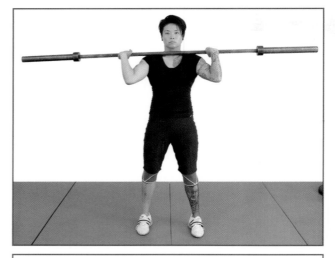

1

Assume the jerk front rack position. To see how to take the bar out of the rack, flip back to the front squat on page 106. To transition into the jerk from the clean, adjust your feet into your pulling stance and lower you elbows into the jerk front rack position.

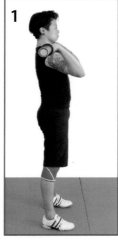
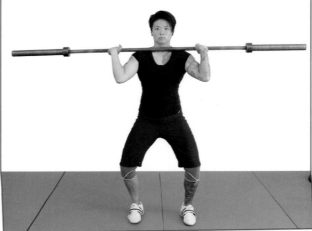

2

Drive your knees out, sit your hamstrings back slightly, and lower your hips between your feet. Keep your shoulders back, back flat, and torso as vertical as possible.

3

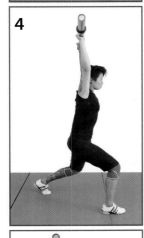

Here you do several things at once. Jump the weight off your chest by extending your knees and hips simultaneously. As you do this, pull your head back slightly to clear your face from the vertical bar path, slide one foot straight back, and slide your opposite foot forward.

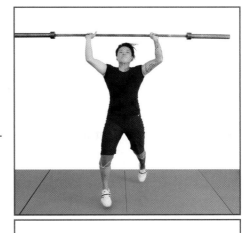

4

Push your head through your arms (not too far) as the bar passes your face, lockout your elbows, and get your armpits forward, catching the bar at its apex height. Notice that Diane is on the ball of her rear foot and her leg is slightly internally rotated. Her lead foot is turned slightly in and her shin is vertical. Both legs have roughly a 45-degree bend. This is the most stable position for your ankles, knees, and hips. The key is to think about driving your lead knee out, your rear knee in—squeezing your rear glute—while keeping your hips square.

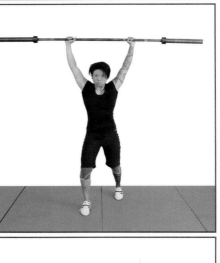

5

Keeping your belly tight, armpits forward, and elbows locked out, slide your lead foot back.

6

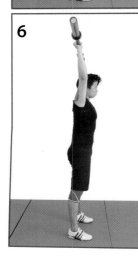

Step your left foot into your start position stance.

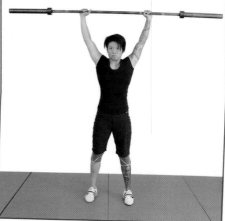

Open Foot Fault

A lot of athletes, especially novices, will turn their back leg out as they drop into the lunge position. This is a huge blow to force production and, as you can see from the photos, puts your back leg into an awful position. Like all movements, start out using a PVC pipe or light weight and drill in the proper mechanics. If you can't get into a good position because you're missing internal rotation of the hip, you know what to do: Flip to the mobility section devoted to hip internal rotation and get to work.

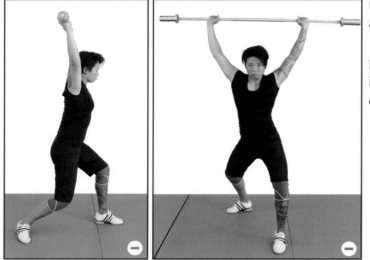

Note: You see this same open foot movement pattern in running. The mobility prescription is the same: Start at the hip and work your way down from there.

Motor-Control Fix:

▶ Focus on internally rotating your back leg with a slight knee bend.

Mobilization Target Areas:

▶ Posterior High Chain (Glute)

▶ Anterior Hip/Quad

▶ Posterior Low Chain (Hamstring)

Knee Fault

Dropping into a lunge position, especially when you're first learning how to jerk, feels unstable to a lot of people. To avoid dropping to depth, athletes will often keep their back leg straight and overextend to keep their torso vertical. As with most motor-control faults, you need to take a step back and drill the movement using a PVC pipe, bar, or bar with a light amount of weight. It's that simple. If, while working on your technique, you realize that the position is unattainable due to limited mobility, figure out what's holding you back and fix the problem. For this particular fault, tight anterior structures surrounding the hip are usually to blame.

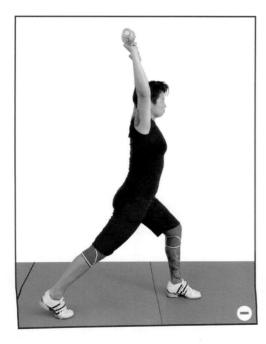

Motor-Control Fix:

▶ Think about bending your right knee and turning it toward the inside of your body. Remember, you want about a 45-degree bend in your legs.

Mobilization Target Areas:

▶ Anterior Hips/Quad

▶ Trunk

SNATCH

Nothing will tell you more about an athlete's range-of-motion and understanding of the midline stabilization and torque principles than the snatch. It's the ultimate assessment tool for the coach and consequently the most challenging category 3 movement for the athlete.

The snatch shares the same setup (bottom-up setup) as the clean, but with a higher degree of motor-control and mobility. You have to pull with a wider grip and receive the weight in an overhead position. In other words, you have to get into a deeper squat and create torque off a wider grip, adding another level of difficulty—screwing your hands into the bar with a hook grip and maintaining that external rotation force as you go from a pull to a stable overhead position is extremely difficult.

This is why so many people struggle to stabilize their shoulders in a good position, keep their torso vertical, and their spine rigid. If you make the slightest error or if you are missing the smallest corner in your mobility, everything falls apart.

Note: What I suggest for the proper width of the snatch grip is this rather critical notion: Grip it so that if things get sketchy you can dump the barbell behind your back and avoid the weights smashing into your skull. Shoulder flexibility is typically an issue when it comes to the snatch grip and ideally you can work with your coach on figuring out what's best and what's safest.

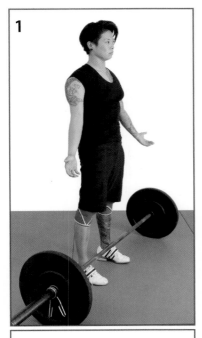

1 Assume your snatch stance (same as your jumping and deadlift stance), pull your shoulders back (with external rotation), and go through bracing sequence.

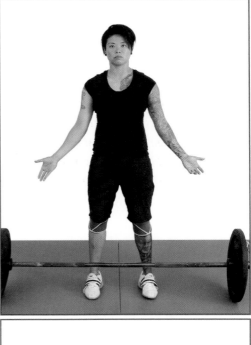

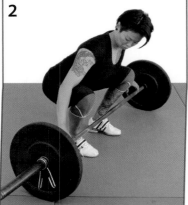

2 Lower into the bottom of the squat—keeping your back flat, shoulders upright and tight, and knees out—and establish a hook grip (see page 120).

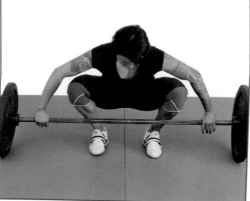

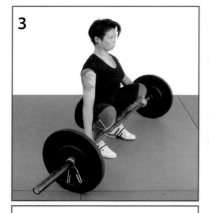

3

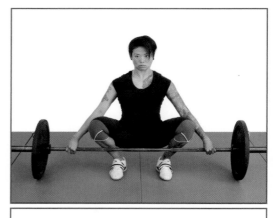

To maximize tension in your upper back and get your torso vertical, screw your hands into the bar—creating an external rotation force—pull your shoulders back, and sit your butt to your heels.

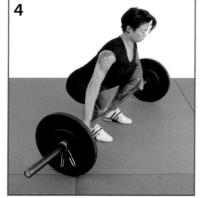

4

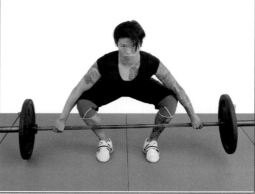

Load your hips and hamstrings by elevating your hips. As you do this, be sure to keep your back flat, shoulders retracted, shins vertical, and knees out. Remember: Take all the slack out of the system before you pull.

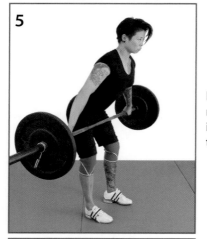

5

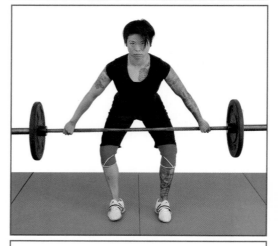

Extend your hip and knees simultaneously. There should be no change in your spinal position as you pull the bar off the ground.

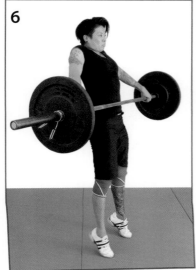

6

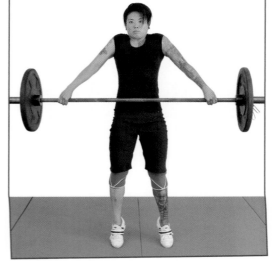

As the bar passes your knees, scoop your hips forward, keeping the bar as close to your body as possible. As you reach triple extension, shrug your shoulders. Notice that Diane's arms are straight and that a hundred percent of the upward energy generated from her legs and hips is being transferred to the bar.

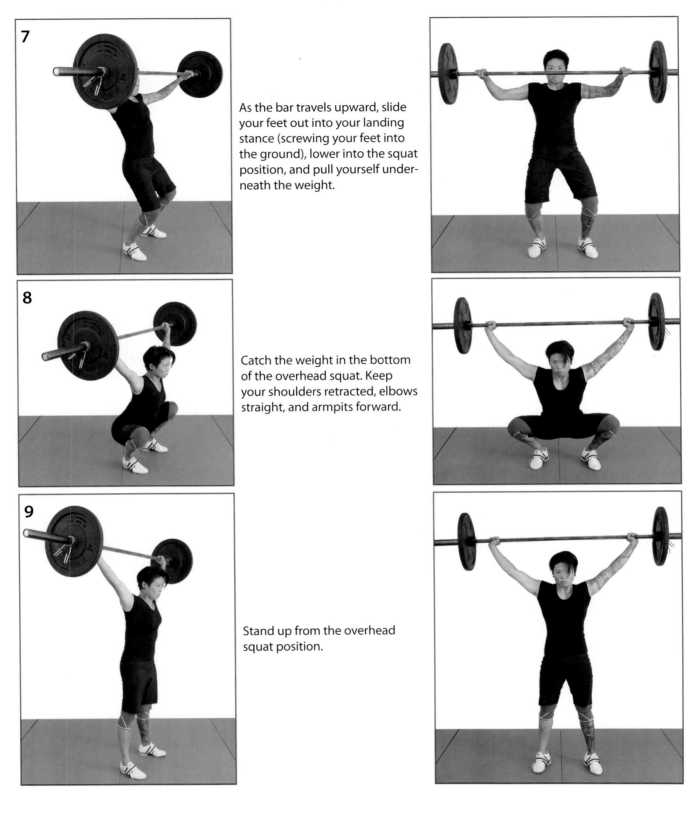

7

As the bar travels upward, slide your feet out into your landing stance (screwing your feet into the ground), lower into the squat position, and pull yourself underneath the weight.

8

Catch the weight in the bottom of the overhead squat. Keep your shoulders retracted, elbows straight, and armpits forward.

9

Stand up from the overhead squat position.

MUSCLE-UP

So you can do a strict pull-up and ring dip without struggle. Most excellent. Can you combine the two movements into one seamless coordinated action? Can you do it while keeping your back flat and your shoulders organized?

The level of trunk and shoulder control required to perform a strict muscle-up is insane. Add a dynamic element like the kip, a dose of fatigue, or string together multiple reps, and the resulting movement will reveal any and all crappy motor-control habits.

By the way, the rings don't do you any favors. You have to cultivate torque and maintain stability as you go from a pull to a press, a sort of motor-control high wire act. It's the equivalent of attempting a snatch while balancing on a pair of rotating, shaking plates. The point is if you don't have a model for generating torque off of an unstable object, you're going to bleed force and get sucked into injury-prone positions.

Just because you have a strict pull-up and a full-range ring dip doesn't guarantee a muscle-up. As with all category 3 movements, the challenge lies in the transition. To shorten the learning curve, we'll often have our athletes practice the transition with the rings low to the ground so that they can use their legs to support their body-weight. We'll also layer in the heaving dip balance, which requires you to remove connection with tension and drop from the top of the dip to the bottom of the dip. This teaches them how to create spontaneous torque in the bottom of the dip and prepares them for the muscle-up transition. In the meantime, we make it a mission to develop shoulder rotational range-of-motion.

Note: The kipping muscle-up is performed in much the same way as the kipping pull-up. (To see how to kip, revisit the kipping pull-up in the category 2 movement section).

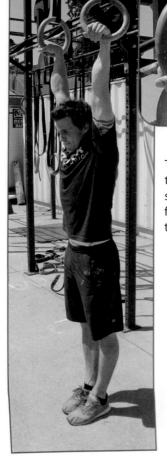

To set up for the muscle-up, establish a false grip by hooking the edge of your wrists through the rings. This grip allows for a seamless transition into the dip and puts your shoulders into a fully externally rotated position. Keep your butt squeezed, legs together, ribcage down, and belly tight.

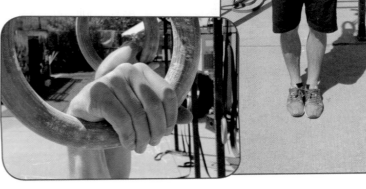

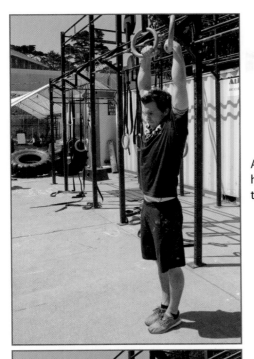

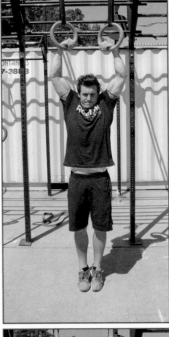

As you initiate the pull, internally rotate your hands—keeping your shoulder blades pulled together—and legs out in front of your body.

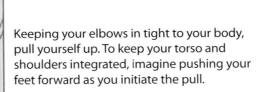

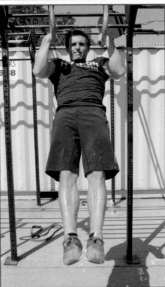

Keeping your elbows in tight to your body, pull yourself up. To keep your torso and shoulders integrated, imagine pushing your feet forward as you initiate the pull.

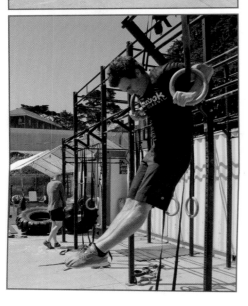

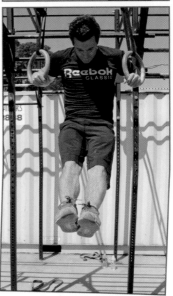

As you pull your chest to the rings, punch your torso forward. Again, think about keeping your toes pointed, legs together, and feet positioned out in front of your body.

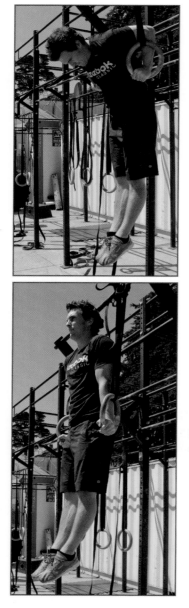

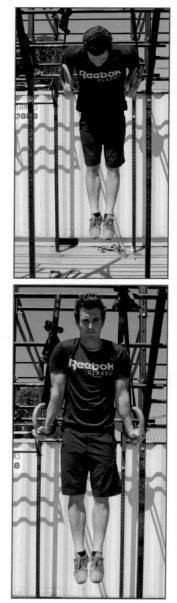

The moment you arrive in the bottom of the dip, actively spin your thumbs toward the outside of your body to create torque in the shoulders.

Still turning your hands out, extend your elbows and establish the top of the dip position.

CHAPTER 6
THE TUNNEL

In the book *The Score Takes Care of Itself: My Philosophy of Leadership*, legendary San Francisco 49ers football coach Bill Walsh described the work ethic and relentless precision of Hall of Fame quarterback Joe Montana. In the months before training camp, Montana could be seen practicing basic drop-back patterns that would "bore a high school football player" to death. He did this day after day, hour after hour, over and over again. He began each drill by paying great attention to his starting position. Then he'd work on mastering each and every crisp, measured step of the pattern, never allowing himself to slide into a compromised stance or take shortcuts. Montana disciplined himself because he knew the importance of each *fraction* of each piece of footwork—from the very beginning of the sequence to the follow-through of a throw—to the success of a play.

Montana employed a conceptual tool I like to refer to as the *tunnel*. Having a tunnel mindset means understanding that you have to start a movement (enter the tunnel) in a good position to finish (exit the tunnel) in a good position. If you don't start right, you won't finish right—end of story.

The tunnel metaphor helps coaches and athletes identify, diagnose, and correct movement and mobility problems. It brings consciousness, intention, and purpose to the principles of movement.

Military trainers use it routinely, even if they don't call it that. For example, recruits are often told, "Pay attention to detail," a mandate they are expected to obey in every phase of every drill. A successful drill must begin with a perfectly executed start. If it doesn't, the soldier earns a "no go" and starts the drill over, preceded perhaps by a set of penalty pushups or a few runs up and down a mud hill. Military trainers know that ingraining this acute focus during basic training can mean the difference between life and death when that soldier is in the heat of battle.

This focus is also at the heart of the tunnel approach. Here's why: Once an athlete is under a load, or has to bring speed or tension to the equation, it's very difficult for him to organize himself into a good position. Let's say, for example, that the athlete loads a barbell onto his shoulders to perform a back squat, but fails to brace his spine in a neutral position before taking the weight out of the rack. With the weight compressing his spine, it's nearly impossible for him to organize his trunk in a braced-neutral position. Similarly, if an athlete with limited range-of-motion or poor motor-control has to compensate during a setup to a lift or mid-movement, his lift is compromised. In short, you can't turn a bad position into a good position once you're in motion. Think about it like this: If Joe Montana began a play with an inefficient stance, he wouldn't be able to execute a perfect drop.

Here's the other takeaway: If a coach notices the error when an athlete is midway through a movement and cues the athlete to fix his position, the athlete is helpless to comply. He may be able to salvage the lift or complete the task, but he'll struggle to assume the safest and most effective stance. Take an athlete whose elbows drop during a heavy front squat or full clean. Telling him to get his "elbows up" is useless. His elbows will remain dropped until he stands up with the weight. Similarly, if an athlete's knees track inward during a heavy squat, you can shout *Knees out* until you're blue in the face, but it's not going to have any impact. By the same token, if someone starts rounding his or her back during a heavy deadlift, it doesn't matter how loud you scream *Flat back!* That back is going to stay rounded for the duration of the lift.

This is why it's so important to prioritize your setup before you start moving. The position in which you enter the tunnel (start a movement) dictates how you will exit the tunnel (finish a movement). If you take the time to get yourself organized—brace your spine in a neutral position, hinge from the hips and shoulders, and maximize torque—chances are good that you will enter and exit the tunnel in a good position. But if you enter the tunnel in a bad position, you have only two options: continue moving in a compromised way or restart in a good position.

Identifying the Problem

The tunnel concept also gives you a place to start your movement assessment. It forces you to go back to your start position and make sure you are setting up correctly. When I evaluate an athlete's movement, for example, I always look at his start position first because I recognize that a poor setup can contribute to finish position faults.

A while back, I worked with a champion Olympic lifter in my physical therapy practice who was having a hard time locking out his arms in the snatch. His coach implemented a slew of drills to help with his finish position, but nothing seemed to work. It turned out that he was missing shoulder internal rotation, causing his shoulders to round forward during the pull. This is why he was having such a hard time stabilizing his shoulders and locking out his arms overhead. He was entering the tunnel in a bad position, which predisposed him to a bad finish. As I've said before: Start out in a compensated position, finish compromised. I cleaned up his shoulders, restored normal range to the tissues that were restrict-

ing the joint, and all of a sudden the problem with his finish position vanished. He could have done a million drills to improve his lockout without ever getting to the root of the issue.

The point is a lot of coaches and athletes mistakenly focus on drills that will improve finish position when the real problem is the start. So when an athlete tells you he's having trouble completing a movement, immediately assess his setup and make sure he's not making a motor-control error or missing key ranges of motion. In the same sense, if you see a good setup, but your athlete is still having problems with his finish, chances are excellent that it is a mobility issue.

As you start putting together mobility prescriptions, use the tunnel mindset to help you focus your time on the areas that require the most attention. The tunnel is a tool that forces you to evaluate position from both sides of the movement. In fact, the start and the finish are the first places to start your diagnosis when you are deconstructing a movement problem. Just to be clear: "Start" and "finish" always refer respectively to the bottom or top position of a movement. I call the start position MOB 1 (mobilization 1) and the finish position MOB 2 (mobilization 2).

Let's say, for example, that an athlete loses his balance and can't maintain a good position when he performs a pistol—single-leg squat. Unless he can't fully extend his hips, you can automatically rule out the start (top) position as the limiting factor. The next step is to see if he can get into a good finish position, which is the bottom of the pistol (squat). He doesn't even have to perform the movement. He just has to squat down and extend his leg out in front of him. If he falls over or can't get into a stable, well-organized finish position, you know right away what the problem is: he's missing range-of-motion in his ankle. Now you can focus on mobilizations that target his position of restriction.

The tunnel also gives you a template for evaluating circular or repetitive movements like running and swimming. Consider a runner who is having problems with his landing—foot contacting the ground. The coach might prescribe any number of running techniques and motor-control drills to improve foot position. And these drills might work for the initial

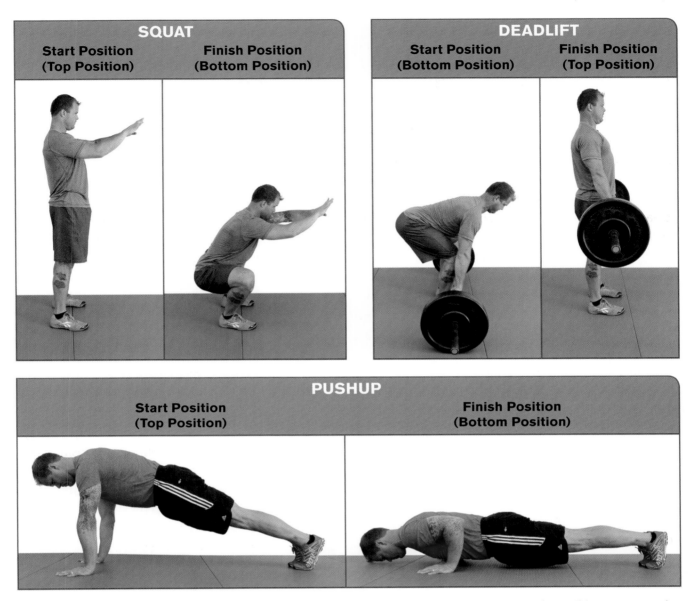

foot contact. But if that athlete is missing range-of-motion in his anterior hip, or his calf or ankle is super tight, his leg will externally rotate into an unstable position. (This is an example of the second law of torque page 54.) He may be able to keep his foot straight at the start, but as his leg swings behind him and externally rotates, he lands with an open foot. He enters a brand new tunnel from a compromised position. In this scenario, it's not a start position problem; it's a finish position problem. The finish position—leg swinging back—dictates how well an athlete will enter his next stride and enter the next tunnel of movement.

This is why when I watch people run, I not only pay attention to initial foot contact, but also to their final foot position.

The kipping pull-up is another perfect example of this. People have difficulty linking kipping pull-ups because they lack full shoulder extension and internal rotation. They will start their swing in a good position—elbows locked out, neutral spine, shoulders back—but as they raise their chin to the bar, their shoulders roll forward, their elbows flare out, and their ribcage tilts. So as they push away from the bar, their shoulders are not in a good position to receive force. Now when they swing underneath the bar, they can't effectively transition into their next rep because they are in such a wrenched position. Here's what this means for you: Your finish position on your pull-up dictates your ability to transition into your next rep, which is your new start position.

Put another way: If you exit a tunnel of movement in a bad position, you will enter the next tunnel in a compromised position.

CHAPTER 7
THE SYSTEMS

"You need to stretch!"

You've heard it a million times before. The perplexing assertion that you're not stretching enough and that it's why you're injured or sore, slow or clumsy. Think of your first coach admonishing you to stretch after practice, or your gym teacher preaching about the importance of stretching. Oh, your back hurts? No problem! Just stretch your hamstrings and it will feel better. You can't get into a good squat position because your quads are tight? Just stretch them out.

Conventional wisdom tells us that if we want to optimize athletic performance, improve flexibility, prevent muscle soreness, and reduce potential for injury, we have to stretch. For a long time, stretching has been a catchall modality for dealing with soreness and pain, for range-of-motion restrictions, and for joint troubles. Just keep stretching. But here's the problem: Stretching doesn't work by itself. It doesn't improve position, it doesn't improve performance, it doesn't make you faster, it doesn't eliminate pain, and it doesn't prevent injury. That's why when you dutifully complied with your coach's order to stretch after class, you didn't become a better athlete or all of a sudden stop getting injured.

Let me clarify: When I say, "stretching," I'm referring specifically to end-range static stretching, or hanging out in an end-range static position with zero intention. I'm talking about purposeless stretching. Consider the classic hamstring stretch: You lie on your back, grab your ankle, pull your hamstring to end-range, and then hang out while you dreamily watch the geese overhead flying south for winter. This type of "stretching" can theoretically "lengthen" your hamstring, but doesn't tell you—or your coach—anything about your motor-control or your ability to get into good positions. In other words, taking your hamstring to end-range and keeping it there is not going to help you run faster or change your capacity to deadlift more weight. Yet when most people have a tissue or joint restriction that prevents them from getting into a good position, they think, "Man, I suck! I need to stretch."

An example by way of analogy: If you pull on each end of a T-shirt, what happens after a minute or so? It becomes all stretched out, right? What do you think happens when you take your beautiful tissues to end-range and keep them there? They get all stretched out like your pitiful T-shirt. Imagine lengthening your hamstrings and then sprinting down a field or attempting a max-effort deadlift without developing the strength or motor-control to handle that new position. You might as well get down on your knees and beg to be injured. "Lengthening" your muscle is not a bad thing if you have the motor-control to support that end-range position and you are expressing those end-range positions with load-bearing, full-range exercises. This is why we deadlift, squat, and practice full-range functional movements in the gym.

The issue is not that static stretching lengthens the muscle. The issue is that it addresses (albeit poorly) only one aspect of your physiologic system—your muscle. It doesn't address motor-control, or the position of your joints, or what's going on at the joints. It doesn't address sliding-surface function—that critical interplay of how your skin, nerves, and musculature react with one another. Any of these things could look like tight musculature. And that's why "stretching it" has been the good, old-fashioned Band-Aid we have always applied. And if "stretching muscles" works so well, why do we still see as much dysfunction and pain as we do?

If stretching is not the answer, what is? In short, we need to systematically deal with each of the problems that prevent us from getting into the ideal positions and keep us from moving correctly. That's what I'm going to cover in this chapter. I want to show you a system for addressing all of the components that limit position and challenge movement efficiency. This way, you'll be able to solve your particular problem(s) and see measurable improvement.

This passage from *Supertraining*, by Yuri Verkhoshansky and Mel Siff, helps put this idea into perspective:

"…the nature of flexibility generally is not adequately appreciated. Flexibility, whatever people mean by that term, differs from joint to joint, displays different properties during dynamic versus static condition, and concerns not only muscles but all components of the muscle skeletal system, as well as the various types of stretch reflex in the neuromuscular control circuits of the body."

Of course, few people think in terms of body systems because the "just stretch it" paradigm remains so prevalent. It's time to move beyond this simplistic outmoded notion of flexibility and start thinking about the aspects that impede position and how position relates to performance. To help people make this transition, I have deleted the words "stretching" and "flexibility" from my vocabulary and replaced them with "movement" and "mobility"—or "mobilization."

I define mobilization as a movement-based, integrated, full body approach which takes into account *all* of the elements that limit movement and performance. These include short and tight muscles, soft tissue and joint capsular restriction, motor-control problems, joint range-of-motion dysfunction, and neural dynamic issues. In short, mobilization is a tool to improve your capacity to move and perform efficiently.

This perspective gives me a clean slate from which to talk about the problems with movement restrictions in a more holistic way. The idea is to get you to stop thinking that stretching is important. Are you truly ready for this? Stretching is not important. Position and the application of position through movement is what matters most. If you can't get into a good position because you're limited or you have a tissue restriction of some kind, stretching alone won't give you the results you want. What will give you results is a system that helps you to figure out which of the variables are compromising your ability to move correctly, and then, once you've diagnosed the problems, effective modalities or techniques to resolve each of them.

A Movement-Based Approach

There's no one-size-fits-all modality when it comes to range-of motion-restrictions or tight muscles. In fact, it's best to combine techniques as often as possible and take a systematic approach so that we can address all positional and movement-related problems, soft tissue stiffness, and joint restrictions.

It's like this: A chiropractor, orthopedist, osteopath, or a joint-nutty physiotherapist cannot solve all the issues in your tissues and joints. Neither can a massage therapist or other body worker. A strength-and-conditioning coach might be a genius when it comes to teaching perfect movement, but that is only one variable in the equation. Does this mean you shouldn't work with a coach, consult a doctor, or get a massage? Absolutely not. You should seek the expertise of professionals in various fields so that you know which modality works for you.

I find that few people have a model for performing basic maintenance on their body. When someone comes to me for treatment, for example, I'll always ask, "What have you done to alleviate the problem?" And nine times out of ten he or she will shrug and admit, "Nothing."

People need a go-to safe plan so that they can take responsibility for their own dysfunctions. And that safe plan starts with position and movement.

To reiterate, you should always go after positional and movement mechanics first, and treat the symptoms after. There are several reasons for this. For starters, if you can get into a good position and move with good form, mechanical inefficiencies automatically disappear, which means that a lot of potential overuse injuries are nipped in the bud. It's like curing a disease without having to treat the symptoms.

Second, when you have good movement and motor-control, your body can deal with tissue restriction and can weather bad mechanics longer. The bottom line is that you can't mobilize—apply a mobilization technique—and resolve all of your problems all at once. It's an all day, every day endeavor. People sit in cars, work at desks, and train as if they were world-class athletes. That's a whole lot of movement to manage. Change takes time. But if you understand how to move correctly, you can at least mitigate movement errors that have the potential to cause injury and buy yourself some time to work on the compromised tissues.

Third, your body adapts to whatever positions and movements you put it in throughout the day—whether you're driving your car or doing burpees. If you move with good form and allow your joints and tissues to assume stable positions—whether you're picking up groceries or deadlifting in the gym—you will ingrain functional motor patterning and have fewer tissue and joint restrictions. However, if you, say, slouch or overextend while doing whatever needs doing in your life, your body will adapt to those poor positions, causing your tissues to become adaptively and functionally short, resulting in some sort of biomechanical compromise. When the joint is in a bad position, the surrounding musculature will adapt to that working position; this is what I mean by adaptively and functionally short. For example, if you sit in a chair every day, your hip flexors, overtime, will become adaptively short and stiff. With that understanding, you can devise an antidote: Implement mobilization techniques that target the front of your hips every day to undo the destructive nature of sitting, or convert to a standing workstation. The latter being a much better option.

Skin-Pinch Test

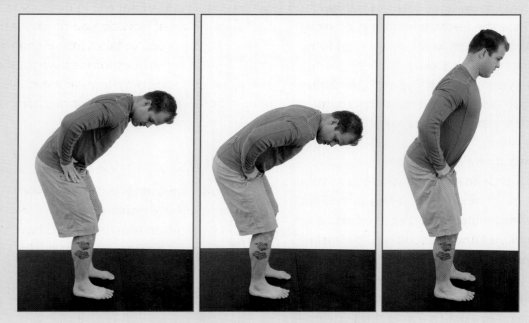

There's a really simple test you can do to illuminate how your body compensates to adaptively short tissues. It's called the skin-pinch test. Stand up, hinge from your hips, and grab a handful of skin around your hip flexors. Now stand up. What happens? You have to overextend and keep your knees bent to lift your torso upright. This is exactly what happens when you sit for long periods of time. Your hip flexors start to reflect your working position, becoming adaptively short and stiff.

By standing in a good position as opposed to sitting, you eliminate the need to mobilize the same stiff tissues over and over again. Instead you can spend your time fixing other positions and addressing other issues (i.e., the bottom of the squat or your deadlift setup).

Let's use a simple example to help clarify my point. Consider an athlete training for a half marathon who experiences hip pain six miles into a run. The fact that she doesn't experience pain until six miles, maybe forty minutes, into her run means that she is either not strong enough to maintain good form for a prolonged period of time or that her body can mitigate her poor mechanics for only six miles. It's not a mobility-related restriction problem; it's a movement problem. Of course, implementing a mobilization technique to address the pain is important, but only in the short term. It might provide immediate relief, but it won't prevent her hip pain from flaring up the next time she goes out for a long run. Simply mobilizing her hip is like taking a pill to mask a symptom but not actually curing the disease.

In this scenario, what this athlete really needs to do is address her running mechanics and make sure she's strong enough to maintain good form throughout the race. Once she learns how to run correctly and develops the strength to maintain good form, her hip won't get tight and pissy. And even if her hip does tighten up (hips inevitably get tight during long runs), she can prolong the onset of pain or maybe even prevent it altogether because she's moving efficiently.

The fourth reason for prioritizing movement and motor-control is that they dictate and guide your mobility program. Put another way, they dictate the position you have to change and the position that you need to mobilize. Otherwise you're just guessing. I call this the press-and-guess model: press or pull on something (without knowing what it does) and hope it works. For example, say you can't get your knees out or maintain a rigid spine at the bottom of the squat. This is what I call a "position of restriction." To improve the bottom of the squat, it makes sense to mobilize in a position that looks like the bottom of the squat. If you're unable to raise your arms overhead, you should probably mobilize in a position with your arms overhead.

You also need to take into account good movement mechanics as you mobilize, which is only possible if you understand what good positions look like. In other words, you will never maximize the benefits of mobility if you don't understand how to organize your body in a good position. For example, say you are missing the capacity to stabilize your shoulders in a good overhead position. To improve shoulder function, you need to not only mobilize your shoulders with your arms overhead, but also cue external rotation. If you mobilize only the overhead component, you'll miss the most important stabilization piece, which is rotation. Similarly, if you understand that your knees should not track inward and that you should see a good arch in your foot, you can carry that idea over to mobility.

Correct human movement is not open to debate. Technique is not some theoretical idea about the best way to move; it provides the means to fully express human movement potential in the most stable positions possible. If you understand what they are, you will incorporate all the elements—joint, fascia, musculature, etc.—automatically engaging several systems at once, meaning that you will address tissue restriction at the joint and in the muscle.

The question is: How do you go about addressing mobility once you've taken motor-control off the table? To answer this question we have to take a closer look at the mobility systems at work. I've broken them into three categories: joint mechanics, sliding surface, and muscle dynamics.

The Mobility Systems

Although most mobilization techniques encompass more than one system (if you address joint mechanics, you will also affect sliding surface), it's helpful to understand how each system works.

This is the mobility checklist:

- Joint mechanics
- Sliding-surface dysfunction
- Muscle dynamics

The idea is to use mobilization techniques that

address each system and work through the checklist until you've corrected your areas of restriction and resolved your pain.

Joint Mechanics

When I treat an athlete in my physical therapy practice, I always make sure that he can get into a good position before I do any kind of mobility work. However, if it's clear that he is missing major ranges of motion—meaning that I've taken motor-control off the table as being a limiting factor—I tend to go after the joint first because if I can set the joint in a good position, a lot of the problems (soft tissue restriction, sliding-surface dysfunction) automatically go away.

Say I'm treating an athlete who has anterior shoulder pain because he doesn't have enough internal rotation, meaning that his shoulders are consistently rounded forward. (When you're missing shoulder internal rotation, you compensate into a rounded forward position.) This puts the external rotators of his shoulders in a state of constant stretch and causes his pecs to become adaptively and functionally short. Now I can mobilize the long, stiff musculature that is overstretched and weak and restore normal range-of-motion to the short tissue of his pecs, but until I resolve the dysfunctional mechanics of his shoulder, weakness and tightness in the tissue will always be an issue.

A much more effective approach is to put his shoulder in a good position. And that starts with thoracic mobility; if I don't fix his spinal position, I will never get to the bottom of his dysfunctional shoulder position. Once I restore suppleness to his thoracic spine, I create the conditions for his shoulder to assume a good position. In most cases, his external rotators will turn back on and his pecs will return to their normal working state. When you put the joint into a good position, all the muscles turn on the way they're supposed to and pain tends to disappear.

The question is: How do you mobilize a joint? There are a few tools that you can use to reset a joint into a good position, which I will discuss shortly. But before I delve into the methods or techniques, let's discuss the component that compromises joint and tissue mobility and ultimately joint stability—the

Bones go where muscles pull them?.

joint capsule.

When it comes to tissue and joint restriction, one of the first things you have to look at is the joint capsule. The joint capsule is a ligamentous sac (thick and leathery fibrous tissue that connects bones and cartilages at a joint) that completely surrounds the joint. This bag of tissue creates an internal environment for freedom of movement. It also helps create stability, keeping the joint itself from overstretching.

What people tend to forget (or don't fully understand) is that this strong, supportive sac can get tight and adaptively short when the joint is put into bad positions for prolonged periods of time. This ultimately affects joint range-of-motion and tissue health. Going back to the previous example, if your shoulders are rounded forward, chances are good that your joint capsule is extremely tight. Similarly, if you sit for an extended period of time, the fronts of your hips will become adaptively short and tight. What happens? You can't pull your shoulders back into a stable externally rotated position, and you can't extend your hips. Now you can mobilize your pecs to feed slack to your shoulders, and you can try to lengthen the fronts of your hips, but that deals only with the musculature; you are not accounting for what is happening in the joint capsule.

To help you understand this, imagine a rubber band that is fat on one end and skinny on the other. If you pull on that rubber band from both ends, what happens? The skinny part stretches, but you get only a little bit of stretch from the thick end. Your tissues will similarly stretch at their weakest point. This is why people feel a big stretch in the back of their knees when they stretch their hamstrings; the weakest end of the muscle is where it inserts behind the knee. Well, your joint capsules represent the thickest part of the rubber band. In order to effect change within the joint capsule, you need to create space within the joint. We do this by creating a banded distraction. Physical therapists have done this manually for a long time, but the band allows you to do it yourself.

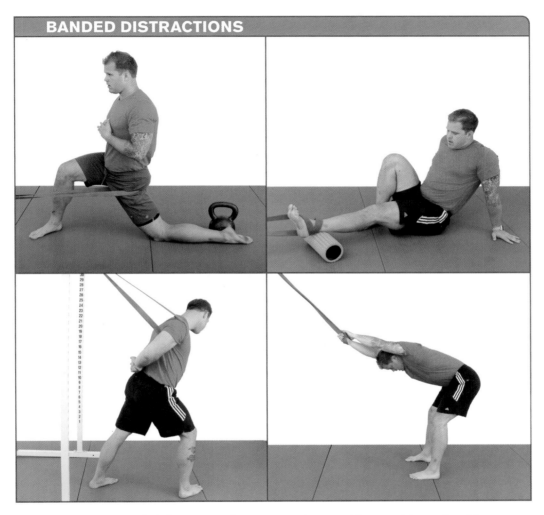

BANDED DISTRACTIONS

You can create a banded distraction from your wrist or ankle, your hip or shoulder.

As you can see from the photos, the band can be used two ways. You can hook it around your wrist or ankle, or you can hook it around your shoulder or hip. The former allows you to pull the joint surfaces apart so that you can reset the joint into a good position; the latter helps encourage motion through the joint capsule so that you can restore intra-joint articulation (meaning, how the joint moves inside the joint capsule) and puts your joint in a good position.

The third way to address joint capsule restriction is to simply force the joint into a good position and then add rotation. For example, if you're having some funky shoulder-impingement pain or restriction, try forcing your humerus into the back of the socket—using a band or a kettlebell—and then externally rotate and internally rotate your arm. This will reset your shoulder into a good position and help you reclaim rotational range-of-motion.

SHOULDER-CAPSULE MOBILIZATION

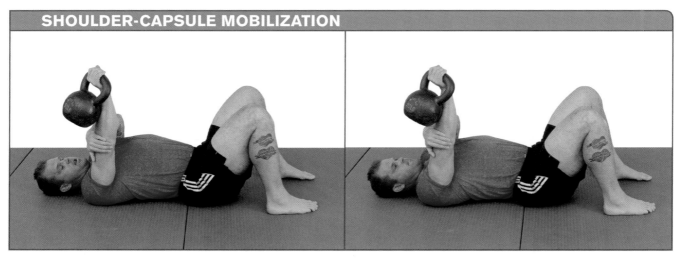

Floor-pressing a heavy kettlebell while actively pulling your shoulder to the back of the socket will help reset your shoulder in a good position. Internally and externally rotating your arm will help restore rotational range-of-motion.

Another way to treat a stiff or painful joint is to create a gapping or compression force around the compromised area. Going back to the hinge analogy, if there's a tight hinge on a door, there will be a little pile of hinge dust. The flexion-gapping method, which is used only at the elbow and knee joints, decompresses some of the joint surfaces and restores motion. Pulling the joint apart helps blow away the hinge dust and resets the joint into a good position. You can also wrap a compression or the dreaded and magical voodoo band around the joints for a similar effect.

FLEXION GAPPING

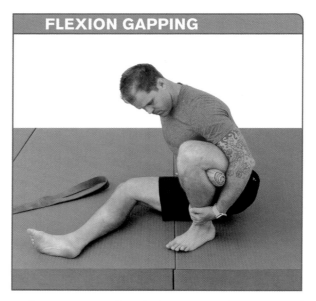

Rolling up a towel and placing it in the crevice of your knee is one way to create a gapping effect to restore motion and decompress some of the joint surfaces that restrict flexion range.

As a quick recap, you can address joint mechanics using three different methods: you can force the joint into a stable position, you can pull the joint surfaces apart by using a band or the gapping technique, or you can compress the joint. Remember, if you are not actively mobilizing your joint capsules, you're leaving a huge chunk of tissue restriction on the table.

Sliding-Surface

After you check joint mechanics off the list, the second system you should address is sliding-surface dysfunction.

Sliding surface is a catchall phrase I use to describe how the different components, structures, and systems of the body relate to one another. To ensure suppleness, your tissue—skin, nerves, muscles, and tendons—should all slide and glide over each other. Your skin should slide over the underlying surface layers (bone, tendon, muscle), your nerves should slide through your nerve tunnels (muscle), and your tissues should slide around your joints.

To test this idea, take your index and middle fingers, press down on the top of your opposite hand, and move your skin around in all directions. What you will notice is that the skin slides over the underlying bone and tissue. To a lesser degree, this is how your skin ought to slide over all the surface layers of your muscle, tendons, and bone.

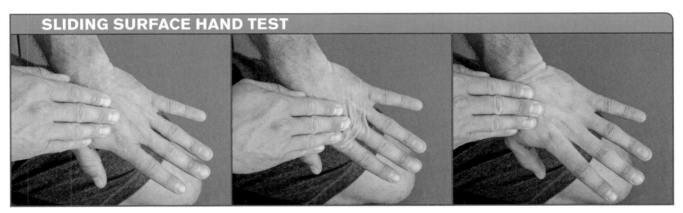

SLIDING SURFACE HAND TEST

Your skin should slide unrestricted over the back of your hand.

For example, if you pull your toes toward you in dorsiflexion, you should be able to pinch or slide your skin over the back of your Achilles tendon. You can also test the sliding surfaces around the outside of your knee, thigh, and ankle, and around the tip of your elbow. If your skin does not freely glide over what's underneath it, you've basically created an external cast—a cast around your system. Isn't that a dreamy image?

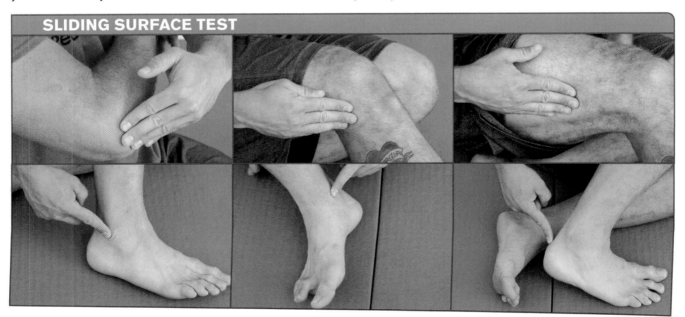

SLIDING SURFACE TEST

Although you don't have as much skin elasticity around your joint, your skin should still slide unrestricted over your elbow, and outside of your knee, thigh, ankle, and heel cord.

Imagine wearing a really tight pair of jeans and then trying to squat to full depth. Not going to happen, right? Your skin is like those really tight jeans. This is exactly what happens to your glutes when you sit down for prolonged periods of time. The bundles of muscle stick to one another and become unresponsive, limiting their ability to contract. This is why when people sit extensively they have trouble fully activating their glutes to stabilize their pelvis and achieve a neutral spinal position.

To restore the slide to surfaces (sliding surfaces), you have to unadhere that skin to the underlying tissue or bone using sliding-surface mobilization techniques (like the pressure wave, smash and floss, and ball whack). There are a number of different tools you can use, the most common being a lacrosse ball, roller, or voodoo band. You can also have a Superfriend smash your quads and big muscle groups by creating shear force—grinding pressures—across the muscle. What you have to remember is that sliding-surface dysfunction can cause a ton of problems down the road, and no amount of stretching will alleviate it. The only way to unadhere matted-down tissue is to unglue the skin and superficial and deeper layers of muscle using large shearing forces across the skin and muscle.

Muscle Dynamics

If I'm running a diagnostic on a patient or athlete and I'm working sequentially through the mobility check-list, by the time I fix his or her motor-control—position or movement error—clear joint capsule restriction, and restore sliding surfaces to overly tight tissues, I've usually already restored normal range-of-motion and I haven't had to stretch anything. This is why muscle dynamics is the last system on the mobility checklist.

Let me say here that the muscle dynamics component uses mobilization techniques that look a lot like traditional stretching shapes. But let me be clear: Muscle dynamics is not stretching as I've classified it. We're not just putting the tissue to end-range and hanging out for a while, hoping that something changes. Rather, we're using an active model—applying tension at end-range—to help facilitate change in the tissue and restore some muscle contraction. And, more important, we're always biasing or emphasizing positions that look like the positions we're trying to correct. If you're restricted in the bottom of the squat, you want to mobilize in a position that looks like the bottom of the squat.

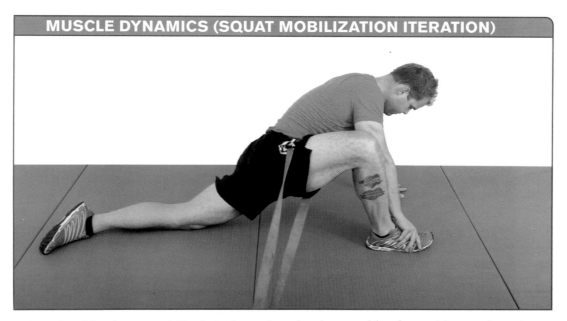

MUSCLE DYNAMICS (SQUAT MOBILIZATION ITERATION)

When possible, always mobilize in a shape that closely resembles the position you're trying to change.

The muscle dynamics system is how we lengthen muscles or increase range-of-motion for athletes who need to get into extreme positions, like dancers, gymnasts, and martial artists. Don't confuse this with growing new muscle. I say this because I've seen people fall into the trap of thinking that they can grow new muscle by stretching. The fastest way to grow or lengthen muscle is to perform full-range loaded movements. If your hamstrings are "tight" for example, deadlifting and squatting will not only stimulate hamstring growth, but also build motor-control and strength at new end-ranges.

When you restore range or function to the joint or tissue, you need to reflect that change back into your motor-control program. If you improve your overhead shoulder range-of-motion by 5 percent, and you use it in the gym, you will more than likely retain that range-of-motion. It's not a mysterious process.

When muscles are working within limited ranges of motion they become functionally short. Consider an elite cyclist who spends half of his day on a bike. His ankles are locked in a neutral position and his hips are stuck in a closed position. By the time he gets off his bike after a long ride, his muscles have adapted to that working position. This is where muscle dynamics and methods like contract and relax—forcing tissue to end-range, contracting the muscle, and then relaxing to get a little bit more range—fit into our paradigm of solving problems. If you're stuck in a car for two hours, undoing the sitting by spending some time at end-range hip extension (using the contract and relax model) to restore normal length to the tissue is the way to go. That doesn't mean hanging out in a static position but actively oscillating in and out of end-range tension and using a band to approximate your hip into a good position.

My rule of thumb is to prioritize motor-control, joint capsule, and sliding surfaces before training, and to save some of the muscle dynamic end-range mobilization techniques for after training. This way, you're warmed up and your tissues are prepped for the mobility work. We hear athletes say that they are afraid of stretching before they work out, and that's a reasonable fear. In fact, static end-range splits before you squat heavy is probably not a good idea.

Now that you understand the mobility systems and you have a blueprint for solving problems, let's take a closer look at the actual techniques or methods that you'll use.

Mobilization Methods

While there are several techniques you can use within the framework of the mobility systems, it's important to realize that there is a dynamic relationship between mobility systems and mobilization techniques. If your joint capsule is altered using a joint capsule mobilization, for example, the soft tissue surrounding the joint will probably also be affected. Similarly, if you restore sliding surfaces to your tissue using a smashing technique, your joint mechanics and muscle dynamics will probably improve.

But just as a carpenter has a tool for a specific job, there are specific mobility techniques for specific systems. There are techniques that focus on improving position and others that are meant to restore length to shortened tissue. In addition, there are mobilizations that offer a more acute pinpoint approach, and some that address an entire muscle group.

You need different methods so that you can cover all the different components of your restriction. So don't limit yourself to just one technique. Most of these methods can be used in combination. Let's say you're working on restoring sliding surfaces to your glutes. You can use the contract and relax method to sink into the deeper layers of tissue, pressure wave across the stiff musculature, and then smash and floss over knotted down tissue. Mix and match in the way that gets the job done and affects the greatest amount of change in the shortest period of time.

Pressure Wave

The pressure wave uses a pinpoint-focused approach for working through deeper layers of muscle and connective tissue like fascia. It's like using a little chisel to pick away at knotted-up pockets of tissue, as opposed to using a sledgehammer to break up large muscle masses.

To correctly execute this technique, lie on a ball or roller while remaining completely relaxed—the goal is to sink into the deepest levels of your muscle tissue. Next, create a pressure wave by slowly rolling the targeted area over the ball or roller using the full weight of your body. This is the equivalent of a structural-integration therapist or Rolfer pressuring an elbow slowly through the length of your hamstrings or quads. Go slow and keep the full weight of your body distributed over the ball or roller, so your tissues have a chance to yield to the ball (relax). As a rule, the slower you move the more pressure you can handle and the more positive effects the tissues will receive. If you move fast and keep your muscles engaged as you roll around, your efforts will be futile.

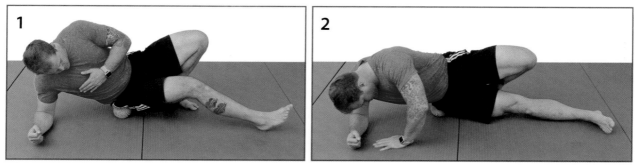

Get all of your weight over the ball or roller and slowly roll the tissues you are trying to change over the object, creating a pressure wave across the knotted-up area.

Contract and Relax

The contract and relax method is based on the scientifically established use of proprioceptive neuromuscular facilitation (PNF) stretching. You can use this method to restore normal range-of-motion to shortened tissue, or to get deeper compression during sliding-surface mobilization. Here's how it works: If you are focusing on muscle dynamics, build tension at end-range for five seconds, release tension, and move into a new range for ten seconds. If you are focusing on sliding surfaces, identify a tight area (an area in which you can't surrender your full weight on the ball or roller) and then engage that muscle for no less than five seconds. After five seconds of tension, immediately relax, allowing the affected tissue to sink deeper into the pressure of the roller or ball.

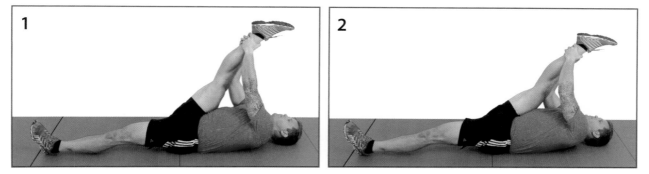

Using your hands to keep your leg in the same place, create tension by driving your leg away from you and hold that tension for five seconds. After five seconds, release tension and move into a new range for ten seconds.

Banded Flossing

The easiest way to deal with muscle stiffness is to put the joint into a good position using a Rogue monster band. Remember, your tissues adapt to your working positions. So if you sit all day, not only will your hip flexors become adaptively short, but the head of your femur will also move anteriorly in the hip capsule instead of remaining in the center of it, where it belongs. Every time you perform deep-flexion-based movements, the head of your femur hits the edge of your acetabulum (hip socket). This is why people feel an impingement or pain in the front of the hip when they squat or mobilize in positions that close that joint. Using a Rogue monster band to create a distraction will pull the head of the femur back to the center of the capsule and effectively clear that impingement so that you can move into newly challenged ranges without discomfort.

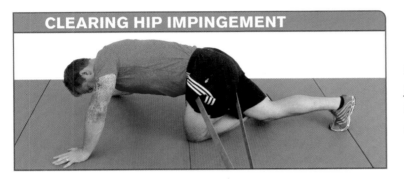

CLEARING HIP IMPINGEMENT

By creating a lateral or posterior distraction, you can effectively clear hip impingements, allowing you to move into deeper flexion ranges, as well as account for joint capsule restriction.

The band also helps you manage joint capsule restriction. Because the joint capsule is so thick and robust, you need a little extra tension to get a stretch through it. Going back to the rubber band analogy, you need to account for the thick end of the rubber band to create an equal stretch throughout the muscle.

Banded flossing is also one of the best ways to prep for dynamic or loaded movements. (Note: "Flossing" refers to movement.) For example, say you're trying to mobilize the front of your hip. The first step is to wrap a band around the back of your upper thigh and create an anterior distraction (pull your hip forward). The next step is to get into a lunge position and perform split squats by lowering and raising your back knee. If you don't feel anything, guess what? You probably have full range-of-motion. But if you find that you can't get your hip into extension or you feel a big stretch in the front of your hip, chances are that your hip capsule is restricted. Although mobility doesn't technically count as a warm-up for movement, banded-flossing mobilizations like the banded split squat is a great prep for loaded and dynamic movements.

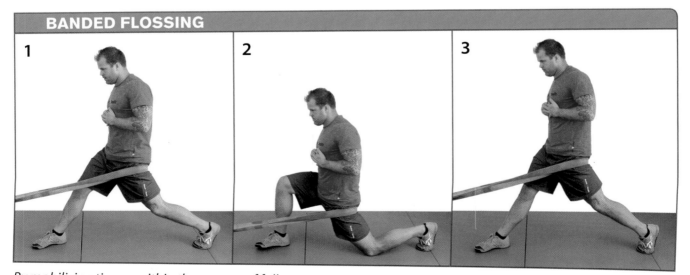

BANDED FLOSSING

1　2　3

By mobilizing tissues within the context of full-range movement, you restore normal range to short and stiff tissues and affect multiple tissue systems.

Smash and Floss

Smash and floss allows you to "tack" down or apply pressure to an area of painfully knotted tissue. Once a "tack" has been applied to the affected tissue, "floss," or move, the limb around in every direction through as much range-of-motion as possible. This method is very similar to active-release treatment (ART), trigger-point therapy, or shiatsu, in that it focuses on trying to restore sliding surfaces by using movement to unglue the deep mechanical restrictions in the tissue.

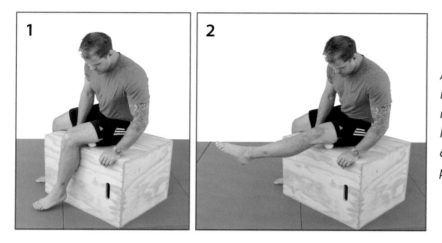

After a tight area has been identified, get maximal pressure (weight) over a ball, roller, or barbell, and then move your limb through as much range-of-motion as possible, thereby flossing the compressed tissues.

Paper-clipping (Oscillation)

Paper-clipping simply refers to oscillating in and out of end-range or peak tension. For example, say you're mobilizing your anterior hip. To get the best results, you want to drive your hip forward into extension and then move in and out of end-range tension. You need to be active at end-range by oscillating in and out of peak tension, not maintaining a static position. It's these small oscillations that really create the most change, especially within the joint capsule. Think about how much bending back and forth it takes to break a paper clip: When tissues are matted-down and as tight as steel wires it takes a ton of movement to get rid of that stiffness and free up the tissues.

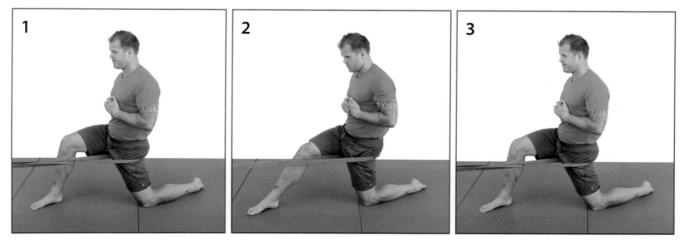

Oscillate in and out of end-range tension by driving your hip forward, hanging out for a second or two, and then retreating back. The key is not to bounce, but to slowly move in and out of peak tension.

Voodoo Flossing (Compression)

Voodoo flossing is an intermittent, compression-based joint-mobilization method that incorporates all the mobility systems simultaneously. In my opinion, it's the most powerful and effective method in terms of restoring position and motion. (Note: A voodoo band is a stretch-band engineered specifically for compression-based mobilization techniques. You can find them at MobilityWOD.com. Another option is to simply improvise by cutting a bicycle tire tube in half.)

To do it, wrap a band around the joint or restricted tissue—creating a large compression force a few inches below and a few inches above the affected area—move your limb around in every direction for about two or three minutes, and then remove the band. What's great about voodoo flossing is that you can mobilize in the position you're trying to alter. Rolling out your quad will certainly improve your position, but you're not mobilizing within the context of functional full-range movement. For example, if you voodoo-band your quads and then squat, you're able to change the mechanics in some of the tissues that may be restricting your squat. If you wrap your knee and then squat, you're loading the joint and encouraging improvement in every system while getting into your position of restriction.

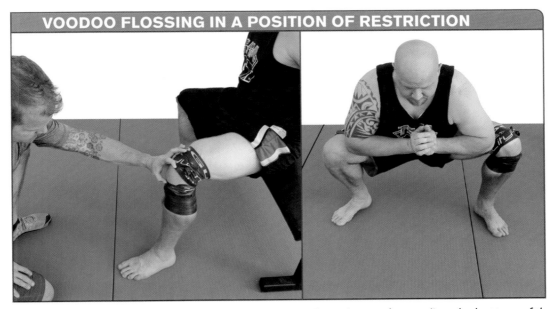

Voodoo flossing allows you to mobilize in the position you're trying to change (i.e., the bottom of the squat).

Here's the deal: You can only hypothesize what you're actually changing because voodoo flossing works on so many different levels. Wrapping a band around a joint or chunk of scar tissue and introducing movement creates a global shearing effect—restoring sliding-surface function to the underlying banded tissues—and the band bulk creates a flexion-gapping force at the joint, which can help restore range-of-motion to the joint. Not only that, but when you release the compression your blood floods into poorly saturated joints and tissues. In short, voodoo flossing will help restore sliding surfaces to matted-down tissue, resolve joint pain, and radically improve muscle contraction. If you're limited by position or have knee or elbow pain (this is my first stop for treating tennis elbow), get a band around the joint or restricted area and force the tissue through a full range-of-motion.

Voodoo flossing also happens to be one of the best methods for dealing with a swollen joint or swollen tissue. Swelling blows out a lot of the proprioceptors, presses on nerve endings, causes acute pain, and degrades joint mechanics. You should take swelling very seriously. By compressing the joint, you push swelling back into the lymphatic system where it can be drained from the body.

It's important to note that the technique for wrapping a joint or tissue and the technique for addressing a swollen joint are slightly different. For example, to flush out the swelling caused by a sprained ankle, start as close to the tip of the foot as you can, wrapping with about a half inch overlap (or half the band overlap), keeping about a 50 percent stretch in the band all the way around the swollen limb. The key points are to wrap a few inches below the swollen area, leaving no skin exposed, and keep the tension even in the band. Once the foot is compressed, move it around for a couple of minutes. Then take the band off for a few minutes to give the tissue a chance to rebound and recover. Then wrap it again. Repeat this process for about twenty minutes, or until you stop experiencing change. It's insanely effective. Using this technique, you can literally restore an ankle the size of a grapefruit to normal size and completely relieve the pain. In my opinion, this is the best remedy for getting rid of inflammation and pain in injured joints.

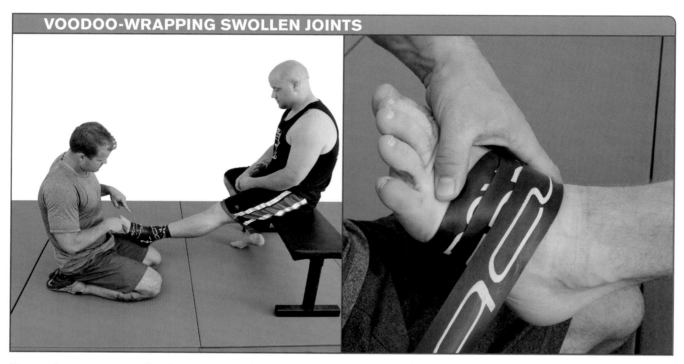

VOODOO-WRAPPING SWOLLEN JOINTS

To voodoo wrap a swollen joint, start as far down on the limb as possible, wrapping toward the heart, and create a 50 percent stretch in the band around the swollen area. The goal is to cover the entire area, keeping a half-inch overlap as you wrap.

The general rule for compressing a swollen joint is to wrap toward the heart. So if you're wrapping an ankle, you start at the toes and wrap up the leg. However, when you're mobilizing a joint or matted-down scar tissue, it doesn't really matter if you wrap from high to low or low to high—just start a few inches below or above the area in question. Typically, I'll put a 75 percent stretch or tension across the area I'm working on and 50 percent around the remaining area. For example, if I'm voodoo flossing the front of my knee around my suprapatellar pouch, I'll put 75 percent stretch over the front and 50 percent around the back. As in wrapping a swollen joint, there should be a half inch (or half the band) overlap. If you've got band left over when you're done wrapping, you can make an "X" over the targeted area for an additional shearing effect.

VOODOO WRAPPING TECHNIQUE

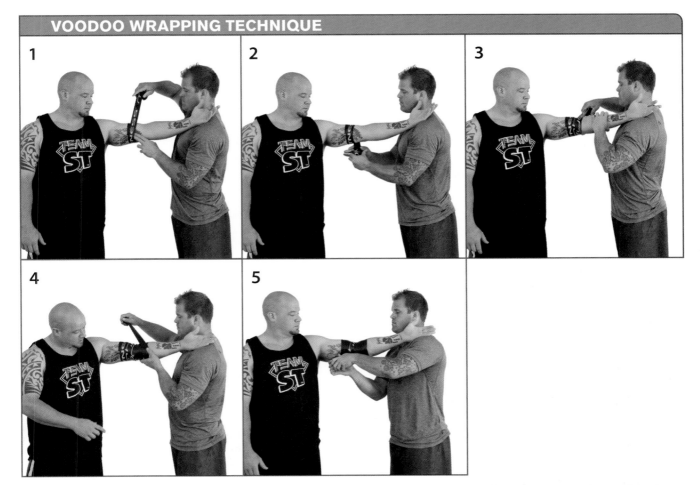

To correctly wrap a joint or section of tissue, start a few inches below or above the compromised area, keeping a half-inch overlap in the band. Continue wrapping until you cover the area you are trying to change. If you have extra band, form an "X" by wrapping across the entire area. On your final loop, create extra stretch so that you can tuck the end piece underneath the band. The tension will keep the band in place. Once wrapped, move the limb through as much range-of-motion as possible.

VOODOO WRAPPING TECHNIQUE

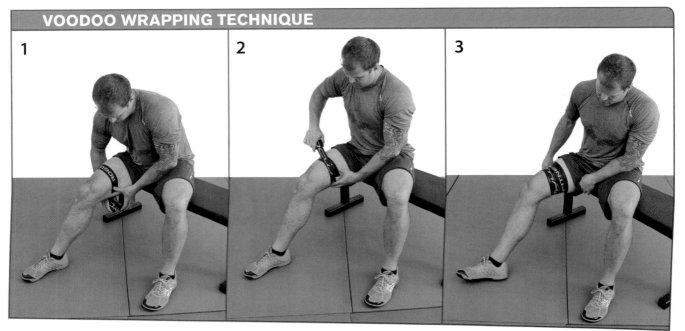

Just so you know, voodoo flossing can be a bit uncomfortable. But don't worry; despite the level of discomfort, it's not sketchy and does not harm the joint or tissue in any fashion. If you end up with some red marks on your skin, which we call leopard stripes, don't panic—that's just the superficial skin layers being pulled on the surface. You'll live.

There are, however, some general guidelines to follow. For starters, if you start to go numb or get a tingly sensation—pins and needles—or your limb turns into a color that makes you think of zombies, take the band off. Usually, that happens at about the two minute mark. In most cases, you will get a tingly sensation before your hand or foot turns white so if you hit this stage you need to act fast. Another warning sign is if you suddenly feel very claustrophobic. You need to respect these sketchy feelings and signs. As with most mobilizations, it's pretty intense but you should be able to differentiate between discomfort and feelings like numbness, tingling, or claustrophobia. And you should be able to recognize skin tone that resembles that of a dead person.

SAFETY CHECK

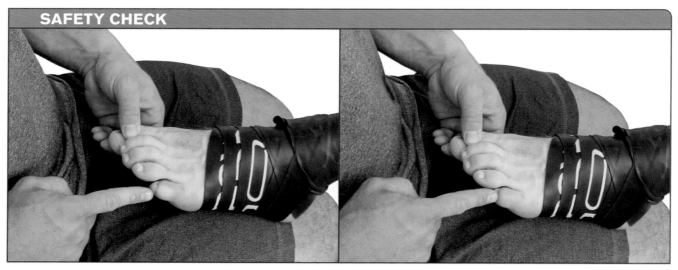

When you touch the skin, it should turn white and then return to normal—like touching sunburned skin. If you touch the skin and color doesn't return, it's time to take the band off.

INCREASED BLOOD FLOW

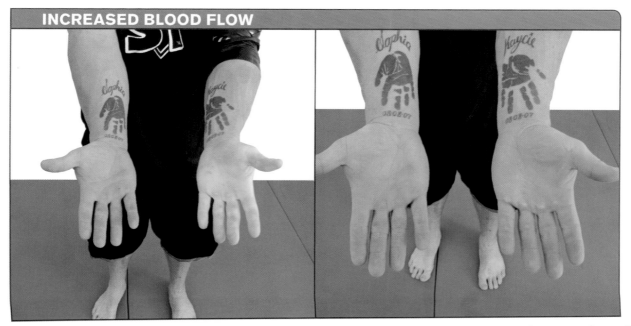

When you take the band off, your skin will turn the color of a dead person. But within a few seconds, you'll notice increased blood flow into the area.

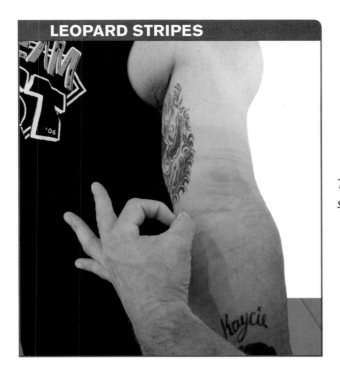

LEOPARD STRIPES

The band will pinch your skin, leaving red lines across your skin. Don't flip out. They will disappear after a few minutes.

Flexion Gapping

Flexion gapping helps to remove joint capsule restriction and restore flexion range-of-motion to the knee and elbow. You should be able kiss your forearm to your biceps and get your calf flush with your hamstring without effort. If you have to move your head toward your hand to feed yourself or turn your feet out so you can drop into a deep squat, you're missing flexion range-of-motion at your secondary engines (knee and elbow). An easy way to blow away the hinge dust and restore normal range to the joint is to roll up a towel, jam it behind your knee or elbow, and then create a compression or flexion force over the fulcrum. You can also use a Rogue monster band or voodoo band to create a gapping effect, as illustrated in the photo.

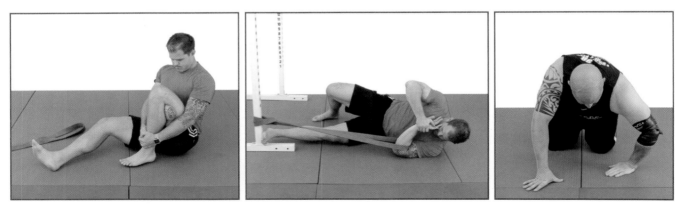

You can create a gapping force by rolling up a towel or by creating a distraction with a band. Voodoo flossing will also create a gapping effect.

Upstream-Downstream Approach

Identifying your position of restriction is the best way to address tissue dysfunction and solve mechanical problems as they relate to movement: If you're struggling to get your knees out in the bottom of a squat, it makes sense to mobilize in that position of restriction.

But what if you are in pain, or tweak your knee or back, or get hurt playing sports?

Even if you maintain good form and move with perfect technique, pain and injury are an inherent reality, especially if you play and train at a high level. Joints get tweaked and tissues get stiff. It's the nature of being a physically active human being. This is why it's important to have a template for not only solving mechanical problems, but also for resolving and treating pain. The upstream-downstream approach serves as this template. It's a simple idea: Mobilize the tissue upstream (above) and downstream (below) of the problem.

What's great about the upstream-downstream approach is that you don't need to know anything about movement or anatomy to take care of yourself. Just target the muscle and tissue above and below the restricted area. It's that simple. And yes, you can certainly mobilize at the site of localized pain. However, where the rats get in is not necessarily where they chew. If you have tight calves and quads, for example, those tissues will pull on your knee, restricting range-of-motion and compromising mechanics. Remember, you are encased in a web of fascia—a layer of connective tissue—that transmits movement throughout your body. So if your calf, quad, or hamstring is tight, the fascia surrounding the musculature will also be tight. And if the fascia is tight, it will pull on your knee, compromising your ability to get into stable positions. By mobilizing the tissues above and below the knee—quad, suprapatellar pouch, hamstring, calf, shin—you feed slack to the tensioned joint and restore normal function to the muscles (and fascia) tugging on your knee.

The only problem with the upstream-downstream approach is that it's predicated on a lagging indicator, meaning that you spent time moving incorrectly before your body started transmitting the pain signal. Ideally, you want to identify and deal with restrictions before they devolve into pain. The problem is that it's easy to circumvent or assimilate bad mechanics until the body starts hurting. So figure out where you are restricted and then work on restoring/improving range-of-motion there before it becomes a problem.

Programming For Mobility

To reiterate, there are two ways to approach mobility. One is to identify your restriction and mobilize within the context of the position you're trying to improve, and the other is to mobilize upstream and downstream of a painful area.

Now that you have a basic template, let's discuss how to program for mobility.

To begin, it's important to understand that there are no days off (see Rules of Mobility, page 223). You need to commit 15 to 20 minutes every single day on mobilizing and working on your mechanics. If you can do more, great, but fifteen to twenty minutes is the minimum requirement. Modern humans are very busy. Yet we still need to carve out time to work on position and improve tissue function. This is why I recommend daily doses of at least 15 to 20 minutes of mobility work. Although this may not seem like much, it accumulates over time. If you mobilize for twenty minutes a day, it adds up to 140 minutes over a week, which is a significant amount of time spent working on correcting tissues and improving position.

What should you do within that 15 or 20 minute timeframe? Here are three general rules to help you devise an individualized mobility program:

1. Always resolve issues with painful joints and tissues first, and then focus on positions of restrictions. If you imagine a target, your pain or restricted area should be at the center of that target every time you mobilize and comprise a good portion of your designated 15-20 minute block of time. Spend the rest of the time focusing on a position that you're trying to improve (bottom of the squat), or undoing any damage you might have incurred from your workday, like being buckled into an office chair.

2. Spend no less than 2 minutes in each position. Research unquestionably asserts that it takes at least 2 minutes to make soft tissue change. This means that 2 minutes is your minimum therapeutic dose per position. For example, if you're doing the couch stretch you need to spend no less than two minutes mobilizing each side of your hip. However, my rule as a therapist is to work on a restricted area until there's improvement or I realize that there's no more to be had in the session. This could mean 2 minutes or 10 minutes. So don't be in a rush to move on if you haven't experienced improvement in the tissue.

3. Choose three mobilization or target areas. Don't get overly ambitious and try to mobilize ten different positions. Most people can handle only three mobilization or target areas per session.

Here's what a sample program might look like:

Mobilize the Shoulder

- Shoulder capsule mobilization: 2 minutes for each arm.
- Overhead banded distraction: 2 minutes for each arm.

Mobilize Bottom of the Squat

- Single-leg flexion with external rotation bias: 2 minutes for each side.

Undo Sitting

- Super-couch mobilization: 2 minutes for each side.

Total time: 16 minutes.

Remember, programming for mobility changes from day to day, depending on your areas of restriction, the movements you are performing, and the positions you're hanging out in. The key is for you to constantly work on your position and spend the necessary time doing basic body maintenance.

Rules of Mobility

To optimize your time and keep you safe, I've laid out six fundamental guidelines for implementing the mobilization techniques.

▶ **Test and Retest**

Everything you do should have observable, measurable, and repeatable results. Otherwise, your time would be better spent watching reality television. Think of testing and retesting as a diagnostic tool for measuring improvement within the context of movement and/or pain.

Here's how it works. Say you're trying to improve your squat. Before you start smashing your quads or mobilizing your calves, get into the bottom of the squat and assess your areas of restriction. Next, perform some mobility therapeutics on the tissues that you think might be holding you back from achiev-

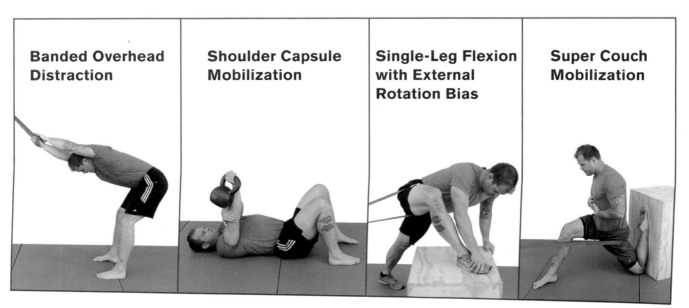

| **Banded Overhead Distraction** | **Shoulder Capsule Mobilization** | **Single-Leg Flexion with External Rotation Bias** | **Super Couch Mobilization** |

ing optimal form. For example, if you think it's your tight calves, do some mobility on them and then retest the bottom of your squat. Can you drive your knees out farther? Can you keep your back flat? If you mobilized the right area and implemented the appropriate techniques, you should experience or observe measurable improvement. If you can't see improvement, then you have irrefutable, the world-is-round evidence that there wasn't any problem in that area, which means you need to start targeting another area.

Mobilizing should improve your ability to get into a good position, optimize movement, and reduce or banish pain. Testing and retesting lets you know if what you are doing is actually working. Also, using your new range-of-motion right away in an actual movement helps your brain keep track of these new ranges.

▶ **If it Feels Sketchy, it's Sketchy**

Mobilizing restricted tissue is uncomfortable—there's no getting around that fact. If you have ever subjected your quads to some smashing on a roller, you know what I'm talking about. But unless your entire quad is as stiff as wood, only certain sections will hurt. When you hit a patch of restricted tissue, it's agony, but as soon as you move past it, the pain is over. That's because supple tissue doesn't elicit a pain response under pressure.

But there's a difference between discomfort, even intense discomfort, and harmful pain. If you think you're injuring yourself, you probably are injuring yourself. If something feels like it's tearing,

something probably is tearing. If you experience hot, burning pain, your body is telling you that something is not right. If you're getting a horrible hip impingement, guess what? You have a horrible hip impingement. Don't keep mobilizing into the problem because it will only make the problem worse.

What am I trying to say? Ungluing stiff and restricted tissues can be uncomfortable, but it shouldn't feel like you're causing more damage than is already there. It's up to you to know the difference and listen to your body. Having a glass of wine can make mobilizing a little more tolerable, but getting drunk and passing out on a lacrosse ball is never a good idea. And if you roll around on that lacrosse ball for an hour (before you pass out!), you're going to bruise your precious tissues.

I often say, "Don't go into the pain cave." People have an immense capacity to hurt themselves, ignore pain, and travel to extreme places of suffering. And that's how they end up hurting themselves when mobilizing. This is what I must say to you: Stand at the entrance of the pain cave, but do not enter the pain cave. Mobility should be uncomfortable but not unbearable.

▶ **No Days Off**

It's important to understand that there is no distinction between lifting heavy in the gym and picking up a pillow from the ground. Both require conscious awareness of positioning and how best to organize your body. So no matter what you are doing throughout the day you should always think about

Don't Make a Pain Face

We have a saying around our gym: Don't make a pain face while mobilizing. We say this for several reasons. For one, it shortens your neck flexors, causing more restriction along the athletic chain.

Secondly, you don't want to associate pain with a weird face because those things get mapped together in the body. If you grimace every time you roll out your quads, what expression do you think you'll make when your quads start burning during a workout? In a competitive environment, you don't want to give away how much you are suffering. Your opponent will see that and use it to his advantage. This is why athletes practice relaxing their face when they're uncomfortable. When you mobilize, you're making a conscious choice to improve yourself, so you might as well embrace it.

Lastly, pulling weird faces while you're lying on a ball can be pretty creepy—you don't want to freak people out.

improving your position and movement mechanics, as well as spend at least fifteen to twenty minutes performing basic body maintenance. Likewise, you don't want to take a day off from good nutrition or miss a night of sleep. Of course, there will be times when you can't eat perfectly, exercise, or get eight hours of sleep. But you should cultivate a habit of always being in a good position, regardless of what you are doing.

The fact is, if you want to play and train at a high level, you cannot slack off for even one day. You have to constantly think about your position, whether you are at work, playing a sport, lifting, or lounging around. This is the basis of the "no days off" rule.

Here's a simple example to help illustrate my point. A DEA agent buddy of mine told me about a friend who used to walk past his trunk every time he got out of the car. It didn't matter if he was on duty or off duty, if he parked at a grocery store, at his house, or at a restaurant—he would walk all the way around the car and past his trunk every single time. He did this because he kept his rifle in his trunk and he wanted to ingrain the pattern of approaching his trunk into his motor program. That way, if he were ever in a dodgy firefight, he wouldn't hesitate or think—he would automatically find himself by his trunk, ready to grab his rifle.

Remember, your body is an adaptation machine. If you spend a few minutes a day trying to improve position, you will improve your position. But if you take a few days off, you will get stiff and your movement and position will reflect that adaptation. Even if you're taking a day off from the gym, you should never take a day off good movement and position or mobilizing. In fact, it's the day after training when a lot of muscle soreness and tissue stiffness aggregates, and those are the days when you really need to make sure that you're working on restoring normalcy to those tissues. For this reason, it's best to break up mobility into short doses. This gives you plenty of time to effect change within the context of movement, and more importantly, it is manageable over the long haul.

▶ **Make Mobility Realistic**

As I said before, the average person isn't going to know what you're talking about if you tell him that he needs to improve hip flexion and external rotation. But if I tell him that he needs to mobilize the bottom of the squat, he can immediately make the connection between the position he needs to mobilize and the position he's trying to change. This makes it really easy to program and start thinking about how to approach mobility. If you're missing overhead range-of-motion, it makes sense to mobilize in a position with your arms overhead and externally rotated.

The key is to prioritize mobilizations that approximate real-life situations. Instead of stretching your hamstrings while lying on your back, for example, get a band around your hip and hinge from the hips while standing up, which looks a lot like deadlifting. The more you can replicate what you're trying to change, the more you will improve your position.

▶ **Always Mobilize in a Good Position**

Committing an overextension spinal fault or mobilizing with your shoulder in an unstable position is not going to get you the results you are looking for. In fact, all you are doing is encouraging bad positions and ingraining bad mechanics. Keep the movement principles in mind as you mobilize. If your ankles are collapsed, your knees cave inward, your back rounds, or you overextend at your lumbar spine, reset and fix your position.

▶ **Don't Get Stuck in One Position. Explore Your Business.**

Think of the mobilization techniques as a basic guide. Although I demonstrate how to perform each mobilization with proper technique, you are not limited to performing them exactly as the photos indicate. You know where you are tight and restricted better than anybody else. As long as you maintain good form and avoid defaulting into bad positions, you should absolutely feel free to explore your dysfunction and move into newly challenged areas. I call this "informed freestyle." If you're mobilizing your anterior hip, for example, you might rotate your body to the side or put your arm overhead. The key is to target areas that feel the tightest.

MOBILITY TOOLS

To best replicate the techniques demonstrated in this chapter, there are a few pieces of equipment that you will need. Understand that if you don't have the listed tools, improvise by using whatever you have laying around the house: wine bottle, dog toys, sports equipment, the list goes on and on. For example, if you don't have a voodoo floss band, cut a bicycle tube in half and you have yourself a functional compression-band. However, everyone should have three lacrosse balls on hand: one for acute smashing, and two for creating a double lacrosse ball (LAX ball peanut).

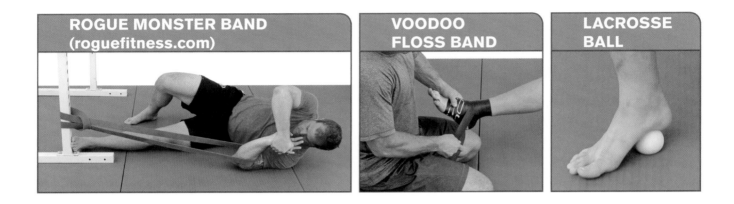

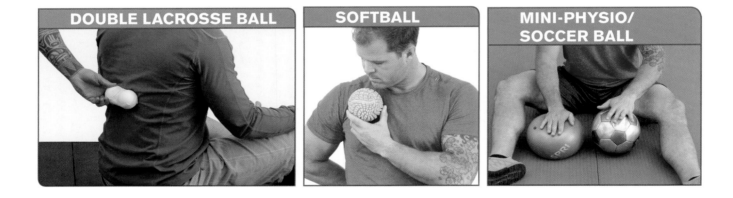

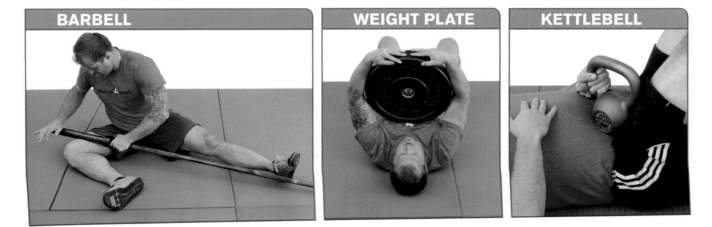

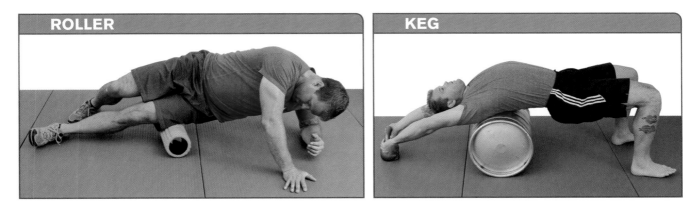

ROLLER

KEG

Double Lacrosse Ball (LAX Ball Peanut)

The single lacrosse ball can be used on pretty much every body part—glutes, feet, hips, suprapetallar pouch, anterior shoulder, ribs, shoulder blades, and other areas of the back (to mention a few)—but not to mobilize the thoracic spine. To restore suppleness to your thoracic spine, you need to block the facet joints—which are the weight-bearing stabilizing structures located behind and between the adjacent vertebrae—using two lacrosse balls. As you can see from the photos, by taping two lacrosse balls together, you can create a very low-tech and inexpensive mobility tool that can be used to restore normal range to the thoracic spine.

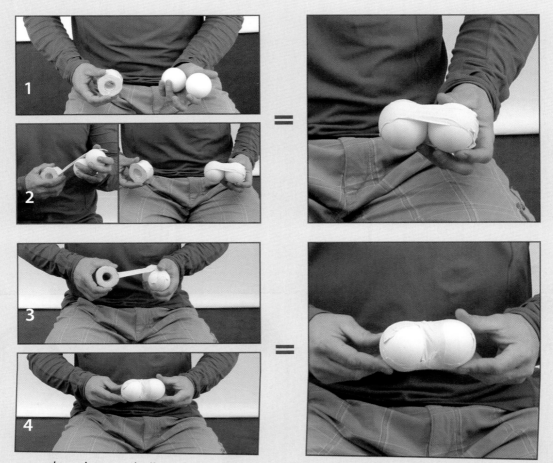

To begin, you need two lacrosse balls and some athletic tape. Next, attach the two lacrosse balls by wrapping a few layers of tape around the outside of the balls. Then wrap another couple of layers around the center. It's that easy.

ANTERIOR VIEW

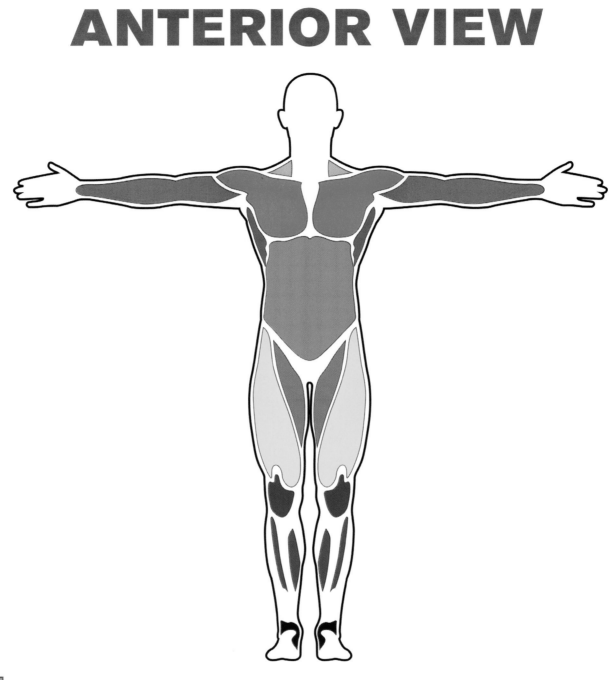

AREA 1: Thoracic Spine (Upper Back, Neck, Scapula)–page 230

AREA 2: Posterior Shoulder (Lat, Posterior Deltoid)–page 248

AREA 3: Anterior Shoulder (Pec, Anterior Deltoid)–page 262

AREA 4: Downstream Arm (Triceps, Elbow, Forearm, Wrist)–page 274

AREA 5: Trunk (Psoas, Low Back, Oblique)–page 286

AREA 6: Posterior High Chain (Glutes, Hip Capsule)–page 298

AREA 7: Anterior High Chain (Hip Flexors, Quadriceps)–page 322

POSTERIOR VIEW

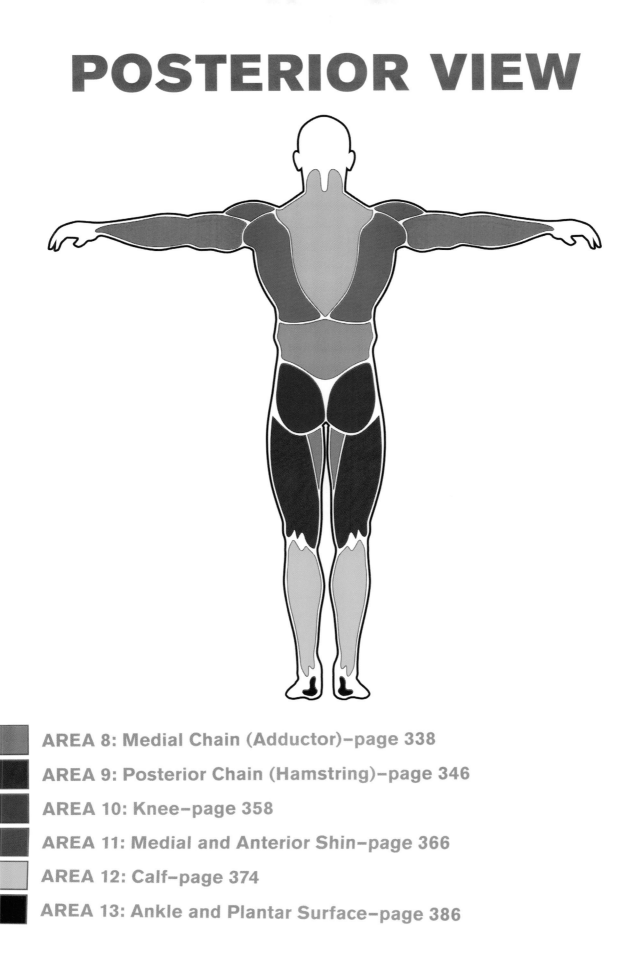

■ AREA 8: Medial Chain (Adductor)–page 338

■ AREA 9: Posterior Chain (Hamstring)–page 346

■ AREA 10: Knee–page 358

■ AREA 11: Medial and Anterior Shin–page 366

■ AREA 12: Calf–page 374

■ AREA 13: Ankle and Plantar Surface–page 386

AREA 1
THORACIC SPINE
(UPPER BACK, NECK, SCAPULA)

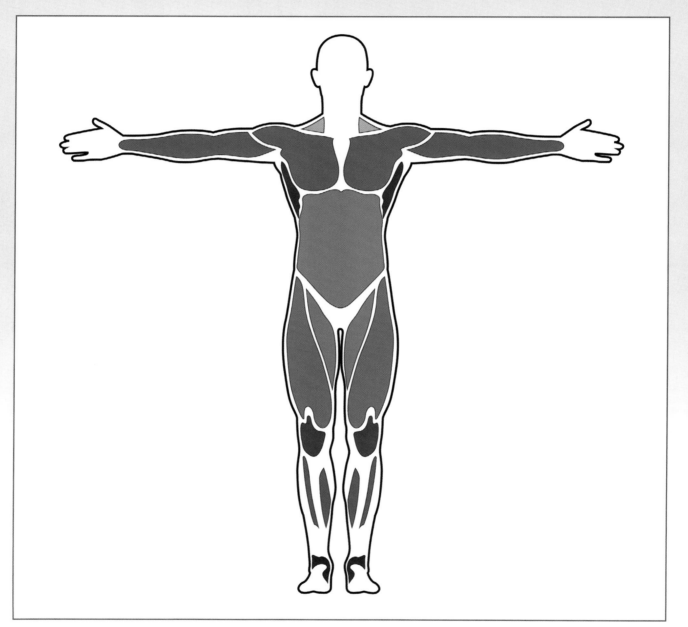

Mobilization Target Areas:

▶ Bottom of the ribcage to the base of the neck and top of the scapula

Most Commonly Used Tools:

▶ Roller
▶ Double Lacrosse Ball
▶ Single Lacrosse Ball
▶ Barbell
▶ Keg

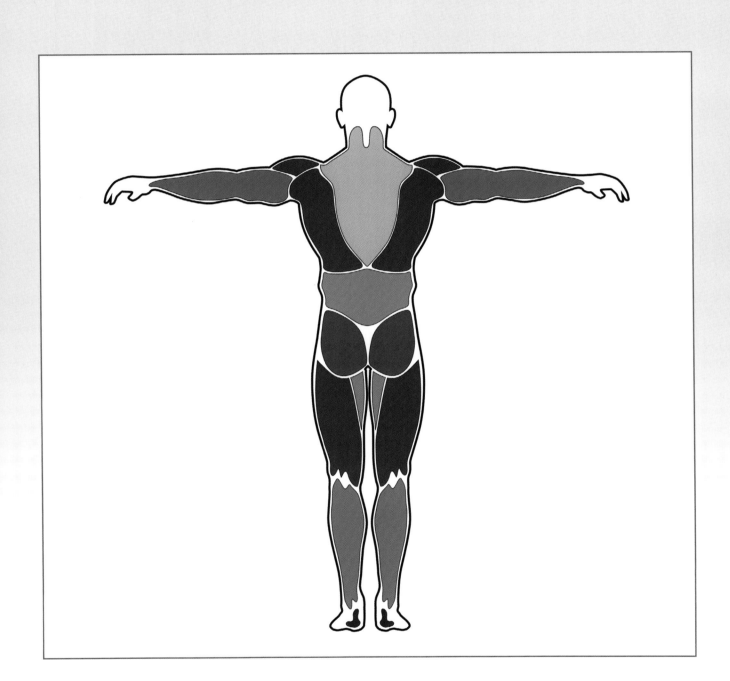

Test and Retest Examples:

- ▶ Overhead Positioning
- ▶ Hanging from the Bar
- ▶ Back Squat Setup
- ▶ Front Rack Position
- ▶ Handstand Pushup
- ▶ Pushup and Bench Press

T-Spine Smash Extension

This is the most basic of all the thoracic-spine mobilization techniques that we use. It is basic thoracic mobility 101.

The t-spine (thoracic) smash is also what we call a "global extension exercise." This means you're not trying to target any one tissue or motion segment as you would when using the double lacrosse ball. Instead, the goal is to open up the entire thoracic system. While a ball is more precise in digging into a tight, nasty spot, the foam roller will tackle two or three motion segments of your back, the rib facet joints, and some soft tissues in the upper back.

The key to this mobilization is to focus on creating large extension forces over the roller by arching back. A common mistake is to mindlessly roll back and forth with zero intention or purpose. This does nothing. At gyms, you often see two people foam rolling aimlessly like this—in the name of a warm-up—while they catch up on a new *Game of Thrones* episode. This does nothing. To make real and lasting change, you have to create as much of a teeter-totter effect and extension force (arching back) over those tissues as possible. When you find a tight area, use the roller as a fulcrum by arching your back. Think about letting the roller break you into extension. You can take a big breath and try to snake your way around, extend back and forth, elevate your hips to add pressure and then lower your butt to the ground. Explore the area, find where your back is tight, and stay on that area it until you've made some change.

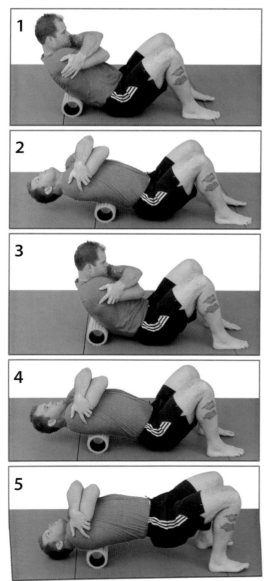

Improves:
- Normal Posture
- Overhead Positioning
- Stable Shoulder Position
- Global Extension and Thoracic Extension

1. To begin, wrap your arms around your chest and position the roller at the base of your ribcage. By wrapping your arms into a big hug, you suck up the slack in your back, pulling all the soft tissue and the scapula out of the way so that you can target the motion segments of your back.

2. With the tissues of the upper back wound up tight, create an extension force over the roller by arching back. From this position, spend as much time as necessary extending over the roller until you feel change in the area.

3. Keeping your arms wrapped tight around your body, sit up as if you were doing a crunch. As you sit up, keep the majority of your weight positioned over the roller, scoot your butt toward your feet, slide your back down the roller, and move on to a new area.

4. Having positioned the roller in the middle of your upper back, arch back and extend over the roller, creating as much extension as possible.

5. As soon as you experience enough change, progress up your spine to the base of your neck. To create additional extension over the roller, squeeze your butt and elevate your hips as you arch back.

T-Spine Smash: Side-to-Side

Sometimes, simply arching over a roller isn't enough to challenge what's most resistant in your signature brand of "tightness." If you stumble across a stiff area that is not responding to the large extension forces, try rolling from side to side across the tissue. This side-to-side smashing allows you to seesaw through some of the soft tissues adjacent to the spine that can limit extension and rotation. If you play golf, tennis, baseball, or engage in any activity that requires you to twist, lock the side-to-side smash into your routine.

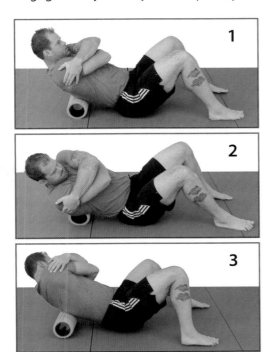

1. Wind up the tissues of your upper back by wrapping your arms around your body, and position the roller at the base of your rib cage.

2. After hunting out a stiff area roll back and forth, making sure to keep your upper back tight. You can twist from your hips or rotate with your entire body. There is no wrong way.

3. Roll across the roller onto your left side. Seesaw back and forth like this until you experience enough change. If you notice that one side is tighter than the other, choose to remain on that side and implement the side roll smash as demonstrated in the next technique.

T-Spine Smash: Side Roll

If you notice one side of your spine is tighter than the other, consider this an alarm that requires urgent response. The stiffer side of your back will impair your ability to rotate on that side. Failure to attack the issue will trigger problems upstream and downstream of the area.

If, for example, you notice the left side of your upper back is tighter than the other, turning onto your side and smashing that area is one way to address the issue. Don't overthink the situation by trying to diagnose the root cause. Just know that the left side should feel like the right side. It's that simple.

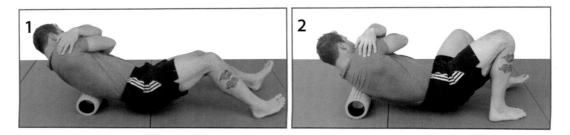

1. If you notice that the left side of your upper back is stiffer than the right, roll onto that side and start slowly rolling up and down the tight area.

2. Roll up and down the side of your back, pressure waving into the tight area. Remember, you're not limited to just rolling up and down. You can pressure wave into the stiffness (which is particularly effective with a rumble roller or double lacrosse ball), or side bend over the area.

T-Spine Smash: Double Lacrosse Ball Variation

Work on the upper back with a roller and you're working the thoracic system in a global way. Working on the upper back with a double lacrosse ball, on the other hand, allows you to localize the target and zero in on one segment at a time. This makes for a more acute thoracic mobilization. What you'll find is that there are usually one or two segments of the vertebra that are responsible for restrictions riddling through the entire back.

There are multiple variations of this technique, as there are with the roller. You can arch your back, elevate your hips and lower them to the ground while arching back, rotate from side to side, raise your arms overhead, or use some combination of all of these. As with all the techniques that I demonstrate, you're not limited to what's shown in the photos.

Improves:
- ▶ Normal Posture
- ▶ Overhead Positioning

Method:
- ▶ Joint Mechanics

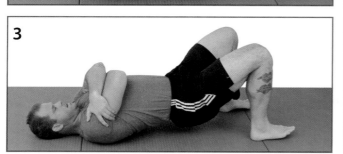

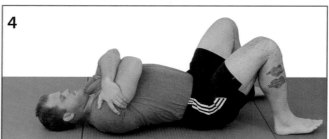

1. Hug your arms around your body to take up slack and move your scapula out of the way. Make sure to nestle the points of the ball in between each vertebral section.

2. After creating tension in your upper back, slowly extend over the lacrosse balls. Because the double lacrosse ball is a more acute fulcrum, you have to keep the base of your ribcage anchored to your pelvis. To avoid overextending your lumbar spine, keep your core engaged.

3. As you arch back, drive your heels into the mat and elevate your hips. To effect change, you can roll from side to side, rotate from your shoulders, and snake around.

4. Still in extension, slowly lower your butt to the mat.

T-Spine Plate Smash

A hard-training athlete is stiff in a more layered and labyrinthine way than your average Joe. So if you're a big strong guy or girl, you probably need to add weight to the double lacrosse ball smash to spur some change. The best way to accomplish this is to position a plate, ideally a 45-pound bumper plate, over your chest and wrap your arms around the outside of the weight. By adding some pressure to your chest, you get the ribs involved, which play a role in t-spine and overhead shoulder mobility. This also forces more downward pressure into the ball, allowing for a more acute and aggressive thoracic mobilization.

Improves:
► Acute T-Spine Stiffness in Athletes

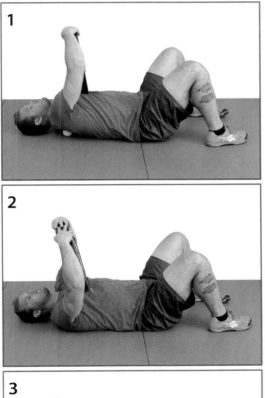

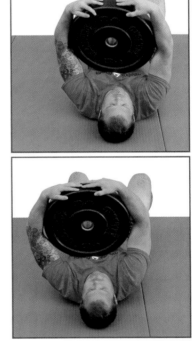

Position a 45-pound bumper plate over your chest and hug your arms around the outside of the weight. By hugging the weight, you pull the soft tissue out of the way, allowing you to focus on the motion segment of your vertebra. Once you have the weight in place and position the lacrosse balls into the motion segments you want to change, arch backward over the balls.

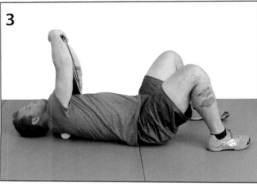

Slowly roll onto your side. Remember, the weight is going to pull you onto your side so you have to go slow and fight that force. For the best results, focus on the motion segments that you're trying to change.

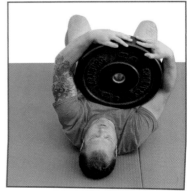

Keeping your arms wrapped tight around the weight, roll toward your right side.

4

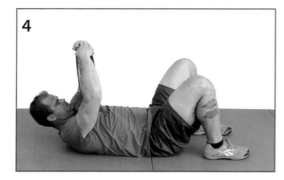

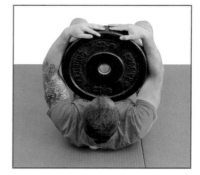

For another stimulus, tilt your ribcage and tuck your chin to your chest as if you were doing a really crappy ab crunch.

5

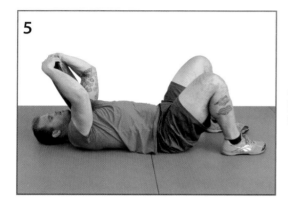

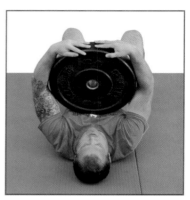

Arch backward. To create additional pressure, tilt the weight toward your face.

T-Spine Smash: Overhead Extension Bias

Although wrapping your arms around your body is a very effective way to improve thoracic mobility, it's specific to your upper back. By reaching your arms overhead, you tie in the shoulder and improve the relationship between shoulder flexion, thoracic extension, and rotation. To help you better understand this, think of a pitcher's fastball, a tennis player's serve, or a volleyball spike. All of these actions require overhead position, thoracic spine extension, and upper body rotation.

Your upper back contains an intricate network of systems that all relate, react, and communicate with each other. Garbled systems in the back can make it difficult to stabilize your shoulders or lift your arms overhead. Hence, if you're trying to improve your overhead position, you need to mobilize around the shape you're trying to change. The t-spine smash with overhead extension bias is a perfect example of this concept.

As a side note, although you can set up for the overhead extension variation from scratch, you don't have to do this mobilization independent of the previous techniques. In other words, you can go from the hug position to arms overhead, back to the hug, back into overhead extension. Just make sure your shoulders are in a stable position and you keep your midline engaged. Be careful that you don't bend your elbows or hinge at the bottom of the thoracic spine. (That's probably the most common error.) Bending your elbows puts your shoulders in an unstable position, while hinging at the bottom of the thoracic spine causes overextension at your lower back. To avoid these faults, you have to fight against the hinge at the junction of your thoracic and lumbar spine by keeping your abs tight and lockout your elbows overhead while actively positioning your armpits forward.

Improves:

- ▶ Overhead Positioning
- ▶ Thoracic Extension
- ▶ Rotation
- ▶ Throwing Mechanics

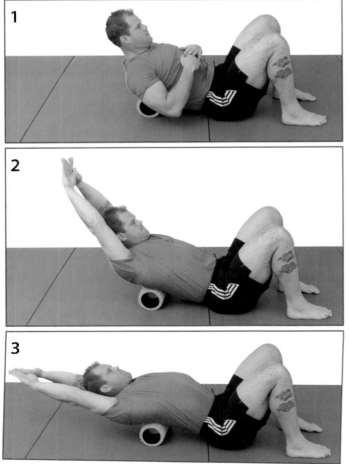

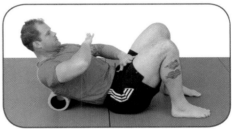

1. Position the base of your ribcage against the roller. While executing this mobilization it's important to remember that raising your arms overhead creates an additional extension force, which can cause you to overextend at the lumbar spine. To avoid this fault, use the two-hand rule to remind yourself to maintain a tight, neutral, and engaged midline.

2. Raise your arms overhead. If you look at the photo, you'll notice that my elbows are locked out, my armpits are forward, and I'm actively reaching toward the ceiling.

3. Keeping your midline engaged and your shoulders in a stable position, arch over the roller.

T-Spine Smash: Lacrosse Ball Extension Bias Variation

This is the same idea in that you're tying in some end-range shoulder flexion with thoracic extension. Instead of mobilizing around multiple motion segments, however, you isolate individual vertebra segments.

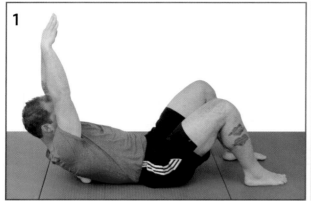

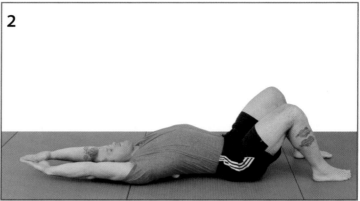

Position the double lacrosse ball into a specific motion segment of your spine and raise your arms overhead. Keep your midline engaged, your elbows locked out, and your armpits facing forward.

Still reaching your arms overhead, extend over the lacrosse ball. From here, you can roll from side to side or elevate your hips to create additional pressure.

T-Spine Smash: Barbell Variation

With the Movement and Mobility System, you're not limited to any one tool. I highly encourage use of everyday items to make good things happen. Enter the barbell. Almost every gym has one lying on the floor so if you don't have access to a double lacrosse ball or pipe, you can use all the variations already demonstrated on the bar. I never want to hear the excuse, "I don't have a lacrosse ball or pipe to roll on so I can't do it." Use your imagination and make use of what's in reach: a dog toy, a rolling pin, whatever. It's all fair game.

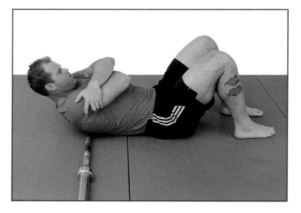

T-Spine Smash: Overhead Extension Bias

If you glance over at the photos, you'll notice that I anchor my hands to a barbell. This can just as easily be the frame of a couch, by the way. Then I lower my hips toward the ground to emphasize extension. Notice I'm using my lower body to create an extension force by bracing my shoulders into a fixed position.

Many people—when they're lying over a roller or lacrosse ball—can't move their arms into a good overhead position and press their hands on the ground due to a lack of mobility. This is why I recommend anchoring your hands to the ground. It facilitates better reach and increases the impact of the exercise.

Let's explore an important concept here. Imagine two exercises that are similar in shape but have a different effect on the system—like the handstand pushup versus the strict-press. Both require a good overhead position, yet each exaggerates a different movement. One begins in the overhead position while the other movement finishes in the overhead position. On paper they appear very similar—but you wouldn't restrict yourself to only one exercise, right? Of course not! All self-respecting athletes and coaches understand the importance of balancing exercises as a means of maximizing performance and health. It's intuitive. However—and here's the message I want you to embrace—when it comes to mobility people tend to get stuck in one dimension.

The point is you have to address both ends of the spectrum in your mobility work. If your goal is to simply improve thoracic extension and bias some arm flexion in the process, the previously demonstrated exercises are great. But if you really want to create change across the entire system, you have to approach your mobilization from both ends—just like you stimulate a multi-dimensional training effect by using both the strict-press and the handstand pushup. For optimal results, you have to balance it out.

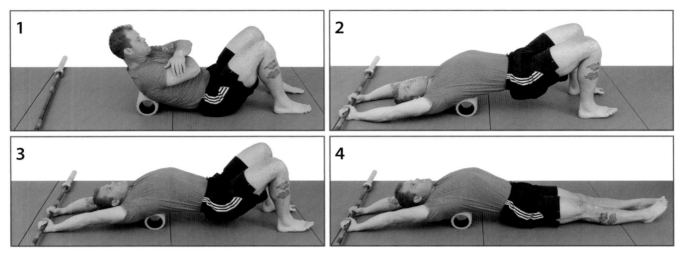

1. To begin, wrap your arms around your body and take up all the slack in your upper back. Once that's accomplished, extend over the roller with your ribcage in line with your pelvis by elevating your hips. Don't arch back into extension.

2. With your hips elevated, anchor your hands to the bar, keeping your elbows locked out and your armpits forward, and then slowly lower your hips toward the ground. The closer you can get your hands together, the better. It's important to notice how this variation allows me to prioritize my overhead positioning and then exaggerate extension with my lower body.

3. Continue to lower your hips toward the ground.

4. As your butt touches down, straighten your legs, anchoring your hips to the ground. From here, you can hang out until you experience some change, or move on to another area. The key is to maintain a good overhead position, keep your midline engaged, and elevate and lower your hips over the fulcrum or hang out in a globally extended position until you effect some change.

T-Spine Smash: Overhead with Extension Bias (Lacrosse Ball Variation)

This is the exactly the same as the t-spine smash overhead with extension bias, but I'm showing it with a double lacrosse ball instead of a roller to better attack specific spots. To get the best result from this mobilization, position the double lacrosse ball in your upper back around the base of your neck.

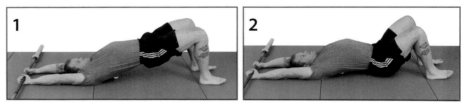

1. Position the lacrosse balls near the base of your neck, elevate your hips off the ground, and anchor your hands to the barbell with your elbows locked out and your armpits forward.

2. Keeping your midline engaged to avoid overextending your lumbar spine, slowly lower your hips to the mat.

T-Spine Keg: Global Extension

Most members of the Supple Legion have a keg lying around the house or gym, which I can appreciate because it serves multiple purposes. You can fill it up with the obvious, or use it as a tool to improve performance: an indisputable double win. For the purposes of this section, you can use it to create a very large global extension of the spine, which is good for two reasons.

First, it allows you to explore global positions that tie in all the motion segments of your vertebra. For example, if you're arching over a foam roller or pipe, you're in global extension, but you're probably only getting two or three motion segments of the spine. When you extend over a keg you're able to explore the relationship of all the motion segments and create a global impact on the spine. A lot of people try to exaggerate this motion in the form of a bridge, which is characterized with sloppy shoulder, back, and hip extension. The keg allows you to focus on the extension without having to strain yourself to maintain a good position.

The second benefit of using a keg is that it opens up the playing field. Often when you're extending over a roller or lacrosse balls, the ground restricts your reach. When you're on a keg or large round surface—like a medicine ball stacked on top of a couple plates—you can get a much larger arch in the tissues you're trying to change.

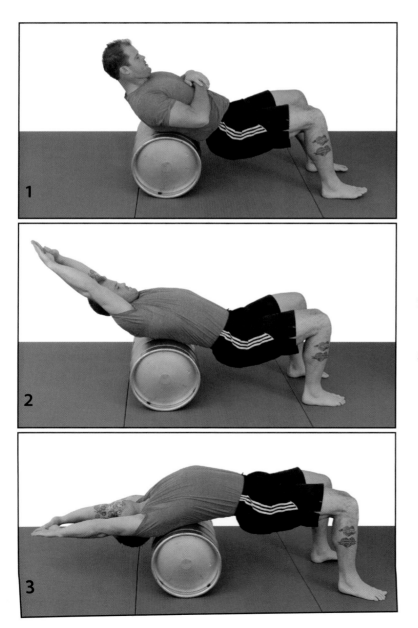

1. Position your back over the keg. Keep your ribcage in line with your pelvis, your midline engaged, and your shoulders in a good position.

2. Reach your arms overhead. (Notice that I place my hands close together, lockout my elbows, and position my armpits forward.)

3. Keeping your shoulders in a stable position with your hands reaching overhead, elevate your hips and extend over the keg.

T-Spine Keg: Overhead Anchor with Extension Bias–Option 1

It's important to remember that you can treat the keg just like the foam roller and implement all the same variations previously demonstrated. So in this sequence, I demonstrate the opposite version of the last technique, which is accomplished by gripping a kettlebell to anchor my hands to the ground and then lowering my hips. Again, because you're a little higher up and not restricted by the ground, you can get a lot more global extension through the spine and shoulders.

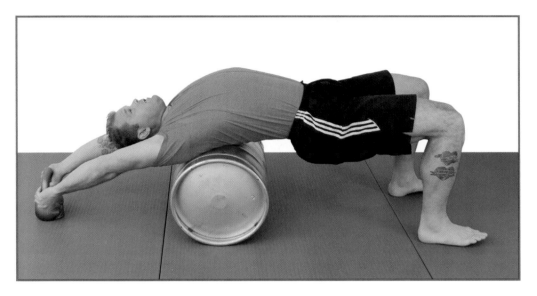

T-Spine Keg: Overhead Anchor with Extension Bias–Option 2

This is the same idea as option 1 but you're adding a little bit of a distraction to the shoulder joint. Although this is a more advanced variation and takes some tinkering to get into the right position, it works wonders. As with all the techniques that require large global extension forces, you have to remain engaged and active. I was working with the Navy, and one of the head instructors (let's call him my big brother) said it best. Pointing to a group of Navy ninjas hanging from a bar with their midline disengaged, he said, "Look at those guys just hanging on their meat." I really think that statement paints a perfect picture of what you *don't* want to do. You never want to hang on your meat. Respect yourself.

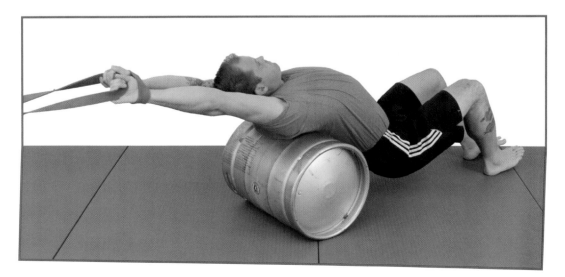

Overhead Rib Mobilization

In addition to restoring motion through your vertebrae, you also want to be sure that your ribs are mobile and supple.

What people forget is your ribs attach on your spine and can have a profound effect on the joint mechanics of the system. So if you have a stiff rib, it not only blocks key motion segments of your thoracic spine, it restricts the resting relationship of your scapula, which dampens the ability to stabilize your shoulders. Here are some very simple mobilizations that can be used to restore suppleness to your ribs.

In the sequence on the next page, I demonstrate one of the most basic and effective techniques for fixing stiff ribs. As you can see from the photos, the mobilization target area is from the second rib up. It extends from the median trap (photo 1) and tracks down the areas bordering the scapula (photo 2). The general prescription is to spend at least thirty seconds or more on each rib and accumulate fifteen to twenty slow arm swings.

As a rule, you always want to spend your time mobilizing the areas that are stiff and restricting movement. However, sometimes you just don't have time to address all of your issues before a workout—like maybe your entire back is a matted-down mess but you only have one minute to warm-up and improve your position for the upcoming workout. In such a situation, it helps to know where you need to spend your time and energy so that you can have the biggest impact on the movement you're going to perform. Naturally, it would be great if you could deal with all of your issues, but you only have so much time to fix yourself. That's why you have to break it up into calculated chunks. Here's what I suggest:

If you're going to do anything overhead, focus your attention on the upper ribs. If you're doing anything that requires extension or internal rotation like the dip, bench press, or pushup, focus your attention on the lower ribs. The reasons are simple. If you have a shoulder impingement that is preventing you from getting your arm into a stable overhead position, chances are good that you're scapula is locked in place, blocking the path of your moving arm. Although all the ribs that border the scapula are implicated, the upper ribs tend to impede upward elevation to a higher degree. In such a situation, starting in the median trap and working your way down is probably your best bet. Conversely, if you're doing a workout that requires a lot of extension and internal rotation of the shoulder, you may want to start lower on the ribcage because stiff lower ribs can act like a strut that limits good scapular positioning.

Organizing the Scapula

A lot of coaches, athletes, and physical therapists seem to think that an impingement of the shoulder automatically means a rotator cuff issue. Here's what's really happening: When your scapula is in a disorganized position, it turns your rotator cuff off. So if someone tells you that your rotator cuff isn't working correctly, that's an indication that you probably need to restore the scapula position so that your rotator turns back on.

If you start at the top of the scapula, place the ball between your shoulder blade and spine. Now bridge your butt up as high as possible, driving the ball deep into your soul, and reach your arm overhead. Keep your elbow locked out. Now draw your arm across your body and try to touch your opposite hip. Those rhomboids, traps, and para-spinals get really tight. Bringing your arm across your body is a great way to unglue them. As you work your way down the border of your scapula, you can continue to swing your arm overhead as described and illustrated in the photos. If you're trying for bias extension and internal rotation, on the other hand, the next technique will have a more beneficial impact on the tissues you're trying to change.

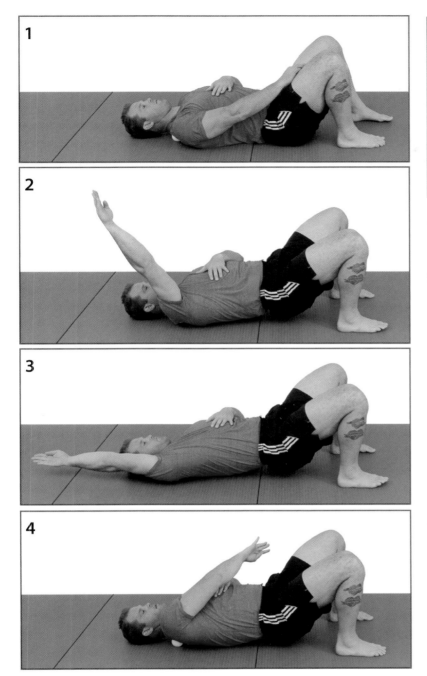

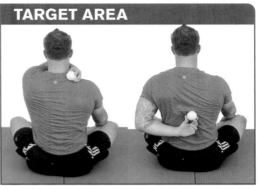

TARGET AREA

1. Position the lacrosse ball in the area bordering your scapula, between your right shoulder blade and spine.

2. To create additional pressure, drive your heels into the mat and elevate your hips. As you do this, reach your hand toward the ceiling, lockout your elbow, and pull your arm overhead. Remember, you want to keep your shoulder in a stable position so don't bend your elbow or internally rotate your arm as you go overhead. If you default into a bent arm, internally rotated position, stop. That's your end-range. Bending your elbow is a pathognomonic cue that you're missing internal rotation of the shoulder.

3. Keeping your elbow locked out, push your arm up overhead.

4. With your hips still elevated, bring your right arm across your body and try to touch your opposite hip. By bringing your hand across your body with a straight arm, you take up the soft tissue slack and bias further excursion (more movement) of your shoulder blade. The idea is to have that shoulder come as far off your scapula as possible so you can to get maximum range in the tissues.

T-Spine Smash: Internal Rotation

Stiff lower ribs have a profound impact on your ability to stabilize your scapula in moments of extension and internal rotation. Think about it like this: If your lower ribs are stiff, that means the tissues between your lower rhomboids are trapped and the tissues between your scapula and spine are not relating well with each other. The result: You experience a diminished capacity to maintain a stable shoulder when you're doing anything that requires extension and internal rotation of the shoulder. For example, if you're bench pressing, dipping, or Olympic lifting (I am referring specifically to the high-hang position) with stiff lower ribs, you'll find it extremely difficult to maintain control of your scapula. Once you lose scapular control, you automatically default into an internally rotated, shoulders-rolled-forward position. You lose power, bleed torque, and increase susceptibility to injury. Not good! To ensure you can maintain control of that scapula to stabilize your shoulders through movement, you have to restore suppleness to those stiff ribs and tissues, which is exactly what this mobilization aims to fix.

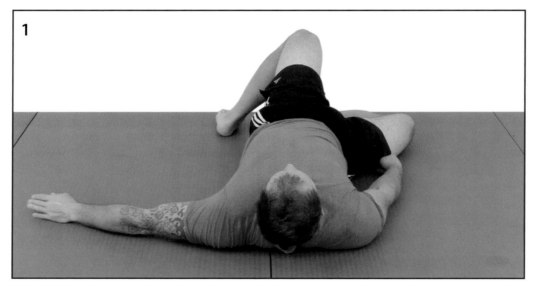

Position the lacrosse ball in your lower ribs between the base of your scapula and spine. Notice that I'm basing out on my left hand and rotating my hips toward my right side.

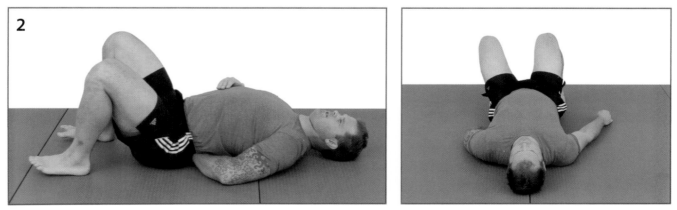

Keeping the ball in place, slide your left hand underneath your lower back and drop your left hip to the mat.

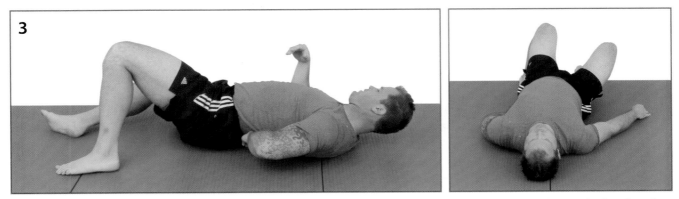

3

With your arm pinned behind your back, rotate toward your right side, focusing on driving the ball into the border of your scapula.

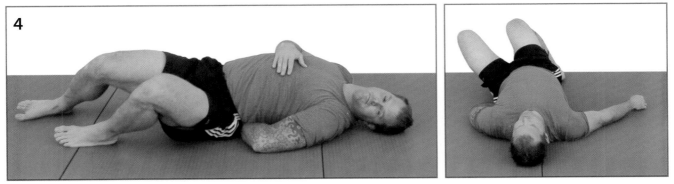

4

Rotate toward your left side. From here, you can hunt around for tight corners by moving your body up and down, driving the lacrosse ball into the border of your depressed scapula. Really work on restoring sliding surfaces to the stiff tissues surrounding the ribs.

First Rib Mobilization

Let's say you're someone who works at a computer all day with poor posture. Or maybe you've been doing some overhead movement with screwy positions. What can happen is your shoulder and surrounding tissues will shorten, causing your first rib to stiffen.

The first rib functions like a pump handle. To go overhead, you need that first rib to glide down as you elevate your arm. If that first rib is stiff, an impingement is created that undermines shoulder stability, making you look like a zombie when you reach upward.

To address this issue, you first have to locate the first rib, which is the bony structure between your collarbone and the base of your trap and neck. Do this by sliding your hand down the base of your neck and pressing straight down into your trap (see photo 1). If you do this, you'll always hit the first rib. Once you've located the target area, pin a PVC pipe or dowel against the wall, lie on the ground, and position an end of the pipe into the first rib. The goal is to create a depression on the first rib by driving your body upward into the pipe. Once you've accomplished that, work to restore suppleness by moving your arm overhead, oscillating your arm back and forth, or by taking in a big breath and driving your body into the pipe. The key is to not just hang out and suffer, but to get as much motion at the first rib as possible.

If you're a tactical athlete who has to pack around 50 to 100 pounds of gear, put a gold star next to this mobilization and place it near the center of your mobility target. Think: The weight of your pack is bearing down on your neck and shoulder, pressing into the first rib. In addition to getting brutally tight, the motion segment gets jammed into the nerves coming out of your neck. No wonder your hands are numb and you can barely raise your arm overhead. By attacking the first rib, you can restore normal function to the scapula.

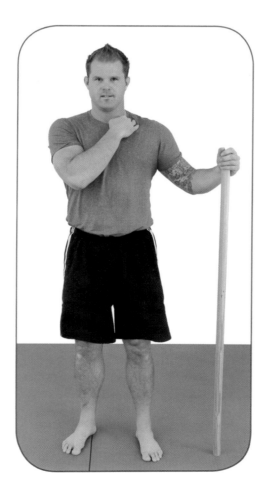

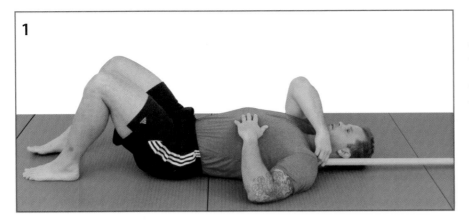

Jam a wooden dowel (you can probably find one of these in your closet) into a corner and position it on your first rib. To create a depression on the area and tack-down your first rib, take a big breath in, drive your heels into the ground, and slide your body toward the wall above you. Alternately, you can also use a PVC pipe with a towel wrapped around the end.

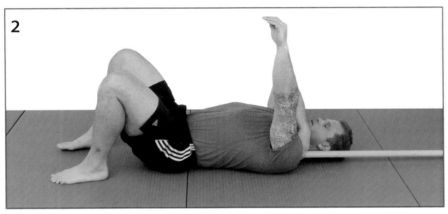

Keeping the dowel pinned in place, straighten your arm over your head. If you run into a barrier as you raise your arm, oscillate back and forth and try to get as much excursion through the tissues as possible.

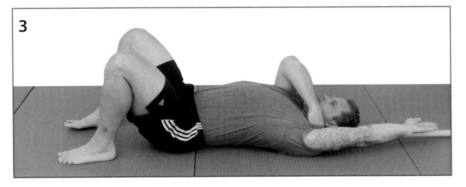

With your elbow locked out, reach your arm straight overhead. From here, you can continue to lower and raise your arm, you can work to elevate your shoulder, or bring your arm underneath your body, as illustrated in photo 4.

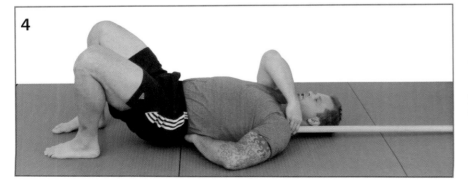

To hit some additional corners, position your hand underneath your body while continuing to scoot toward the wall.

AREA 2
POSTERIOR SHOULDER
(LAT, POSTERIOR DELTOID)

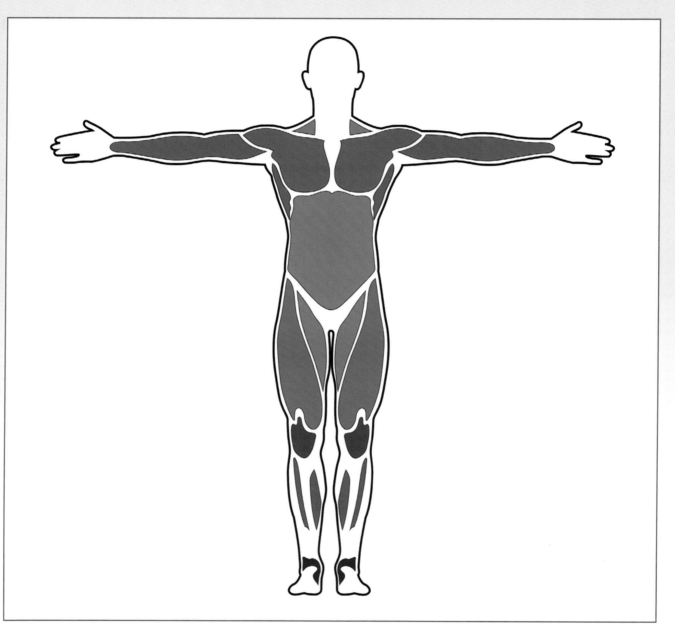

Mobilization Target Areas:

▶ The back of the shoulder, border of the scapula, insertion of the lat

Most Commonly Used Tools:

▶ Single Lacrosse Ball

▶ Rogue Monster Band

▶ Roller

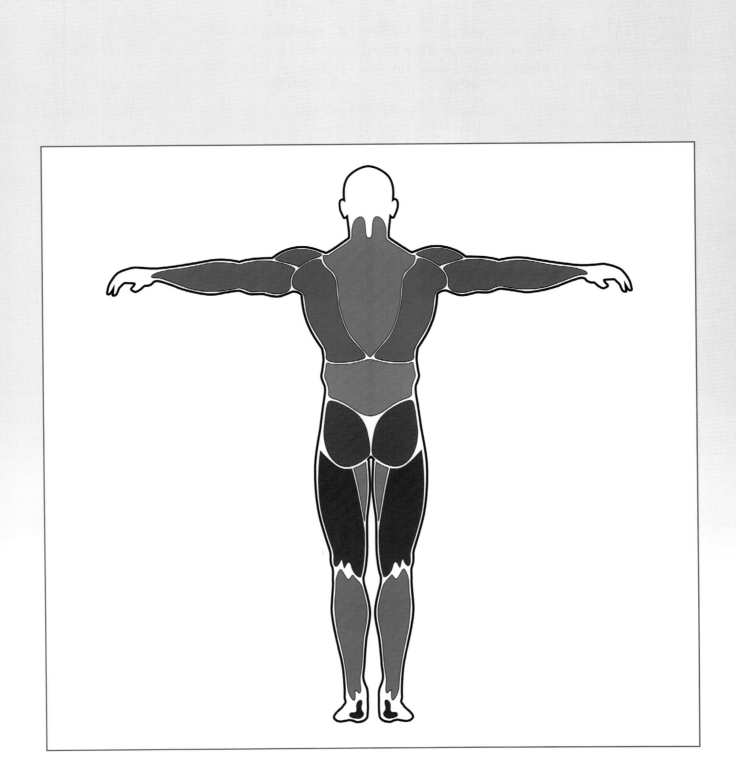

Test and Retest Examples:

- ▶ Overhead Press
- ▶ Hanging from the Bar
- ▶ Back Squat Setup
- ▶ Front Rack Position
- ▶ Pushup and Bench Press

Shoulder Rotator Smash and Floss

If you've tuned into Mobilitywod.com or attended one of my seminars, you've inevitably heard me refer to the forward-rolled shoulder as the dreaded douche bag shoulder position. Why? Have you ever seen "that guy" walking around with his shoulders forward and his chest puffed out in an attempt to look jacked and tough? Of course you have. And I'd be willing to bet that the first thing that ran through your mind was probably something along the lines of: "Damn that guy looks like a giant douche bag." Hence, douche bag shoulders.

It's important to mention that if your shoulders are rolled forward because you sit at a desk all day with bad posture, or you're a cyclist who is constantly stuck in a rounded position, it doesn't mean you're a douche bag, it just means you have douche bag shoulders. The problem with douche bag shoulder syndrome is that a forward-rolled shoulder is an unstable position that limits your capacity to create external rotation torque, which, as you know, is a mechanism for dysfunctional movement patterns, force dumps, torque bleeds, etc. Not only that, when you hang out in an internally rotated position, the external rotators of the shoulder get overstretched, brittle, and extremely stiff, which can lead to acute shoulder pain.

Fortunately, restoring suppleness to the area and relieving pain is very simple. All you need is a hard ball, ideally a lacrosse ball, and you can effectively unglue these tissues that are compromising your mechanics, causing you pain, and making you look douchey.

What you have to remember is the human body has a lot of big muscles that have an internal rotational effect. Very few have an external rotation effect. You cannot afford to put those external rotators into a position where they become ineffective. Put another way, if you've rendered your external rotators impotent by your douche bag shoulder position, you're going to have shoulder pain and probably injure the rotator cuff. This is why when someone comes up to me and says, "I have shoulder pain," I'll immediately ask them if they've smashed the back of their rotators yet. If the answer is No, I tell them, "Go and hit this mobilization and tell me how you feel." In most cases, just a few minutes of smashing will relieve shoulder pain and reduce the douche-ness of your shoulder position. It makes a gigantic difference.

Improves:
▶ Internal and External Rotation
▶ Torque Capacity
▶ Douche Bag Shoulder Syndrome

Methods:
▶ Smash and Floss
▶ Contract and Relax

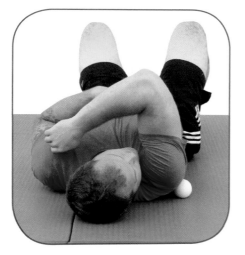
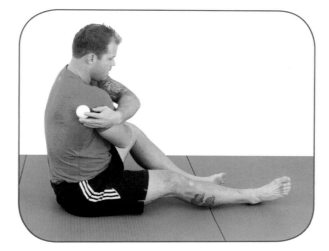

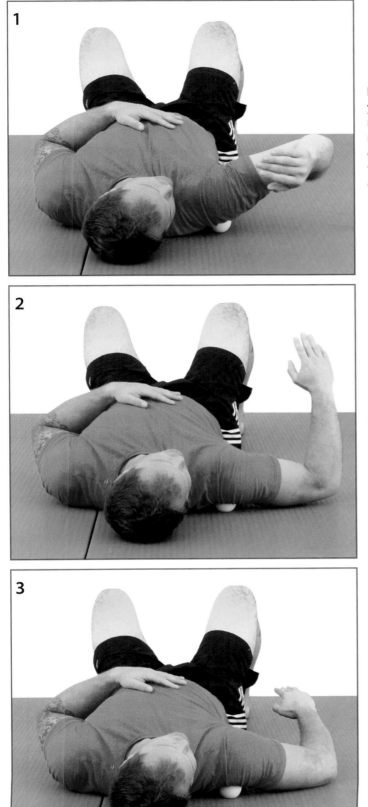

1

Position a lacrosse ball right above the insertion of your lat near your armpit. This is where the external rotators insert behind your shoulder. It's important to note that there's no right or wrong way. The goal is to get some pressure on the ball so if you want something a little bit more aggressive, roll onto your side to get some additional weight over your shoulder.

2

With the tissue behind your shoulder tacked-down, rotate your hand toward the ground.

3

Internally rotate your arm until you reach your end-range. From here, you can continue to move you hand back and forth.

Shoulder Capsule Mobilization

One of the issues of being a modern human is that we end up living in the front of the shoulder capsule. If you're someone who spends any amount of time driving, working in front of the computer, or doing anything that the typical modern human does, chances are good that your shoulders have been resting in the front of your capsule to such an extent that your posterior shoulder capsule gets extremely tight. This not only makes it difficult to pull your shoulders to the back of the socket, but also causes you to lose the capacity to generate effective rotation of the shoulder. To fix this issue, you have to set the shoulder to the back of the socket so that you can effectively mobilize the posterior capsule.

It's important to note that people have been trying to solve this issue of posterior stiffness for some time. The classic shoulder stretch where you pull your arm across your body is something that you always see athletes do, almost instinctually, as a way to mobilize their posterior shoulder capsule (photo 1). What they're really doing is just causing an impingement in their shoulder, which leads to more problems. Do you really think that rolling your shoulder forward into a crappy position and then pulling it across your body is going to help you? Of course not! Mobilizing in a compensated position is never okay. If you want to make change in the posterior capsule, you have to set your shoulder in a good position first, and then pull across (photo 2).

The problem is this: If you've been hanging out in the front of your capsule, or you strained or tweaked your shoulder, there's a good chance that your posterior capsule is tight. In such a situation, setting your shoulder to the back of the socket, which is the stable position of the joint, is difficult. This is where the shoulder capsule mobilization comes into play. By using a heavy kettlebell, you can effectively drive that shoulder to the back of the socket and then bias or encourage the tissues into external rotation. This resets the shoulder into a good position, stretches the posterior capsule, and accounts for the passive accessory motion of the joint. In addition, the act of externally rotating gives you some neuromuscular cuing (think breaking the bar), which transfers over to many of the midrange pressing skills (bench press, pushup).

Improves:

▶ Shoulder Position   ▶ Recovery After a Shoulder Tweak   ▶ Midrange Pressing Mechanics

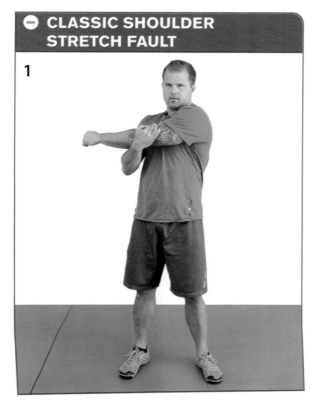

● CLASSIC SHOULDER STRETCH FAULT

1

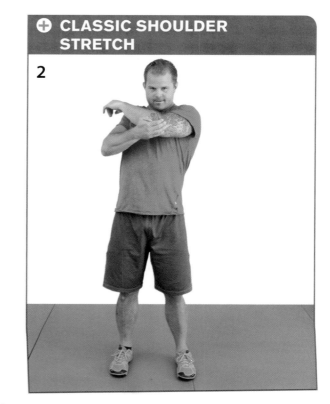

⊕ CLASSIC SHOULDER STRETCH

2

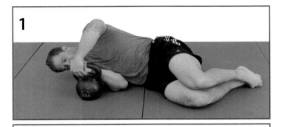

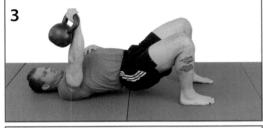

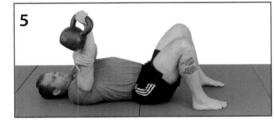

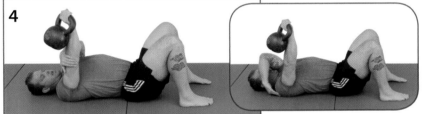

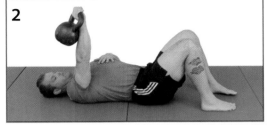

1. Position the kettlebell next to your right shoulder and latch on to the handle with your knuckles facing the ground. Notice that I'm gripping the top of the handle with my left hand.

2. Roll onto your back and pull the kettlebell over your right shoulder while simultaneously pressing it into extension.

3. To set your shoulder to the back of your socket, elevate your hips, move your shoulder blades out of the way, and pull your right shoulder to the mat. This is very similar, if the not the same setup, that you would do for a bench press or floor press.

4. Keeping your midline engaged and your shoulder positioned to the back of your socket, lower your hips to the ground. Note there should be no space between your shoulder and the mat. To keep your elbow locked out and your arm straight, reach your left arm across your chest and cup the back of your elbow.

5. With your shoulder pulled to the back of your capsule, externally rotate your hand. Continue to internally and externally rotate your arm to restore normal function to your shoulder.

If your posterior capsule is extremely tight, it can be difficult to fully reset your shoulder into a good position using the classic mobilization. In such a situation, add a lateral distraction to open up the tissues so that you can let your shoulder sink into the back of the capsule.

DISTRACTION VARIATION

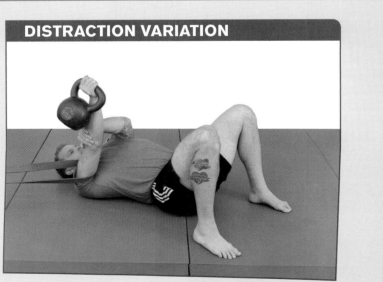

Super-D Shoulder Capsule Mob

This is a variation that I stole from Donnie Thompson, the world's mightiest powerlifter. It emphasizes setting your shoulder to the back of the socket, like the other techniques in this section. But what's great about Donnie's piece is the simplicity. Manipulating a heavy kettlebell into the press position can be sketchy if you don't know what you're doing. With Donnie's variation, you can safely and effectively handle much larger forces without lifting any weight. This is particularly useful if you're really tight or you're a big strong guy like Donnie who needs several hundred pounds of tension to get the shoulder to drop into the right position.

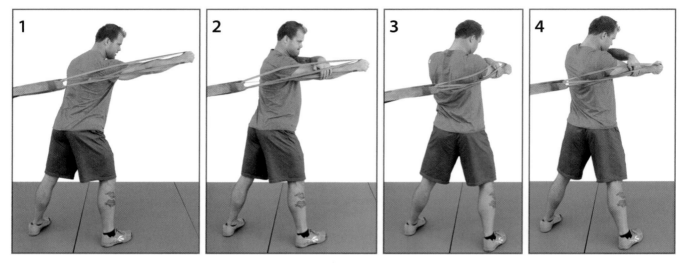

1. Punch the Rogue monster band out and create tension by walking forward.

2. After you've created a monster amount of stretch in the band, reach across your body and cup your left hand over the back of your right elbow. This prevents your arm from bending. Then, let the tension pull your shoulder into the back of your socket. Note this may take some time. Your instincts tell you to fight against the band, but you have to get your shoulder blade out of the way and let your arm sink back.

3. With your shoulder pinned in the back of your socket, rotate your body 90-degrees in a counterclockwise direction, wrapping the band around your body. This adds additional pressure and locks your shoulder into a good position.

4. From here, add rotation by externally and internally rotating your hand. Remember, you want to keep your arm straight and your shoulder back. Don't fight against the band. Just let it pull your shoulder into the right position and then add some rotation.

Overhead Tissue Smash–Option 1

Whenever possible, you want to mobilize in a position that looks similar in shape to the movement or position you're trying to change. For example, if you're trying to improve your overhead position, it makes sense to put your arm overhead and mobilize anything that might be limiting your range. In most cases, what you'll find is that the underarm region, which is where the lat and rotator cuff insert into the armpit, is really stiff and grotty. The approach is simple. If you can't get your arm overhead, or you're having overhead pain, just ask yourself: What are the tissues that are limiting that overhead position? Put your arm overhead, lie on a ball, and start hunting for tight corners. Chances are, you'll find something that is really stiff and painful.

Improves:
- Overhead Positioning
- Shoulder Pain

Methods:
- Contract and Relax
- Pressure Wave
- Smash and Floss

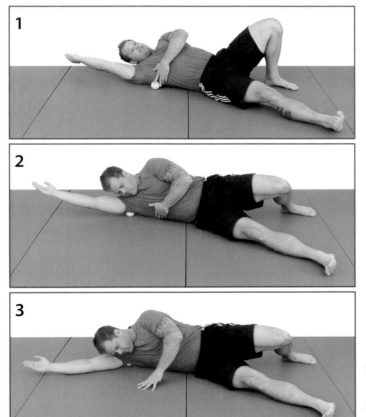

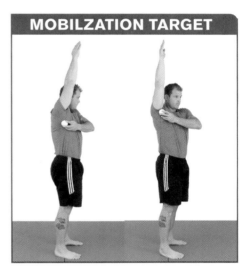

1. Position the lacrosse ball in your armpit near the insertion of your lat and rotator cuff.

2. Roll slowly onto your right side, smashing the underlying tissues.

3. Pressure more weight into the ball and slowly oscillate around the armpit area.

Overhead Tissue Smash–Option 2

Another way to bias the overhead tissue smash is to pin a lacrosse ball or softball against a wall. The target area is the same, but executing the mobilization from the standing position allows you to get deeper into the tight tissues of the lat. In addition, standing gives you a little more range to flex the arm, which not only takes up soft tissue slack, but also allows for a different flossing stimulus.

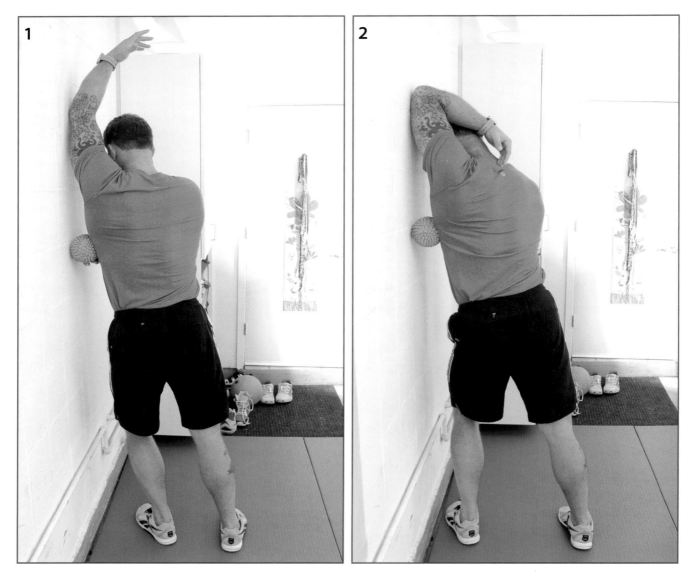

1. Straighten your arm overhead, place the ball on an area of stiff lat tissue using your opposite hand, and pressure your weight into the ball to pin it in place.

2. From here, you can pressure wave from side to side, contract and relax, and smash and floss by bending your arm.

Overhead Tissue Smash–Option 3

There are two main templates when it comes to dealing with sliding surface dysfunction. One is to go after it with a ball, which is the equivalent of having someone drive a thumb, knuckle, or elbow into the tissue. The second is to implement a roller, pipe, or larger object, something comparable to a palm or fist. The former is more of a trigger point approach that targets specific tissues, and the latter is a broad compression surface that ties in larger sections. Both are useful, but they have a different impact on the tissue you're trying to mobilize. In this sequence, I attack the overhead position with a roller for a global smash effect.

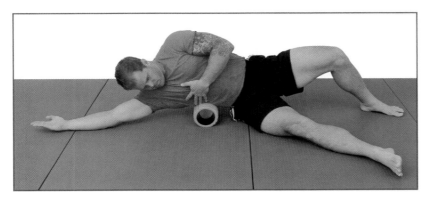

Position the roller on your lat. To mobilize the tissue, slowly slide your body down the roller until you encounter a tight spot. From there, you can contract and relax, roll from side to side, and flex your arm overhead.

Banded Overhead Distraction

If you've ruled out motor-control as a limiting factor in going overhead, you automatically know that you have a mobility obstacle working against you. The template for improving the overhead position is a no-brainer: Simply mobilize the tissues you're trying to change while practicing the movement. Although this is an easy enough concept to grasp, people still seem to get it wrong. If you ask someone who is missing overhead range how much time they've spent mobilizing overhead, they can usually only count the seconds, not the minutes, that they've accumulated in that position.

An example:

Athlete: "Coach! I'm having trouble in the bottom of the squat."

Me: "Did you mobilize in the bottom position?"

Athlete: "Sure, I did some air squats. That counts, right?"

Me: "Your butt only touched the bottom position for .1 seconds for every squat. So no, that doesn't count. Maybe try this: Drop into the bottom position and actually spend some real time mobilizing in the position that is giving you trouble."

Although this would seem obvious, it's not intuitive to people. When I see someone who is missing overhead range, this is one of the first mobilizations I prescribe because it forces him or her to spend a great deal time under tension while working at end-range.

To correctly perform this mobilization, make sure you create external rotation torque by turning your palm up prior to loading up the shoulder. You can do this by either grabbing your thumb and forcing your palm up, or having a Superfriend do a jiu-jitsu wristlock on you, putting your wrist into an externally rotated position. Far too many people just grab the band and distract their arm overhead. This does not account for full range-of-motion! You're just hanging on your meat. Remember, full-range is not putting your arm overhead. That's still an unstable position. Full range-of-motion means you can put your arm overhead to its end-range with rotational capacity.

Improves:

▶ Overhead Positioning

▶ External Rotational Capacity

Methods:

▶ Contract and Relax

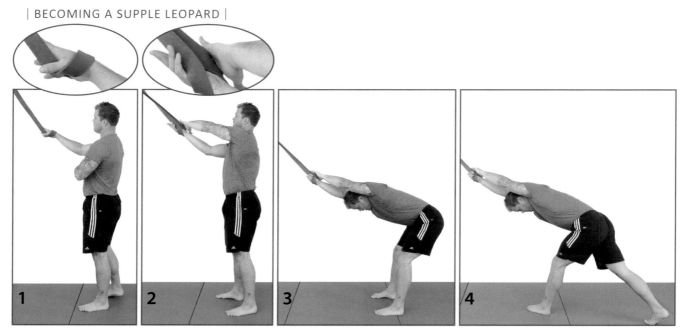

1. Hook your wrist through the band and grab both ends. Don't make the mistake of latching on to the end of the band!

2. Use your opposite hand to bias your right arm into external rotation so that your palm is facing up and your thumb is pointing toward the outside of your body.

3. Keep your arm locked in an externally rotated position. Create tension by sinking your hips back and lowering your torso toward the ground. With your arm externally rotated in the overhead position, contract and relax and try to distract the shoulder into new end-ranges.

4. After spending some time in the first position, start hunting around for some stiff areas. For example, I start by throwing my right leg behind me, which lengthens that fascial line, increasing the aggressiveness of the stretch. The key is to keep your right palm up and your thumb out as you explore.

Overhead with External Rotation Bias

This mobilization is a companion piece to the Banded Overhead Distraction. As you can see from the photos, your elbow is fixed and being held with the band, allowing you to plumb a deeper range of shoulder flexion as compared to the banded overhead distraction. Put simply, you change the dynamics of the shoulder by changing the position. It's like one of them is a barbell push-press and the other is a handstand pushup. They're very similar, but give you a very different stimulus.

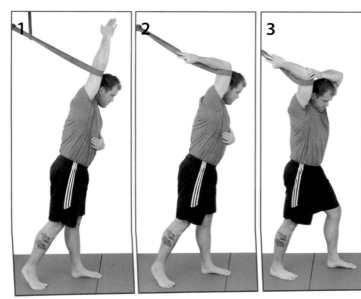

Improves:
- Overhead Positioning
- External Rotation Torque of the Shoulder

Methods:
- Contract/Relax

1. Punch your arm through the band and hook the strap around your elbow.

2. With the band distracting your arm, latch on to the outside of the band using your right hand. The key here is to keep your ribcage down with a tightly engaged midline.

3. To add more tension and increase the aggressiveness of this mobilization, grab the back of your elbow, pull it toward your head, and lower your elevation. As you do this, fight to maintain external rotation torque.

Bilateral Shoulder Flexion

This is another fantastic mobilization that improves your overhead positioning as well as midrange flexion movements like the bench press or pushup. What's different is you're bringing your arms closer to your center-line and then adding external rotation. The rotation helps tie in the posterior shoulder capsule. So unlike the previous mobilizations, which highlight end-range flexion and then add external rotation, you bias end-range external rotation first and then add flexion as a tensioner.

To hit the ugly corners of your external rotators, you want to create as much torque as possible, which is accomplished by keeping your elbows close together.

Here's why: As you apply tension to the load, your elbows spread apart. You can't help it. There is so much torque that when you apply tension to the position, your elbows go wide and torque is lost. To help you make the connection, imagine someone pressing a heavy load overhead with his or her elbows out. If you've read the previous chapter, you know that this is a huge torque dump. The same thing is happening here. As your elbows go wide, you bleed out torque and the stretch becomes less intense.

To prevent your elbows from spreading, have a Superfriend block your elbows together, or wrap your arms up with a band—see banded distraction variation.

Improves: Methods:

▶ Overhead Positioning   ▶ External Rotation Torque   ▶ Contract and Relax

▶ Bench Press and Pushup   ▶ Front Rack Position

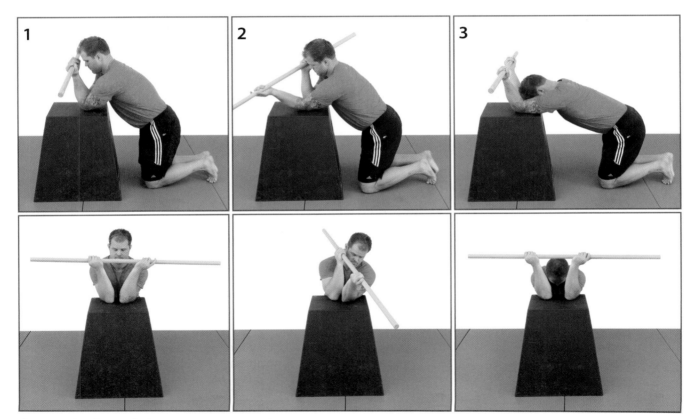

1. Kneel in front of a box with your palms facing toward your body and your elbows positioned next to each other.

2. Keeping your elbows as close as possible, rotate the dowel and spread your hands apart until you reach end-range external rotation.

3. With your shoulders wound up into an externally rotated position, apply tension to the load by pushing your body back and dropping your elevation. This hits all the big soft tissue of the lat, as well as the external rotational features of your shoulder.

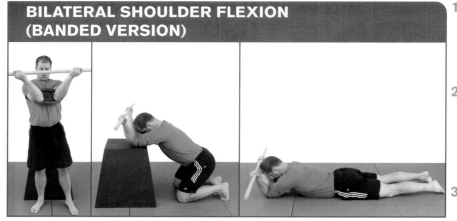

BILATERAL SHOULDER FLEXION (BANDED VERSION)

1. Wrap a band into three loops, hook it around your elbows, and then bias external rotation by twisting a dowel and spreading your hands apart.

2. With the band preventing your elbows from spreading, you can implement the same strategy with the box by sinking your hips back and punching your head through your arms.

3. You can do the same mobilization on the ground.

Super Front Rack

The super front rack is my go-to mobilization for improving the overhead position and more specifically (to state the insanely obvious) the front rack position. The key to this technique is to keep your hand up and your elbow in while you're in the position. You'll find as you step through and create tension, your hand will turn down and your elbow will fly out to the side, which are two ways you lose torque. This fault also makes it difficult to maintain a neutral position. When you try to create tension off an unstable shoulder, it's much easier to break into overextension. The exact same thing happens in the front rack position, when athletes fail to create a stable platform. They can't get their elbows up because their shoulders are douched, so they have to overextend to maintain an upright position. To avoid these faults, try to exaggerate the hand up position, use your opposite hand on your elbow to prevent it from flying out, and stay integrated as you walk out to create tension.

Improves:
▶ Overhead Positioning ▶ Front Rack Positioning

Methods:
▶ Contract and Relax

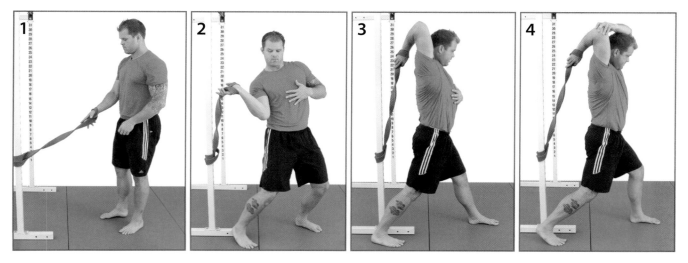

1. Hook your wrist through the band.

2. Turn your palm up and wind your shoulder into external rotation. As you do this, step through, rotating your body underneath the band as if you were setting up for a Judo throw.

3. Keeping your palm up, maneuver your shoulder underneath the band and stand upright to create tension. Note that I squeeze my right glute and keep my abs turned on to avoid breaking into overextension.

4. Still fighting to keep your right palm up, grab the outside of your right elbow using your opposite hand (this prevents your arm from flying out to the side) and shift your weight forward.

Classic Triceps and Lat Stretch

Let me ask you something: When is the last time you spent a significant amount of time smashing and mobilizing your triceps? Wait. I already know the answer. Never.

This is a classic triceps stretch that hits the long head of the triceps and the lats, and some of the structures that limit overhead movement across the shoulder. To make this mobilization even more effective, wrap a voodoo band around your upper arm and floss your triceps as demonstrated below. Guaranteed, voodoo banding and flossing your triceps will bring new life into an area that has probably been neglected for your whole life.

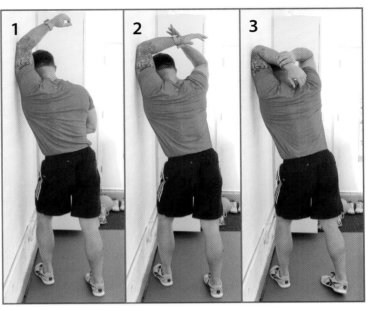

1. Position your distal triceps and elbow against the wall.

2. Drive your weight into the wall, creating a stretch through the long head of your triceps, and latch on to your left wrist with your right hand.

3. Still leaning into the wall, force your left arm into flexion by pushing your left hand toward your left shoulder. **Note:** If you can do this with a voodoo band, it increases the mobilization's effectiveness by a hundred, maybe more.

Reverse Sleeper Stretch

We all have busy lives so we have to find ways to mobilize and improve positions when we're jammed into a 737 window seat, or sitting at the office, and so on. In this sequence, I demonstrate a very low-tech and highly versatile way to work on the internal rotation of your shoulder. This is my car/airplane/trapped-in-a-chair internal rotation stretch. It's something I've done for a long time and still do to this day. An oldie but goodie.

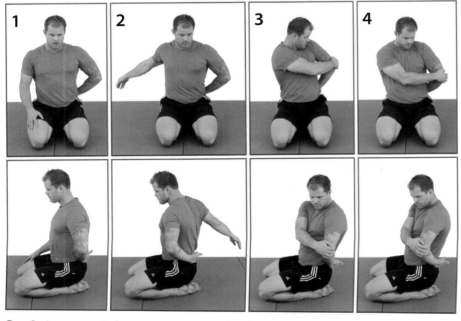

1. To begin, pull your left shoulder into a tight position and then place your left hand with your palm facing away behind your lower back.

2. Cock your right arm back. Sometimes reaching across your body is difficult with your arm behind your back. If you feel you're going to round forward and compromise your posture to grab your shoulder, cock your arm back and swing it across your body as demonstrated here.

3. Swing your right arm across your body, grab your left elbow, and pull it toward your centerline to bias more internal rotation. As you pull your arm across, really focus on keeping your shoulder back. If you let your shoulder roll forward into a compensated position, you'll create an impingement and lose the effectiveness of the stretch.

AREA 3
ANTERIOR SHOULDER
(PEC, ANTERIOR DELTOID)

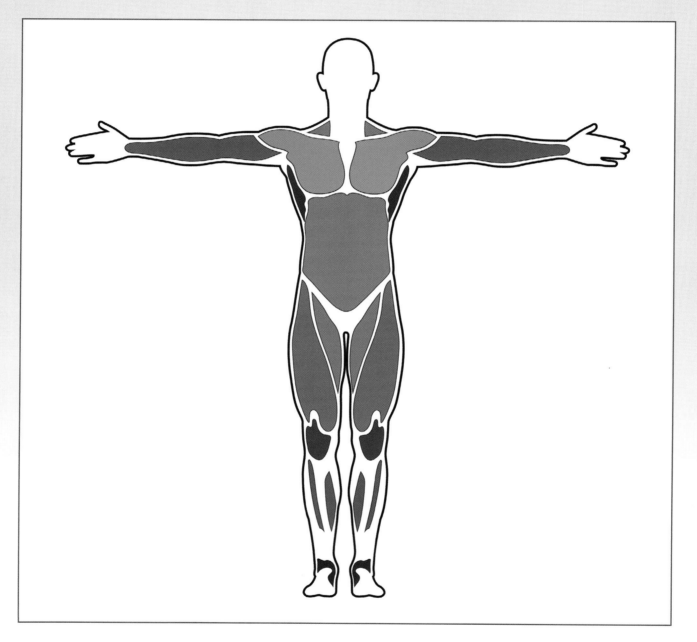

Mobilization Target Areas:

▶ Anterior and lateral shoulder, deltoid, chest, biceps.

Most Commonly Used Tools:

▶ Single Lacrosse Ball
▶ Softball
▶ Voodoo Band
▶ Rogue Monster Band
▶ Barbell
▶ Roller

Test and Retest Examples:

▶ Dip
▶ Overhead Press
▶ Hanging from the Bar
▶ Back Squat Setup
▶ Front Rack Position
▶ Pushup and Bench

Anterior Compartment Smash

Athletes report to me all the time that they still have a hard time getting their shoulder into a good position, even after attacking the thoracic spine and posterior structures. What they forget is that the condition of the anterior compartment can do as much to limit a good shoulder position as the condition of the scapula, ribs, and thoracic spine. It's an interconnected system. If any of the tissues that attach to the shoulder blade get tight and short, it will restrict your ability to put your shoulders in a stable position. For example, if you sit at a desk all day, or spend a lot of time in a car, or you're a cyclist, or you're simply missing internal rotation, chances are good that you spend a lot of time in a forward shoulder position. While this compensated position wreaks havoc on the thoracic spine, scapula, and ribs, your pec minor, which goes from your shoulder blade to your sternum, gets brutally stiff, effectively locking your shoulder into an unstable position.

This is a huge problem because now your arm has to internally rotate as a way to stabilize your shoulder and rectify your limited range. It's your body's way of dealing with the open circuit of an unstable shoulder. Internally rotating is less of a liability than having your shoulder flop around in the socket. So if you spend any amount of time under load or tension in that compensated position, your pec minor has to work really hard to keep your shoulder stable, causing it to get chronically tight as a result.

In the subsequent mobilizations, I demonstrate a couple of methods for restoring suppleness to the area. It's important to note that you can also perform the anterior compartment smash in a doorway. This variation gives you a slightly different stimulus because you're free to the move your arm in some new vectors, allowing you to hit some nasty corners that are unavailable to you using the techniques demonstrated below.

Improves:
- ▶ Douche Bag Shoulder Syndrome (Stable Shoulder Position)
- ▶ Overhead Positioning
- ▶ Midrange Pressing (Bench, Pushup)

Methods:
- ▶ Pressure Wave
- ▶ Contract and Relax
- ▶ Smash and Floss

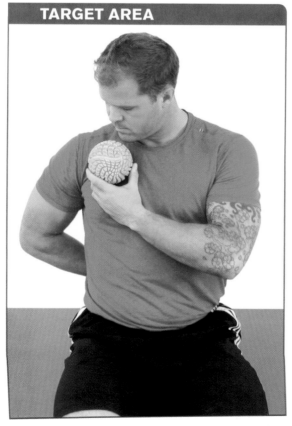

TARGET AREA

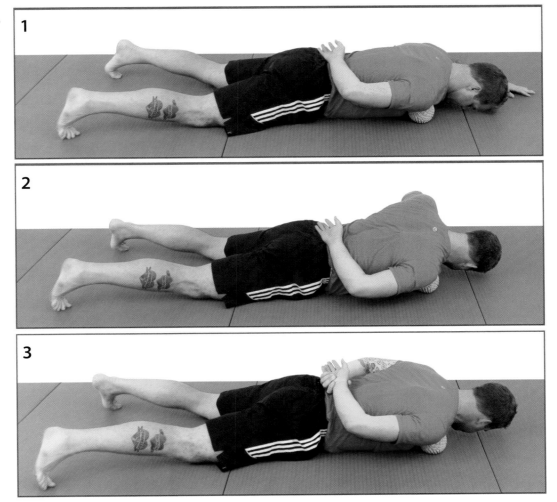

1. Position a large ball on your pec minor and apply pressure. Notice that my right hand is behind my back. This is an easy way to not only bias the tissue into internal rotation, which is the motion you're working to restore, but also gives you the pressure you need to make change in the area.

2. Push off the mat using your left hand, rotate toward your left, and pressure wave the tissues.

3. After hunting out a stiff spot, throw your left arm behind your back, and grab your right hand. This puts additional pressure into the area you're trying to change and allows you to kind of floss your arm further into internal rotation by pulling your right arm up and across your back.

ANTERIOR COMPARTMENT SMASH VARIATION

The doorway pec smash is a way to add a flossing element into the equation. Also note that you can use a lacrosse ball in place of softball for more a targeted effect.

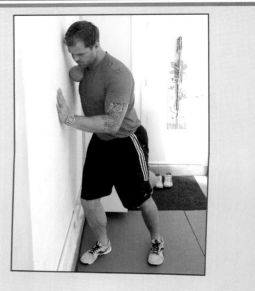

Barbell Shoulder Smash

If you're missing internal rotation, your entire shoulder complex has to compensate. Put in enough duty cycles from an unstable position and you will end up with shoulder pain or worse, an injury. In my practice I treat a lot of athletes who are missing critical internal rotation range. One of the first things that I clear is the anterior deltoid in the area of the upper shoulder. By cleaning up this area, I can effectively fix a lot of the dysfunctional shoulder mechanics that are typical of most athletes.

The simple fact is most of us live in a shoulder-forward position. And the problem is most of the demands of daily life and training involve loading up the anterior deltoid complex, causing it to get extremely tight. One of the most effective and easiest methods to unglue matted-down tissues in this area is to employ the barbell smash or Superfriend internal rotation smash. When you perform it correctly often enough, you may feel you've been blessed with a new shoulder. I've yet to find anything else that unglues the ugliness and restores

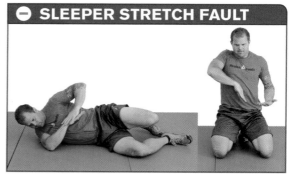

SLEEPER STRETCH FAULT

internal rotation faster than these two pieces, specifically the Superfriend variation with a voodoo banded shoulder. It's like magic.

The key to this mobilization, whether you're implementing the barbell or Superfriend variation, is to lie on your back and avoid getting into a sleeper stretch position by rolling onto your side. The problem with the sleeper stretch is that it is ultimately trying to fix internal rotation from a poor position. You don't need to fix internal rotation with your arm across your body. That doesn't look like anything! What you need to do is mobilize in positions that look like athletic movements. Think of the high-hang position, the recovery phase of the swimming stroke, the dip, or jumping. You get the idea.

Improves:		Methods:
▶ Internal Rotation Capacity ▶ Shoulder Mechanics		▶ Smash and Floss
▶ Shoulder Pain		

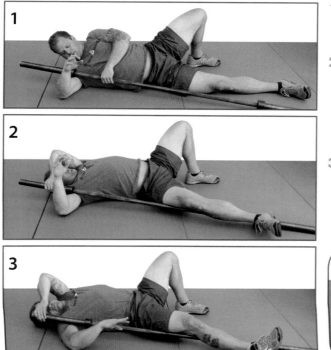

1. To set up for the barbell shoulder smash, lie on your back and position the notch of the barbell in the anterior deltoid area.

2. Next, throw your right leg over the bar. This not only helps pin the barbell in place and adds additional pressure, but also helps push your shoulder to the back of the socket. As you do this, lie back to put your right shoulder in a good position and grab the sleeve of the barbell with your left hand.

3. After you've tacked the anterior tissue down, internally rotate your hand and push down on the barbell using your left hand. The combination of these actions creates a lot of shear, which allows you to un-laminate the tissues of your anterior shoulder.

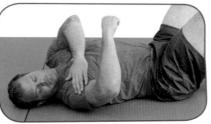

Voodoo Floss: Superfriend Variation

This is an excellent variation to implement if you have a team of athletes. You can have one group wrap the arms of the people in the second group and step on their shoulders, and then switch after a couple of minutes. It's literally the fastest and easiest way to improve and restore internal rotation to the shoulder.

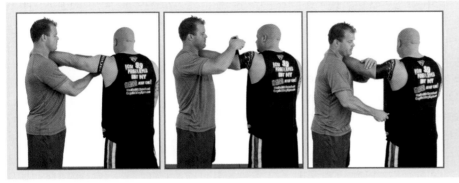

Starting from the top of the shoulder, I wrap Jesse's shoulder with the voodoo band to create a compression element. To see more on how to correctly wrap using the voodoo floss band, revisit the introduction to this chapter (page 219).

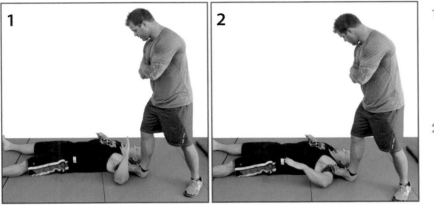

1. After wrapping his shoulder, Jesse lies on his back and positions his arm at a 90-degree angle. To ensure his shoulder is in a good position and help tack-down his laminated tissues, I step on the front of his shoulder with the ball of my right foot.

2. With my foot tacking down his shoulder, Jesse internally rotates his arm past my foot, effectively ungluing all the matted-down tissue of his shoulder.

Bilateral Internal Rotation Mobilization

The bilateral internal rotation mobilization is a quick and dirty way to work on extension and internal rotation. As with the voodoo floss Superfriend variation previously demonstrated, this is another excellent mobilization that you can throw into a big group of athletes in a class setting.

What's important to note is that you can't relieve truckloads of muscle stiffness or restore a lot of motion to the joint with just a static stretch. For optimal results, you have to tie in the contract and relax element and try to work in and out of end-range tension. In addition, you really have to focus on keeping your shoulders pinned to the mat and avoid compensating into a forward-rolled position as you lower your hips into your hands. This can be very difficult to do, especially if you're missing some of these key internal rotation and extension corners. The best way to deal with this issue is to have a friend press down on your shoulders. This not only ensures that your shoulders remain in a good position, it allows you to hit some more extreme vectors.

Personally, I only like doing this mobilization when I have a Superfriend on hand because it's so difficult to keep your shoulders back. However, even if you don't have someone to help you out, this is an excellent mobilization to see just how your body compensates for its lack of range. You can really feel what's happening. Sometimes when you're descending into a dip, it's less obvious. You can't feel when you compensate. Setting up in this position, on the other hand, will tell you exactly if it's motor-control or a mobility issue. It makes the invisible, visible.

Improves:
▶ Extension and Internal Rotation (Dip)   ▶ Midrange Pressing (Bench, Pushup)

Method:
▶ Contract and Relax

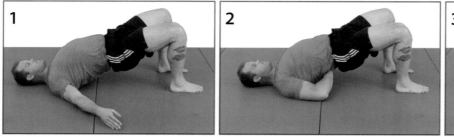

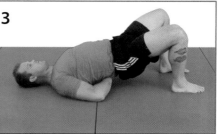

1. To set up for the mobilization, drive your heels into the mat, bridge your hips, and drive your shoulders to the back of the socket.

2. Maneuver your hands underneath your lower back.

3. To add a tension force, slowly drop your hips toward the mat and lower your back into your hands. From here, you can contract and relax as well as oscillate in and out of end-range tension. It's important that you avoid compensating into a forward-rolled position as illustrated. You have to fight this force and control the tension.

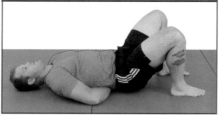

⊖ COMMON FAULT

SUPERFRIEND VARIATION

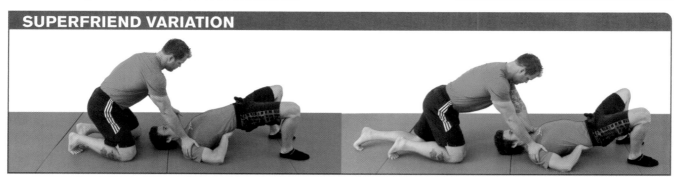

1. I've positioned my hands over the front of Carl's shoulders with my palms facing away from my body. Before Carl starts to lower his hips, I load some pressure into the front of his shoulders.

2. As I keep Carl's shoulders pinned to the ground, he lowers his hips into his hands to apply a tension force.

Banded Bully

It's not easy to improve extension and internal rotation without ending up in a weak shoulder position. This is why I recommend the Superfriend variation of the previous entry. It prevents you from blowing off torque, dumping tension, and defaulting into a crappy forward shoulder position.

If you don't have a Superfriend in range, the banded bully is good alternative. As you can see from the photos, the band pulls my shoulder to the back of the socket, which not only allows me to mobilize from a stable position, but also intensifies the work.

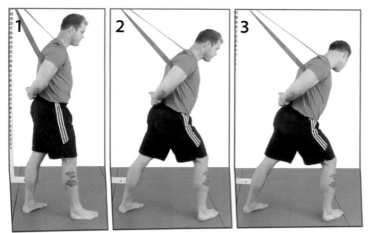

1. Hook your right arm through the band over your anterior deltoid and position your arm behind your lower back. To keep your right arm in place, latch on to your right wrist using your left hand.

2. To create tension in the band, lean forward and allow the band to pull your shoulder into the back of the socket.

3. With your right shoulder locked into an ideal position, start hunting for stiffness by pulling your right arm up and across your body using your left hand. This helps bias internal rotation with extension. You can also tilt your head to tie your neck into the mobilization.

Triple Bully

The bully sequences look a lot like a cop restraining a purse-snatching suspect with a behind-the-back arm lock. If you've ever been winched into this position you know how much it hurts, especially when applied correctly and with the right amount force. The lock is effective because it forces your arm into red-hot corners that you never really explore on your own time. Not to mention the fact that you're probably missing serious internal rotation. No wonder you submitted so easy!

The triple bully is designed to hit these corners using three key motions. With your hand fixed to a pole or rack, first step away to create extension; second, twist away from the arm you're mobilizing to bias a little bit more adduction (moving toward your centerline); and third, drop your elevation and pull your fixed arm up and across your back to add more internal rotation.

As with any mobilization, you have to use a combination of motions to bring the most change. Thinking in terms of singular motions, like flexing for example, is a mistake. You're never going to express the true nature of the joint and how it moves. But the triple bully—that's another story. The combination of these three motions allow you to wind up your shoulder in a tight position and floss in and out of some really stiff and painful vectors of the joint that rarely get attention. It's an easy way to mobilize your shoulder into some crazy positions without having a cop put you in an arm lock and push you into the back of a squad car.

Improves:
▶ Extension and Internal Rotation (Dip) ▶ Midrange Pressing (Bench, Pushup)

Method:
▶ Contract and Relax

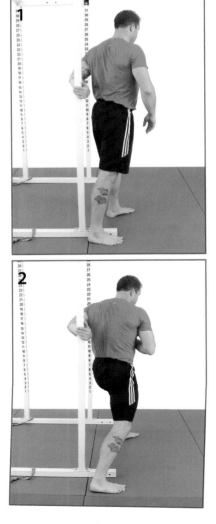

To set up for this mobilization, grip the rack at about hip level with your left hand so that your thumb is pointing up. Next, actively pull your shoulder into the back of your socket and create extension by stepping forward.

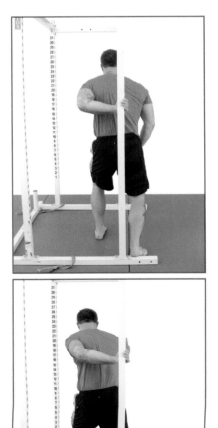

Having created tension in your shoulder with your previous action, as well as biased extension of the joint, twist your body in a counterclockwise direction and lower your elevation. The former biases more adduction while the latter biases more internal rotation. From here, you can keep your hand fixed in the same position while continuing to twist lower and pull your body away in an attempt to find some untapped corners of the shoulder. The key is to keep your shoulder in an idealized position as you explore its ugliness. The moment you feel your shoulder dump torque, release the tension force and reestablish a stable position.

Bully Extension Bias

There is considerable overlap among the shoulder mobilizations. That's a good thing because they all have a slightly different stimulus. Ultimately I want you to play around and use the mobilizations that give you the best results.

With the bully extension bias, you're still working on internal rotation and extension of the shoulder, but in this particular mobilization you exaggerate extension first and then add internal rotation as a tensioner. In addition, because your hand is fixed to the band, you can distract the joint into the back of the socket, which allows you to put a little bit more love and attention into the extension of the shoulder. This gives you a slightly different feel than if your hand is fixed in the same position as in the triple bully.

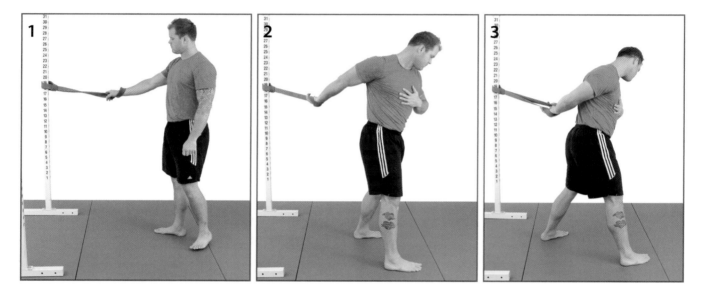

1. Hook your right hand through the band.

2. Wind up your right shoulder into extension by turning your body 180-degrees in a counterclockwise direction so that your back is facing the structure. As you step through with your right foot, rotate your right hand so that your palm is positioned toward the ceiling. This helps bias more internal rotation of your arm. With your banded hand exaggerated into extension, you can contract, relax, and go hunting for some tight corners by lowering your elevation and twisting your upper body.

3. After spending some time in some deep extension, go hunting for some new corners by twisting away from your arm as if you were trying to wrap the band around your body. This adds more internal rotation into the mobilization. You can also tilt your head to the side to tie in the components of the neck/shoulder complex.

Sink Mobilization

The sink mobilization is a non-specific mobilization, meaning it doesn't really bias the joint, but rather attacks anything that is tight or limiting your shoulders in extension. It's a global mobilization. However, the fact that it's not a very sophisticated means you can use it just about anywhere, anytime. If there's a fence pole, railing, or sink, you can work on improving your shoulder extension.

The sink mobilization is especially useful for runners because it improves pulling the elbow straight back during the running stride. If you're missing extension range, you will hit an extension wall as you pull your arm back during the stride, causing your elbow to fly out, which in turn forces you into a compensated shoulder position. Here's what most people do in that situation: Instead of swinging front to back, which is the proper technique, they go around the body, which slows them down, accelerates fatigue, and aggravates tissues. That, and it looks really weird. Don't be that person. Learn how to run correctly.

Improves:
▶ Shoulder Extension

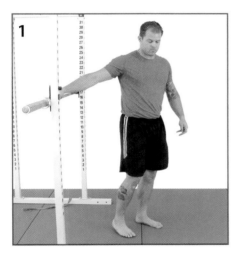

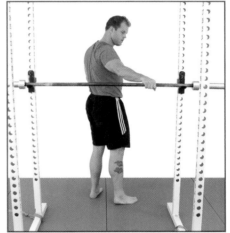

Using your right hand, latch on to the barbell with your palm.

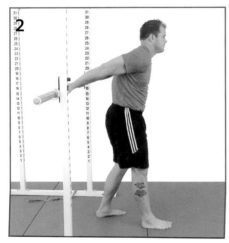

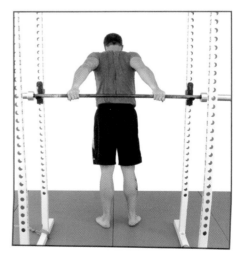

Grab the bar with your left hand, positioning your hands as close together as possible without losing shoulder position.

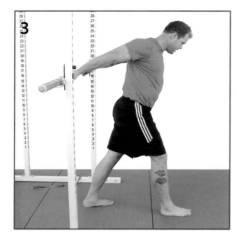

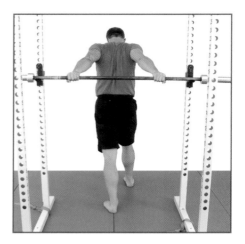

Keeping your shoulders back, apply tension by straightening your arms and leaning forward.

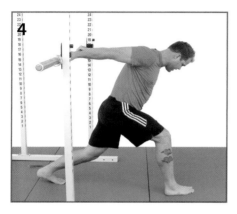

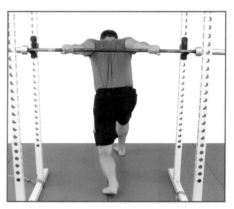

Still leaning forward, increase tension by dropping your elevation. The goal is to position your hands on the same horizontal plane as your shoulders without having to compensate.

Banded Lateral Opener

The banded lateral opener is another global mobilization that exaggerates extension of the arm. But instead of opening the shoulder into internal rotation, this distracts the shoulder into external rotation and ties in the front of the chest and puts the pec into a full stretch. It's quick, easy, and a beautiful prep for any kind pressing motion, specifically pushups and bench press iterations.

Improves:
► Midrange Pressing (Bench, Pushup)
► Shoulder Extension

Method:
► Contract and Relax

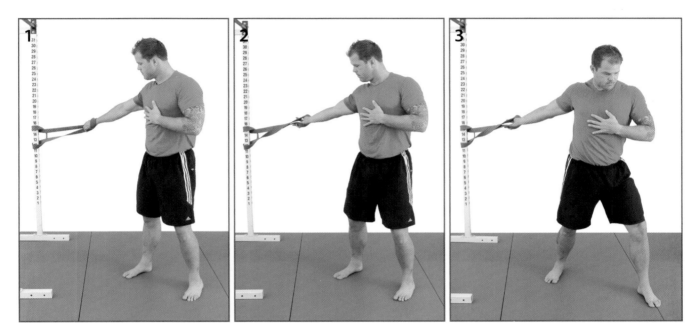

1. Hook your right hand through the band and create tension.

2. Rotate your palm up, biasing external rotation of your shoulder.

3. Keeping your arm externally rotated and your shoulder back, turn away from the band and twist your upper body in a counterclockwise direction. This opens up the chest and arm and allows you to capture the connective and soft tissues along those fascial planes.

AREA 4
DOWNSTREAM ARM
(TRICEPS, ELBOWS, FOREARM, WRIST)

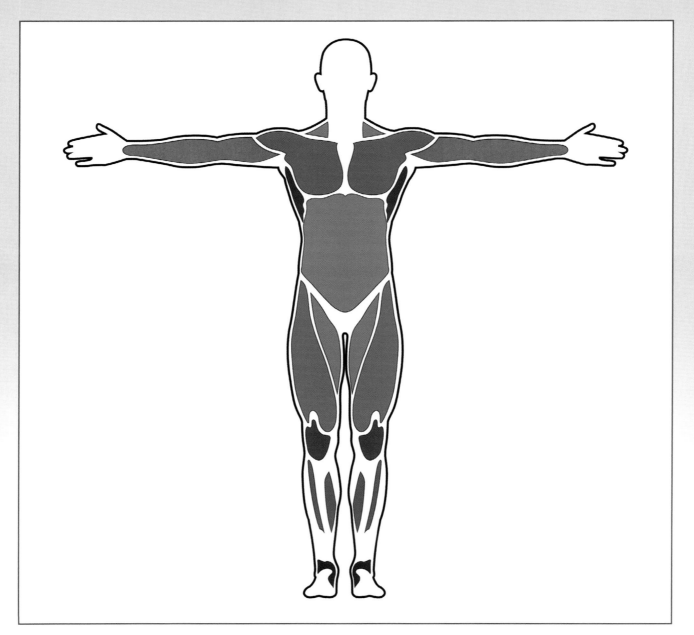

Mobilization Target Areas:

▶ Triceps, elbow, forearm, and wrist

Most Commonly Used Tools:

▶ Voodoo Band
▶ Barbell
▶ Single Lacrosse Ball
▶ Rogue Monster Band
▶ Roller

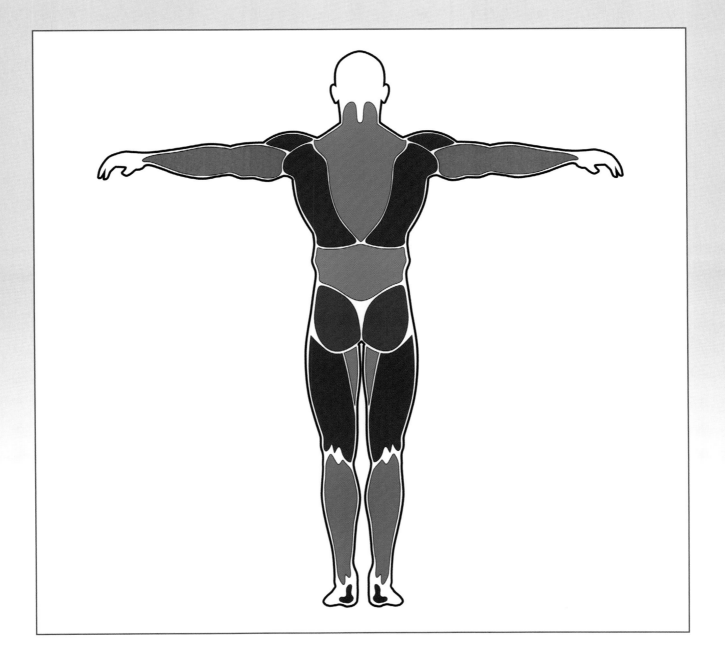

Test and Retest Examples:

▶ Overhead Press   ▶ Back Squat Setup

▶ Hanging from the Bar   ▶ Pushup and Bench

▶ Front Rack Position

Triceps Extension Smash

Your triceps are wicked strong and account for two thirds of the mass of your arm. Consider a powerlifter like Mark Bell who can bench press over 800-pounds. Most of that is triceps. If you are someone who lifts weights or does CrossFit, you can probably remember a time when your triceps were so sore that you couldn't extend your arm. It just hurt to move. I'd be willing to bet that rather than address the stiffness, you waited for the soreness to go away or continued to work out with stiff muscles. Sound familiar? Of course it does. You are an athlete and that's what athletes do. But that doesn't make it right. When your triceps get tight and nothing is done, they get adaptively short, causing you to lose extension in your arm.

If you don't have the full length of your triceps, creating external rotation torque and locking out your elbow is difficult. Elbows tend to chicken flap out into a compromised position. The same thing happens with your legs in the squat when you have stiff quads. You end up missing external rotation and dumping torque by collapsing your knees inward. Restore suppleness to your quads and you can solve this problem.

These big tissues, whether it's the triceps or quads, dictate your capacity to generate stability in your primary engines. The triceps affect your shoulders and the quads affect your hips. If these regions get stiff, it's going to reflect in your movement mechanics and eventually express itself in the form of pain. That means you have to address the ugliness by smashing away the stiffness so that you can reclaim stable positions. And the triceps extension smash is one of the best ways to accomplish that.

Improves:
- ▶ Elbow Extension
- ▶ Front Rack Position
- ▶ Midrange Pressing Mechanics
- ▶ Overhead Position
- ▶ Elbow Pain

Method:
- ▶ Contract and Relax
- ▶ Pressure Wave
- ▶ Smash and Floss

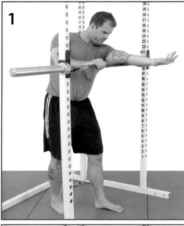

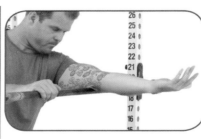

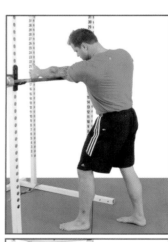

Position the head of your triceps (right above the elbow joint) on the barbell with your arm in extension. Apply downward pressure with your arm to tack-down the underlying tissue.

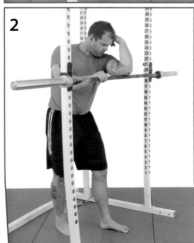

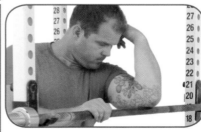

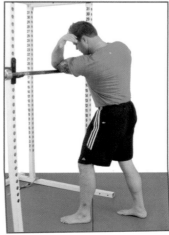

Having tacked-down a stiff area of tissue at the base of your left elbow, pull your left hand to the left side of your head.

3

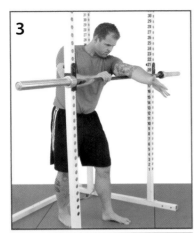
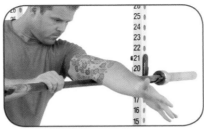
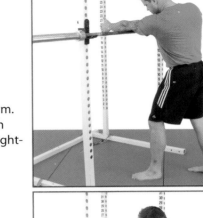

Staying on the stiff tissue, straighten your arm. The idea here is to find a tight spot and push and pull past that spot by bending and straightening your arm.

4

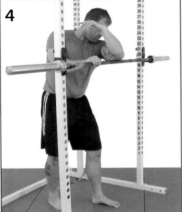
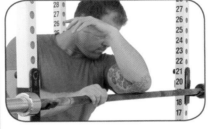
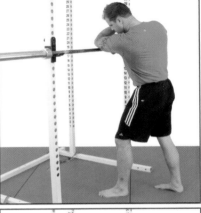

To get full excursion of the tissue, bend your left arm to the opposite side of your body.

5

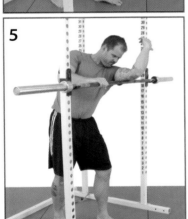
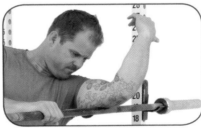
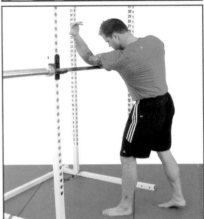

Keeping your arm bent, continue to smash the tissue by moving your arm toward your left side. The idea here is to pressure wave back and forth, smashing the tissues laterally.

TRICEPS SMASH—ALTERNATE OPTIONS

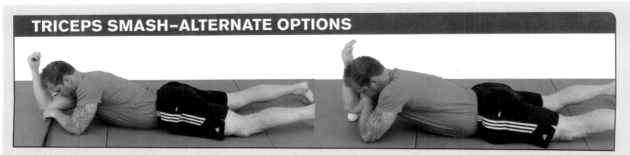

If you don't have a rack, don't panic. You can do this on the ground using a barbell, lacrosse ball, rolling pin, wine bottle, or whatever you have at your disposal. Find something to smash your triceps on and get some work done.

Voodoo Elbow Mobilization

Wrapping a voodoo band above and below your elbow and then spending a few minutes moving through a full range-of-motion is one of the fastest and most effective ways to address elbow pain and restore suppleness to your triceps. If your elbow aches, or you're missing key corners in your mobility—elbow extension or flexion—this should be one of your first stops. In fact, if I have an athlete that is suffering from epicondylitis (tennis elbow), this is the first thing I have them do. Seriously, nothing I've seen, experienced, or been taught solves "hot elbow" problems as quickly and effectively as the voodoo elbow mobilization. To learn more about proper wrapping technique, revisit the introduction to this chapter.

SUPERFRIEND TORTURE

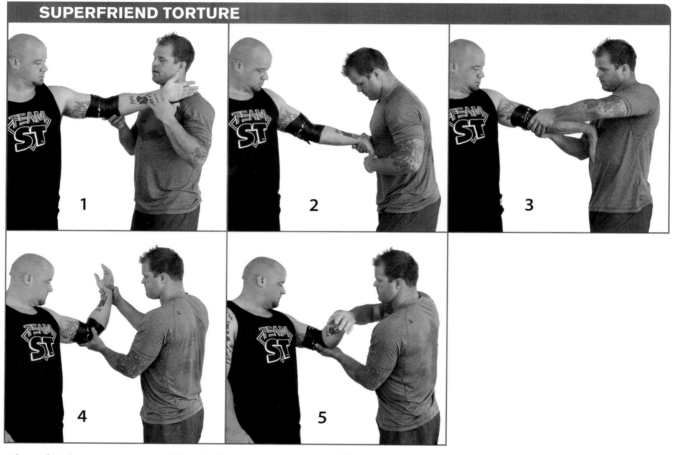

After I finish wrapping an athlete's elbow, the first thing I'll do is rotate his elbow toward the ground, position his palm flush against my chest, and then pull his arm into full extension. As I do this, I'll externally rotate his arm to capture all the corners of the joint. The role of the Superfriend is to force the elbow into as much range-of-motion as possible while making sure your partner doesn't pass out. As with most of the highly effective mobilization techniques, voodoo flossing your elbow is not a pleasurable experience. This is why having a Superfriend manipulate your arm into key ranges is ideal, because he or she is not limited by your pain. However, like all Superfriend mobilizations, you probably need to pick and respect the use of a safe word.

FORCED FLEXION AND EXTENSION

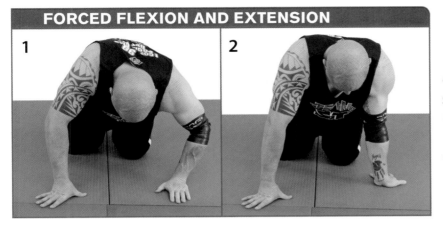

Placing your palm on the ground is a great way to encourage flexion and extension movement through the elbow. The idea is to explore different positions and accumulate 15 to 20 arm bends.

MOBILIZE THE MOVEMENT YOU'RE TRYING TO CHANGE

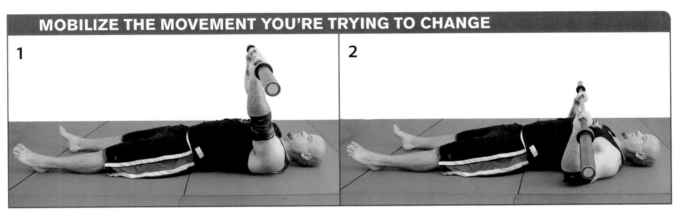

One of the best aspects of voodoo flossing is that you can mobilize in the position you're trying to change. For example, if you're benching, pressing, or doing a workout with a lot of pushups, wrap your elbow and perform the movement you are about to perform.

HANG FROM A BAR

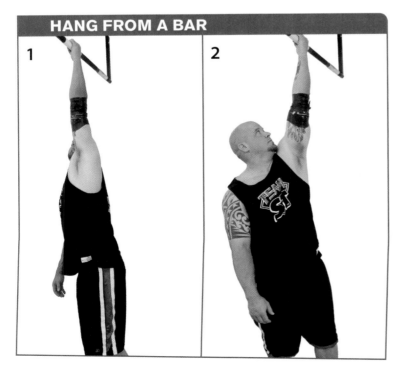

Anchoring your hand to a bar and twisting your body is a great way to tie in the rotational components of your elbow. The key is to spend some time in both hand positions: supinated (chin-up grip) and pronated (pull-up grip).

Banded Elbow Extension

The elbow is a workhorse. It's insane. Think about how much you use and count on the work flowing through your elbows. Flexing and extending your arms are a big part of daily life. So it's no great mystery that arms and elbows get stiff and painful, and full extension of the arm comes with a grimace (if at all).

The trouble tends to spread. Consider an athlete—with limited range-of-motion in the elbows—pressing a barbell overhead. As he nears locking out with his elbows, he flares his elbows out and rolls his shoulders forward. He's risking more pain and injury to make the lift.

People tend to think of the elbow as a simple joint that just bends and extends. But there's a rotational component that contributes to generating shoulder stability. This goes back to the idea that the smaller structures dictate the capacity to create stability in the primary engines. In this case, it's your shoulders.

Think of the front rack position. Being able to externally rotate your shoulders into a good position to create a stable platform is predicated on having full range-of-motion in your downstream joints like your elbows and wrists. In other words, missing extension doesn't just affect your ability to lock your arms out, it also messes with your ability to create the rotation in your elbows that helps stabilize your shoulders.

People think they can get away with missing a little bit of extension in their elbows. They can't. To get an idea of what I'm talking about, try this simple test:

Get in the pushup position, bend your arms slightly, and then externally rotate your arms to create a stable shoulder position. Then, lock your arms out and do the same thing.

As you will find, locking out your arms creates a much stronger and stable position. If you don't have full extension in your elbows, perform this test using the squat. Stand with your knees slightly bent, and then create external rotation force by forcing your knees out. Then, do the same thing with your knees locked out. What you'll find is that when your knees are locked out, your butt turns on and you can really feel the stability of your position. Per the one-joint rule, the same thing happens in the shoulders.

So let's go after restoring full range-of-motion to the elbows.

As you can see from the photos, I work the elbow from two different positions to account for the rotational component of the structure. The key is to floss in and out of extension by bending your elbow into the band and then, with control, slowly straighten your arm into extension, really allowing the band to distract the joint to the end-range of the capsule.

Note: For the best results, execute the following mobilizations with a voodoo banded elbow. As a case study example, Sarah Hopping—All American hammer thrower and CrossFit phenomenon—came to my practice at San Francisco CrossFit seeking to correct her elbow position and fix the concurring pain. She had broken the head of her radius, a catastrophic injury, and couldn't lock out or extend her elbow to end-range. This dramatically restricted overhead positions. I saw her for one session and essentially focused on voodoo flossing her elbow using the techniques below. With just a little bit of voodoo love, we managed to restore full-range to the joint. She ended up winning the snatch ladder at the NorCal CrossFit 2012 Regionals shortly after. Her physicians were left in disbelief. The moral of the story is this: If you can wrap a compression band around your elbow and voodoo floss using the below techniques, do it. It will work miracles!

Improves:
▶ Elbow Extension
▶ Rotational Capacity
▶ Overhead Positioning
▶ Pushup and Bench

Method:
▶ Flossing
▶ Voodoo Flossing

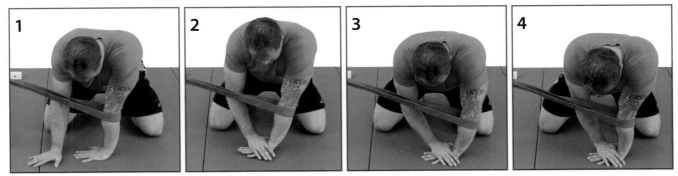

1. Hook a band around your elbow and create tension by sliding your arm back. Notice that my fingers are pointed in the direction of the band.

2. Staple your palm to the mat by placing your right hand over your left hand.

3. Keeping your shoulder in a stable position, flex your elbow into the band.

4. Controlling your arm into extension, allow the band to pull your elbow to its end-range position. From here, flex and extend your elbow until you have full range-of-motion or you can feel change in the joint capsule.

BANDED ELBOW EXTENSION (VARIATION)

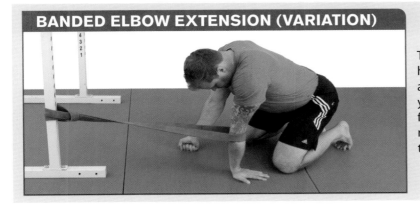

To capture the entire capsule, you have to hit the elbow from an open palm position and a closed palm position. In other words, you're working from a full pronation and full supination. This helps account for the rotational components of the elbow and ties in the forearm and wrist structure.

Banded Elbow Distraction

The banded elbow distraction is another way to solve poor mobility in your elbow and treat pain. This technique also works on improving full flexion of your elbow. As you can see from the photos on the next page, the band distracts your elbow joint and creates a gapping force in the crook of your elbow. This distraction force puts your elbow in a good position with the capsule, which clears any impingement in the joint and allows you to floss unrestricted. The key here is to focus on moving your arm in different directions. Doing so will account for the rotational component of your elbow structure and accumulate as many bends in your elbow as possible.

Think about the paper clip concept. You're never going to get anywhere just bending it back and forth a couple of times. To break the paper clip, you need anywhere from 30 to 60 bends before it breaks. That is exactly what you want to do here. To make any kind of change, you need to oscillate in and out of end-range flexion, as well as explore the full excursion of your elbow by turning your palm toward and away from you. It's not a fixed position mobilization. By turning your hand and scouring all the ranges of your elbow joint, you completely change the dynamics of how your elbow is mobilized. Not only that, switching hand positions helps account for common grips such as chin-ups (palm in or supinated) or a rack and pulling position (palm away or pronated).

Improves:
- Full Flexion of the Elbow
- Pulling Positions
- Hanging Positions
- Joint Dynamics
- Elbow Pain

Method:
- Distraction with Gapping Bias
- Flossing (Paper-clipping the Joint)
- Voodoo Flossing

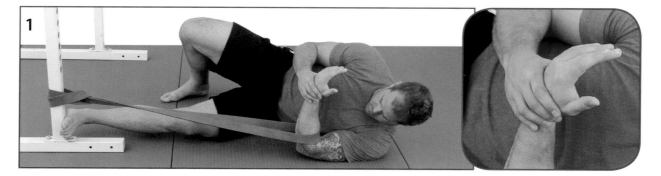

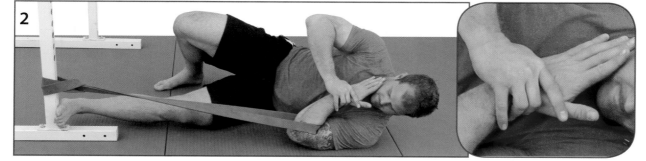

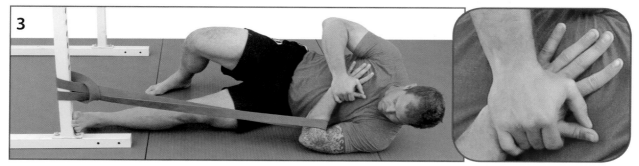

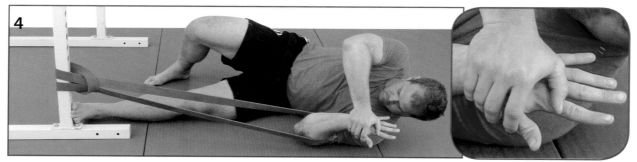

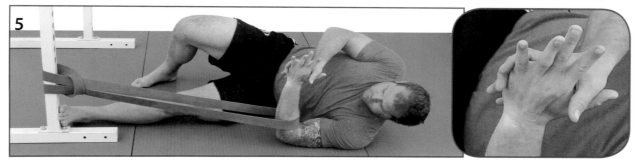

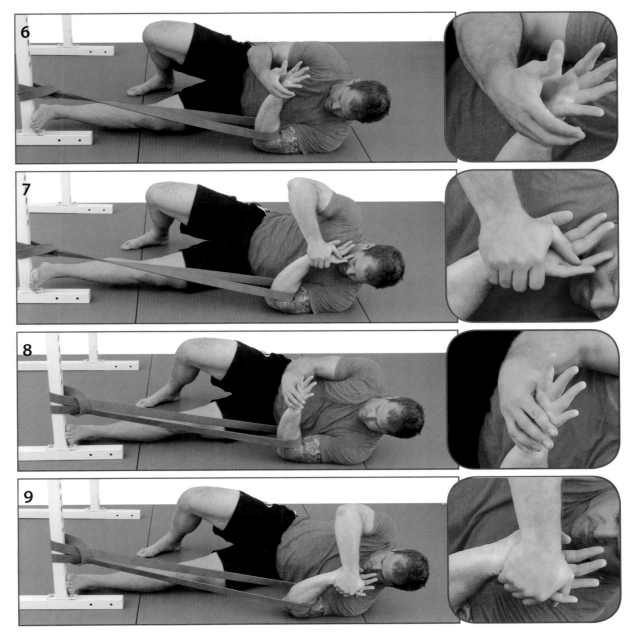

1. Hook the band on the bottom of your forearm, near the crook of your elbow, and then push yourself away from the rack to create tension in the band.

2. Pull your left hand toward your face using your right hand. I'm not going to lie: This hurts. Stay out of the pain cave and break your elbow like a paper clip until you effect change.

3. Reposition your right grip on your left hand, hooking the web of your right hand around your left thumb and over the top of your hand.

4. Using your right hand, force your left arm laterally toward your left side while twisting your palm toward the ground.

5. To ensure you hit all corners, reposition your grip on your hand, this time gripping your left palm.

6. Twist your palm away from your body.

7. Pull your left hand to your face, keeping your palm facing away from your body.

8. Reset your position.

9. Still scouring the full ranges of your elbow, force your left arm into flexion while pushing your left hand toward the outside of your body with your palm facing away.

Double Lacrosse Ball Smash

If you're one of the unfortunate people who are stuck in static positions at work all day, stretching is not going to do all that much for you. When your muscles mold and adapt to the positions you are in—meaning they get adaptively short and stiff—the restoration of elasticity requires ungluing.

For example, wrist pain is a common problem of deskbound athletes. So what do they do about it? Stretches like flexing and extending the wrist. You need a better plan. To treat the problem, you not only have to address the positions you're in, but also implement a combination of smashing, flossing, and distracted joint mobilizations.

A much better option is to look upstream of the wrist and attack the tissues that are pulling on your elbow and hand. Your forearms do an unbelievable amount of work for your hands and you probably do nothing for them. No wonder you have tennis elbow or you can't assume a good front rack position. The strings that control the hands have turned into steel cables.

Here's the bottom line: If you have elbow or wrist pain, your forearms probably need some love. You can work on these tissues using the double lacrosse ball smash, which is demonstrated below.

Improves:
▶ Wrist and Elbow Pain
▶ Wrist and Elbow Joint Dynamics (Extension, Flexion, and Rotation Capacity)

Method:
▶ Smash and Floss
▶ Pressure Wave
▶ Contract and Relax

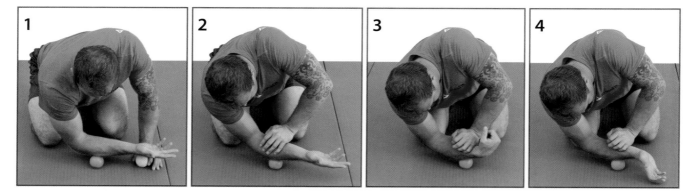

1. Position your forearm over a lacrosse ball with your palm facing the ceiling. Note: You can place the bottom ball anywhere in the meat of your forearm, ideally on a stiff spot.

2. Position another lacrosse ball directly over the bottom lacrosse ball and drive it into your forearm using your opposite hand, effectively sandwiching the tight tissue.

3. Maintain downward pressure using your left hand while flexing your right wrist.

4. From here, make circles, flex, extend, and try to move your hand around in all directions. Once you feel some change, move on to another tight spot.

Banded Wrist Distraction with Voodoo Wrist Sequence

The banded wrist distraction is similar to the ankle mobilizations in that you really just work on oscillating in and out of range to improve the dynamics of the joint. It's a simple mobilization that is very effective for treating wrist pain. It's also a great way to prep for any kind of front rack demanding exercise. For the best results, wrap your wrist with a voodoo band and work your way through the voodoo wrist sequence mobilizations.

Improves: **Method:**

▶ Joint Mechanics   ▶ Wrist Pain   ▶ Flossing   ▶ Voodoo Flossing

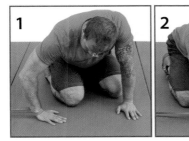
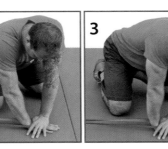
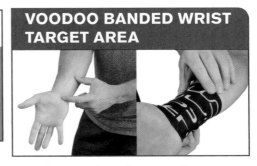

VOODOO BANDED WRIST TARGET AREA

1. Hook a band around your wrist.

2. Slide your hand across the mat to create tension in the band. This distracts your wrist joint into a good position. Once accomplished, staple the base of your hand to the ground with your left hand.

3. Blocking your right wrist with your left hand, lockout your elbow, extend your right arm over your right hand. From here, floss back and forth in and out of end-range until you feel some change in the joint.

Start the wrap from the base of your hand and work your way up your forearm. At about a quarter of the way up your arm, you can cross the band back and forth over the banded area, or work your way back down the arm. The key is to cover the area shown in the photo.

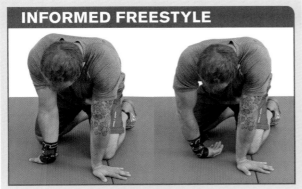

INFORMED FREESTYLE

Once you've wrapped your wrist, try playing around with different mobilizations by forcing your wrist into common positions.

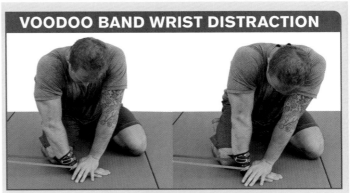

VOODOO BAND WRIST DISTRACTION

Combining a distraction with a voodoo band is always a good idea. As with the elbow extension, block your wrist, lockout your elbow, and extend your arm over your planted hand, flossing in and out of end-range.

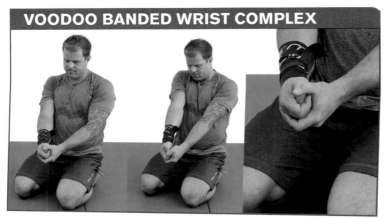

VOODOO BANDED WRIST COMPLEX

This voodoo band wrist mobilization gets a gold star for effectiveness. This should be the first stop for keyboard warriors who suffer from stiff thumbs and wrists. To execute this technique, make a fist over your thumb and then lockout your arm while bending your wrist toward the ground. This will help unglue the laminated tissues that surround your thumb and wrist complex, restoring sliding surfaces to that region.

AREA 5
TRUNK
(PSOAS, LOW BACK, OBLIQUE)

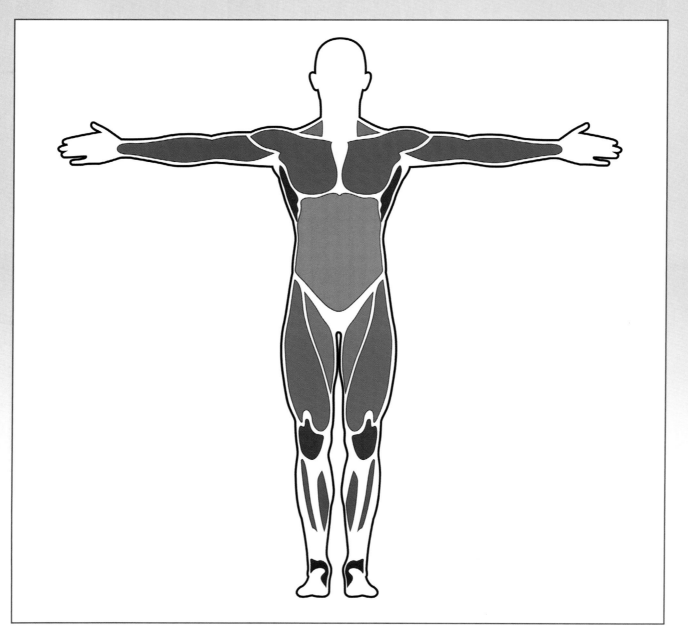

Mobilization Target Areas:

▶ Psoas, low back, abdominals, obliques, and QL

Most Commonly Used Tools:

▶ Single Lacrosse Ball

▶ Double Lacrosse Ball

▶ Large Ball (Softball, Small Deflated Soccer Ball, Kids Ball, etc.)

▶ Roller

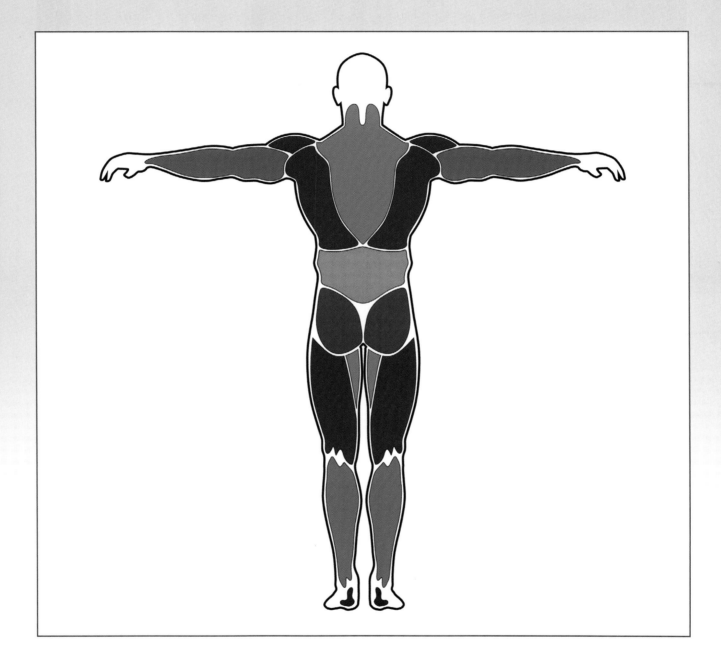

Test and Retest Examples:

▶ Global Extension

▶ Overhead Press

▶ Hanging from the Bar

▶ Squat and Overhead Squat

Low Back Smash: Single Lacrosse Ball

If you have low back pain, put this mobilization at the top of your list. By sticking a single lacrosse ball in the low back and upper glute region, you can effectively unglue the matted-down tissues that cause low back pain and restrict movement and positional mechanics.

It is better to perform this mobilization with your feet elevated, either on a box or a chair. There are three reasons for this. First, it's easier to mobilize in a good position without breaking into overextension. Second, you can get more pressure into the ball, which is necessary for effecting change in the tissue. And third, it takes the slack out of the musculature of your trunk and low back. You take up the soft tissue slack in your lower back, making it easier to maintain a neutral spinal position.

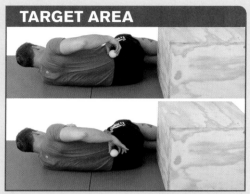

TARGET AREA

The goal is to work back and forth from the side of your hip to your spine, trying to stay on the crest of the pelvis and superior glute.

Improves:

▶ Low Back Pain and Stiffness

▶ Position Mechanics (Neutral Posture)

▶ Rotational Capacity

Method:

▶ Pressure Waving (Side-to-Side)

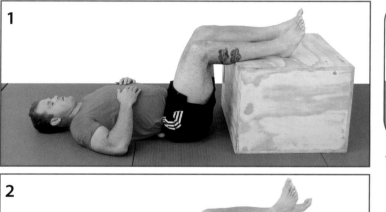

1

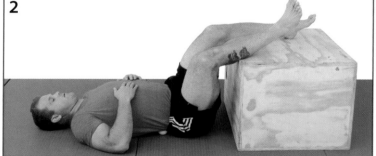

2

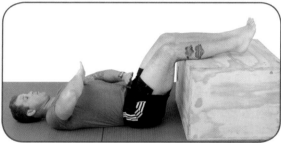

1. Place the lacrosse ball on your lower back just above your pelvis and position your feet up on a box. It's important that you focus on keeping your midline engaged so that you can maintain a neutral spinal position. If you overextend by tilting your pelvis, which is a very common fault, you will only make your low back pain worse.

2. Slowly shift your hips toward your left. The goal is to grind back and forth against the grain of the muscle and slowly smash the tissue using the pressure wave technique.

Back tweak? Reset your pelvis!

Low back pain either stems from long hours of sitting with poor posture, or moving and lifting in a compromised position. Once you ingrain dysfunctional movement patterns or adopt a poor position while in the seated position, low back pain turns into a real problem. You can treat the issue using mobilization techniques, but the moment you default into your bad positions, it flares up again. That is why I say things like, "The number one predictor for low back pain is a previous history of low back pain." Once you burn out your duty cycles, the issue persists. Unless you address your position and perform constant maintenance on the problem areas, it's always an issue.

If you don't have a previous history of low back pain, on the other hand, the number two predictor of back pain is having a pelvic rotation obliquity stemming from a back tweak. For example, if you were to tweak your back playing sports or doing whatever, chances are good that one side of your pelvis has been rotated out of position, creating side-to-side differences in your mobility. So if you have one hamstring that is a lot tighter than the other pulling down on one side of your pelvis and you try to lift a large load, it creates a rotational shear on your hips and pulls your pelvis into a bad position, which in turn tweaks your low back. You don't even have to be lifting a heavy load for this to occur. Sometimes low back tweaks happen when you're not braced and you rotate or move the wrong way. Regardless of how it happens, there's a really simple technique that you can use to reset your pelvis into a neutral position.

The idea here is to use rotation and counter rotation by pushing on one knee and pulling on the other. This action fires your hamstring and hip flexor at the same time for the purpose of resetting your pelvic position. The general prescription is to hold both positions for five seconds while resisting the pressure with your legs, switch sides three or four times, and then finish by squeezing a ball between your knees as hard as you can. This last step helps reset the pubic symphysis.

To put it in simple terms, you're using your muscles to restore a normal pelvic position. Often times, you'll hear a pop or feel the pelvis 'clunk' into position.

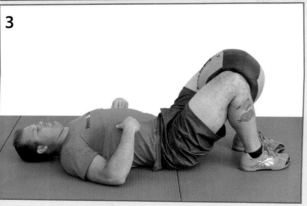

1

To reset your pelvis, push on your right knee using your right hand while countering the pressure with your right leg, which fires your right hip flexor. At the same time, pull on your left knee using your left hand while countering the pressure with your left leg, which activates your left hamstring.

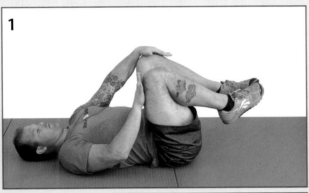

2

After holding the previous position for 5 seconds, switch your hand positions and apply the same push-pull pressure, counter pressure to your knees. Repeat this sequence, going back and forth between positions and resisting for 5 seconds.

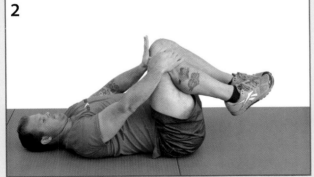

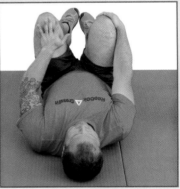

3

Once you've completed a few rotations, and then a few counter rotation cycles on your legs, position a medicine ball between your knees and squeeze as hard as you can for five seconds. Repeat this process for three to five sets until you feel or hear a clunk.

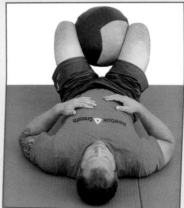

Low Back Smash: Double Lacrosse Ball

If you have a stiff lower back, chances are good that you're missing normal motion in your lumbar spine. This makes you highly vulnerable to back tweaks. In this sequence, I show a really simple mobilization to restore basic spinal motion and relieve stiffness to your low back. It's very similar to the low back smash, but instead of working on the muscles that tie into the area, you target the motion segment vertebra of your lumbar spine. The former deals with muscles stiffness, while the latter addresses joint mechanics. But unlike using a single lacrosse ball, you don't have to worry as much about overextending because the ball supports both sides of your spine. However, that doesn't mean you can put your abs to sleep. You want to keep enough tension to maintain a neutral position and avoid tilting your pelvis as you drop your knees from side to side.

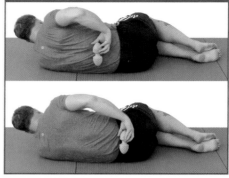

TARGET MOBILIZATION

The idea is to hit each motion segment of the spine stretching from the base of your ribcage to your pelvis.

Improves:

▶ Relieves Lower Back Pain
▶ Global Rotation
▶ Lumbar Joint Mechanics
▶ Unlocks Stiff Lower Back

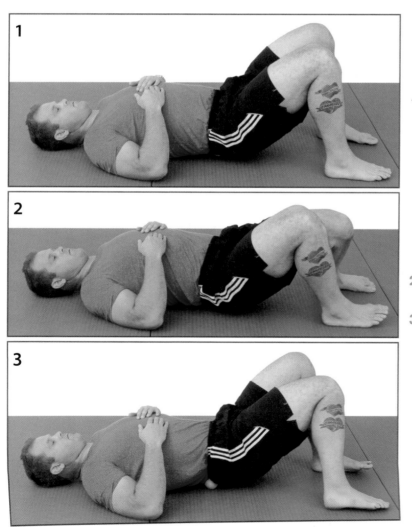

1. Position a double lacrosse ball on your lower back between the motion segments of your vertebra. To avoid breaking into overextension, keep your midline engaged and your hips off the ground. A helpful cue is to think about creating a long spine as you drop your knees toward the ground. Also, if you want to increase the pressure, you can post your feet up onto a box or chair or lift your legs into the air.

2. Drop your left knee toward your right side and rotate your hips slightly.

3. With your motion segments still blocked, rotate your hips and drop your right knee toward your left side. It's important not to over rotate and lose shoulder contact with the ground. Rotate back and forth from side to side until you feel some change and then move up or down to the next motion segment.

Oblique Side Smash

If you're walking around with a tight low back, you need to make sure you address all of the tissues that tie into that lumbar region. One of the biggest mistakes that you can make as an athlete is to only mobilize the area of localized pain and stiffness. While you obviously want to address any ugliness in the areas where you feel most restricted, you also have to work on the surrounding structures so that you can feed some slack to those tight tissues. For example, in this sequence I demonstrate a very simple side smash that targets the oblique and other lateral units that tie into the low back structure like the high glute and tensor fasciae latae. In most cases, these tissues are very restricted and need to be unglued with some smashing. The best way to accomplish that is to pressure wave back and forth over a Rumble Roller (MobilityWOD.com) between your ribcage and hipbone. Although the Rumble Roller works the best, you can also use a lacrosse ball or anything that digs into the ropey tissue.

Improves:
- ▶ Low Back Pain   ▶ Global Rotation   ▶ Lateral Extension

Method:
- ▶ Pressure Wave

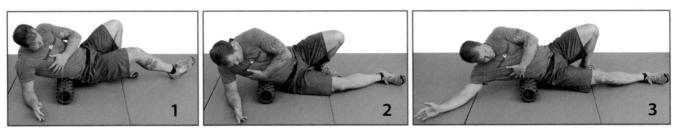

1. Start on your side with the rumble roller positioned between your ribcage and hipbone.

2. Roll toward your right side and twist your torso over the roller, smashing your oblique, QL, and high glute.

3. To make this mobilization more aggressive, you can lengthen the tissues by stretching your arm overhead.

Classic Spinal Twist

The classic spinal twist is a global mobilization that catches anything that is tight in your lower back region. It's not the first stop you want to make when addressing low back and lumbar spine issues, but it's an easy way to relieve stiffness to anything that is tight in that area.

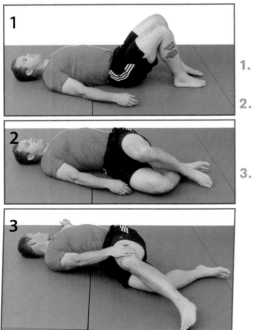

1. Lie on your back with your feet on the mat.

2. Keeping your left shoulder flush with the mat, drop your knees to your right side.

3. Cup your right hand over your left knee, pulling it toward the mat, straighten your left arm, and turn your head toward your left side.

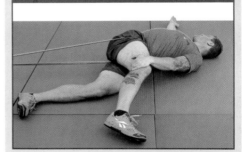

BANDED DISTRACTION

Obviously, if you can attach a band to your hip and distract toward your feet, it makes it a hundred times more effective.

Lateral Hip Opener

Athletes with lower back pain will often attack things from the front and the back, but omit work from the side. You must approach the issue from all angles. Performing this basic lateral side bend is just you being responsible for your global stiffness. What you'll find is that your obliques, ribs, and QL are tacked-down and really tight, which contributes to your pain and restriction. This is a very basic mobilization that you can drop in after a workout, or as you're watching television. It's simple. The key is to keep your hips planted on the ground and your torso and arm on the same vertical plane as you fall to the side. Imagine that there are two parallel planes of glass in front and behind your body that prevent you from folding forward or falling backward.

Improves:

▶ Global Rotation

▶ Low Back Pain and Stiffness

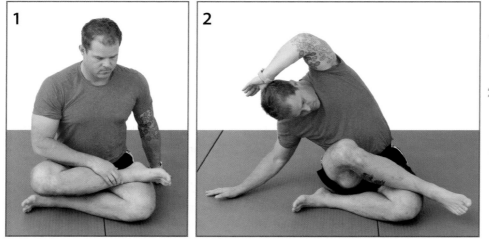

1. From the crossed-legged position, pull your right foot over your left knee.

2. With your right leg holding down your left hip, bring your left arm over your head and fall to your right side. Keep your torso and arm on the same vertical plane as you lean over your right hip.

Lateral Side Opener

This is just a variation of the previous technique, which mobilizes the lateral compartment encompassing the oblique, QL, ribs, and hip. It's important to note that this mobilization can be performed on a keg, physioball, or a medicine ball stacked on some plates. Just like the previous technique, you want to avoid twisting as you bend over your side. Adding rotation will cause you to overextend, which is never okay.

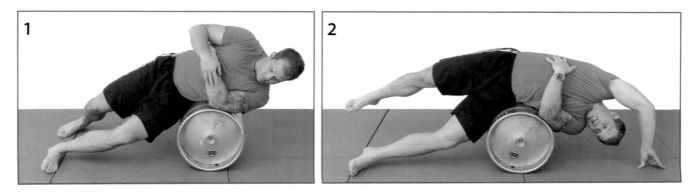

1. Bend over the keg.

2. Keeping your midline engaged to avoid rotating, reach your top arm over your head and bend over the keg.

VARIATION

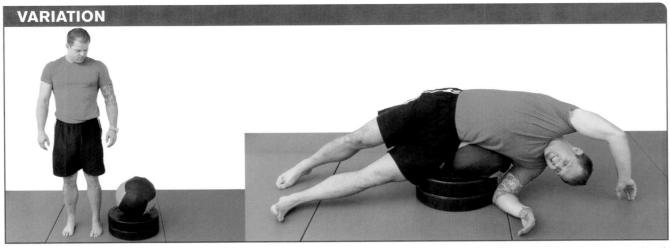

If you don't have a keg or physioball at your gym or house, you can still perform this mobilization by stacking a med ball on some bumper plates.

Targeted Gut Smash: "The Jilly"

This is one of my absolute favorite mobilizations. I teach it to everyone. It comes from the wonderful and twisted brain of Jill Miller of "Yoga Tune Up" fame.

The trunk is a hardworking system that is bound to get tight, regardless if you're organized or disorganized. The simple fact is you spend a lot of time and energy maintaining and creating stability through your midline, which causes the layers of your abdominal structure, particularly your psoas, to get tacked-down and stiff. If you're hanging out or moving in dysfunctional positions, the psoas and surrounding musculature has to work extra hard to stabilize your spine.

The psoas is a big bastard of a muscle that crosses from your diaphragm and lumbar region of the vertebral column to your pelvis and leg. It has the supreme responsibility for stabilizing the spine, flexing the hip, as well as powering rotation. So if it gets tight and tacked-down to the surrounding structures, it's going to cause a lot of problems—like an inflamed lower back or cruddy movement patterns. This is another reason why you want to avoid sitting for extended periods of time. With your hips closed and muscles of your primary engine turned off, your psoas has to work really hard to keep your spine stabilized.

Think about it like this. Imagine bending your arm 90-degrees and then having someone pull on your hand, putting a low-grade tug on your biceps, for six hours. What do you think is going to happen to your biceps? It will get brutally tight, causing acute pain at your elbow and shoulder. This is exactly what happens to your psoas when you sit for a long time. Your psoas is under constant tension to maintain an upright position, causing your hips and low back to hurt. This is one of the reasons I encourage people to use some kind of lumbar back support that forces you into a neutral position. In a neutral position your psoas isn't overburdened trying to maintain normal lumbar curves.

Always prioritize optimal spinal mechanics by enforcing good positions. You also have to feed some love to the large muscle that supports these structures; otherwise you will end up in pain. In the following sequences, I demonstrate a few different options that you can use to restore suppleness to your psoas. Please note that these are acute targeted approaches aimed at releasing the superficial layers of stiffness. To get the biggest impact on psoas, as well as hammer the surrounding abdominal tissues, use the *global gut smash* demonstrated in the subsequent sequence.

Improves:
- ▶ Low Back and Hip Pain
- ▶ Optimal Spinal Mechanics
- ▶ Stabilization of the Spine
- ▶ Flexion and Extension of the Spine and Hip
- ▶ Rotation Capacity

Method:
- ▶ Smash and Floss
- ▶ Pressure Wave
- ▶ Contract and Relax

Psoas Smash and Floss–Option 1

Although this mobilization represents the lowest form of psoas smashing, it's not a bad place to start, especially if you've never smashed your psoas before. Executing this first option will help prepare you for the more tortuous mobilizations, as well as tap into some of the superficial layers of the muscle.

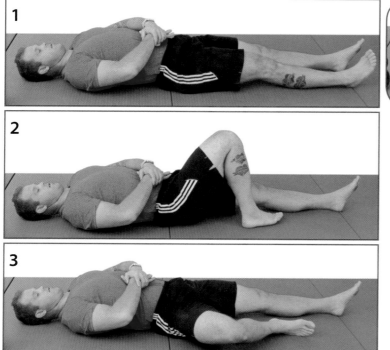

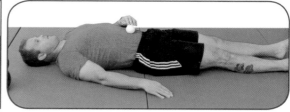

1. Position a lacrosse ball a couple of inches to the outside of your belly button, and then use both of your hands to push the ball into the lateral structures of your abdominals.

2. Having tacked-down a piece of your psoas, bring your knee up and try to floss around the underlying belly tissues underneath the ball.

3. Drop your right knee out to the side, keeping downward pressure on the ball. From here, you can move your knee from side to side, straighten your leg, or move on to another area of your psoas. The goal is to just find an area that feels painful, tack-down the tissue, and then apply a flossing element.

Psoas Smash and Floss–Option 2

This is the same idea as option 1, but instead of using your hands, you position a kettlebell over the lacrosse ball to get more acute pressure into the area.

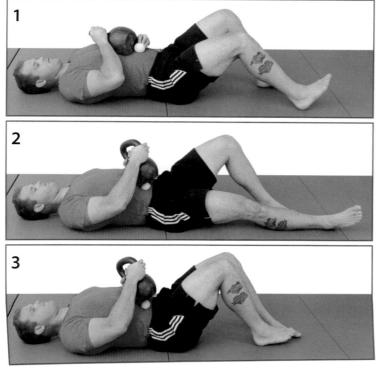

1. Position a lacrosse ball a couple of inches to the outside of your belly button, targeting your psoas, and then position the base of a kettlebell over the ball.

2. With the kettlebell smashing the ball into a stiff spot on your psoas, straighten your leg and begin flossing around the tacked-down tissue.

3. Elevate your knee. From here, you can externally and internally rotate your leg, as well as flex and straighten your knee until you feel some change in the tissue.

Psoas Smash and Floss–Option 3

This option gives you a slightly different stimulus by placing your legs up on a box. This takes a bit of tension out of the psoas, which allows you to penetrate deep into the pelvic area. The idea here is to just extend and flex your leg and pull tension into some of the neural tissues—like the sciatic nerve—to ensure the nerves are flossing smoothly through the psoas meat tunnel.

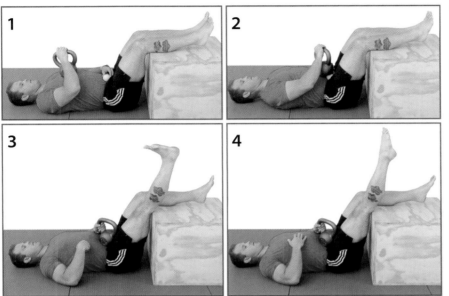

1. Position a lacrosse ball into your pelvic area just to the inside of your hipbone.

2. Next, add pressure by positioning the base of the kettlebell over the ball.

3. With the weight of the kettlebell driving the ball deep into your pelvic area, straighten your leg and flex your foot. This allows you to floss around some of the stiff, tacked-down tissue of your psoas.

4. Continue to floss around the tacked-down neural tissues by extending your right foot.

Targeted Gut Smash

The targeted gut smash allows you to penetrate deeper into the superficial layers of the psoas and surrounding abdominal tissue. Although you're tying in some of the musculature that relates to the psoas, it's still a targeted approach because you're using the point of the lacrosse ball or softball to tack-down tight tissues. You can use a smash and floss approach by moving your leg around, or you can roll from side to side and explore the outside and inside layers of your abdominal musculature.

Basically anything that makes you feel like vomiting is probably worth spending some time crushing.

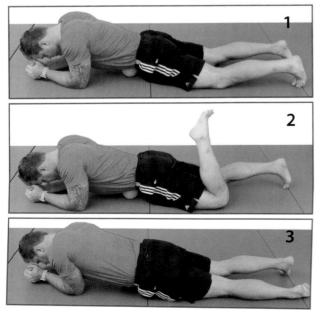

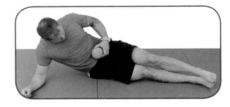

1. Lay down over the ball, positioning it just to the outside of your belly button.

2. After finding a stiff spot, take in a big breath, hold it for a few seconds and then exhale, relaxing into the ball. With your psoas and surrounding tissue tacked-down, floss around it by curling your left heel to your butt. You can also move your leg from side to side.

3. Still pressuring your weight into the ball, straighten your leg and then rotate your body slowly to the side to get a pressure wave effect across the tissue.

Global Gut Smash

As the name implies, the global gut smash hits all of the abdominal musculature surrounding your psoas. Think of it like this: Using a lacrosse ball targets one piece of your psoas like a chisel attacks stone; the global gut smash is like taking a sledgehammer to all the abdominal musculature and tissue surrounding the psoas, your illiacis and iliopsoas. Remember, you need these muscles to slide and move over one another unrestricted. If they are matted-down and adhered, the entire kinetic system is compromised.

The fact is that we not only rely on these muscles to stabilize, flex, and rotate the spine in our day-to-day lives, we spend a ton of our strength-and-conditioning efforts learning to create and maintain maximum trunk stiffness. Yet we do nothing to "unstiffify" the area. To be a fully functioning elite warrior leopard, that tissue needs to be like a filet mignon, not a grisly piece of beef jerky.

This mobilization is especially important if you've had any kind of abdominal surgery. Procedures like a C-section or appendectomy leave a lot of scarred layers of tissue that need ungluing. Moreover, if you have a history of lower back pain, or if you have to sit down for long periods of time, this mobilization gets a gold star and should be placed near the center of your mobility target.

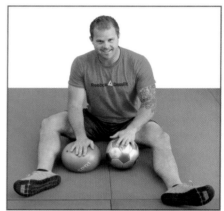

To correctly execute the global gut smash, use a large ball that has some pliability. You can use a kid's ball, which is like a mini physioball, a soccer ball, whatever. The harder ball should be reserved for voodoo leopard Jedi's. As you will realize, this mobilization is not pleasant. So don't pass out in the back corner of the pain cave or vomit on your living room floor. That's not cool. Remember, if the layers of your abdominal muscles are sliding, as they should, you will have little pain or visceral symptoms, achiness, pulling, or burning sensations. It will just feel normal. However, if you're a tacked-down mess, expect some pain and discomfort. Ten minutes is the minimum commitment to effect change, so pony up.

Note: Don't do this mobilization before any serious heavy lifting. The last thing you want to do is monkey around with your spinal mechanics before you max deadlift. While I don't think it would cause injury (in fact, you may experience great exercising after this mobilization), it's better to be safe and save it for after the workout.

Improves:

▶ Low Back and Hip Pain

▶ Sliding Surfaces in Abdominal Musculature

▶ Optimal Spinal Mechanics

▶ Stabilization of the Spine

▶ Flexion and Extension of the Spine and Hip

▶ Rotation Capacity

Method:

▶ Pressure Wave Smash from Side to Side

▶ Contract and Relax. (Take a big breath in, hold it, and press the ball deeper into the tissue.)

▶ Smash and Floss

TARGET AREA

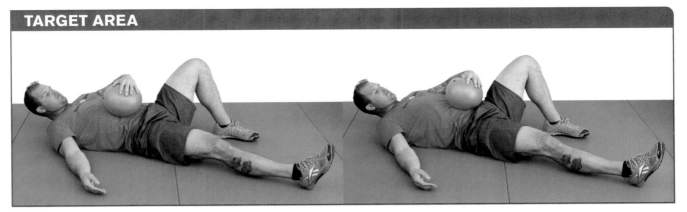

The target area for the global gut smash covers the region from the top of your hipbones, around your pelvis, up to your diaphragm, and around your ribcage (basically your entire abdominal section).

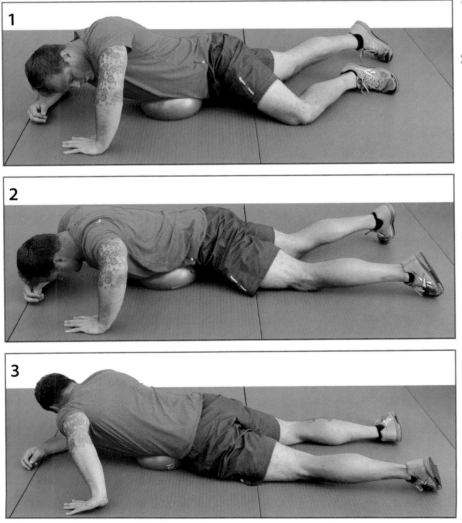

1. Lay over the ball, positioning it between your hipbone and ribcage.

2. To get the best results, you need to penetrate into the basement level of your tissues by sinking all of your weight into the ball. To accomplish this, take a big breath in, hold it for a few seconds, and then exhale. As you breathe out, relax your weight over the ball and sink deeper into your gut as if you were a piece of melted cheese.

3. After getting your full weight on the ball, slowly pressure wave. If you find a tight spot, you can contract and relax by holding in air and then exhaling to sink further into the bottom, or implement a smash and floss technique. The key is to spend at least 10 minutes on the area—5 minutes on each side.

AREA 6
POSTERIOR HIGH CHAIN
(GLUTES, HIP CAPSULE)

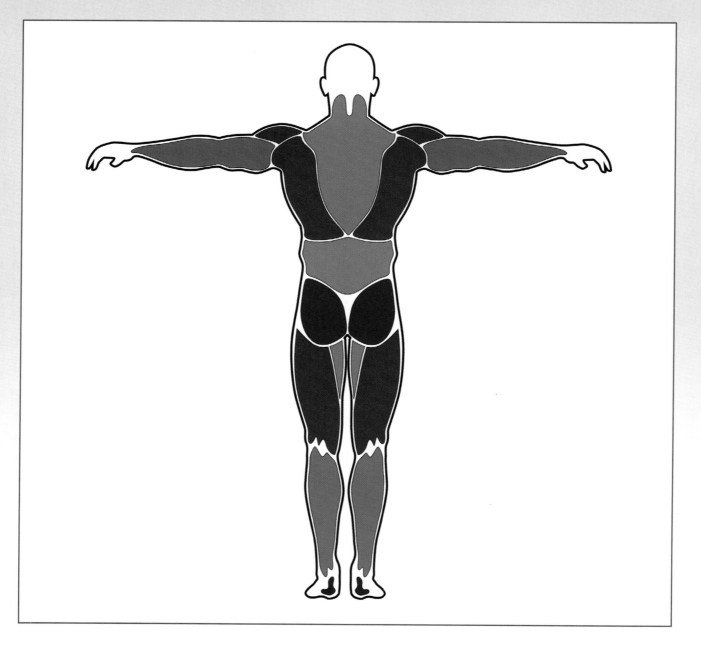

Mobilization Target Areas:

▶ Hip (glutes) and hip capsules

Most Commonly Used Tools:

▶ Single Lacrosse Ball
▶ Rogue Monster Band
▶ Roller

Test and Retest Examples:

▶ Squat and Pulling Position
▶ Lunge and Split-Jerk

Glute Smash and Floss

Although there are several habits that create stiffness in the high posterior chain, there are two that really mess you up: sitting is one, and assuming an open foot stance is the other. Sitting creates an inordinate amount of ass lamination, so if you take a long flight, drive in a car for extended periods of time, or sit at a desk for a living, you have to constantly work on restoring sliding surfaces to the tacked-down quagmire that is your butt. The second issue, which can run parallel or separate to the sitting paradigm, is if you stand or walk around with your feet turned out. If you're in a fully externally rotated position with your feet angled out, the tissues of your posterior high chain are permanently trapped in a shortened state. The result: Your hip external rotators get smoked and a lot of full range movements become untenable.

Want one of the best methods to unglue the laminated tissue of your butt? Jam a lacrosse ball in the side of your glute and find an ugly area of trashed tissue. Then use the three sliding surface techniques—pressure wave, smash and floss, contract and relax. Don't feel like you need to overcomplicate this mobilization by targeting specific muscles. People like to tell you, "Hit your glute mead or short hip rotators." If your last anatomy lesson was dissecting a frog, this one might leave you a tad clueless. What's important is that you find your business and put in some qualitative work, staying on the tight area until you make change. Fundamental stuff.

As with other large muscle group mobilizations, you don't need to cover the entire glute region in one session. Set a timer for 5 minutes a cheek and put in some work. You'll be surprised what a difference it makes. To test and retest, employ the butt acuity test. It's easy to do and illuminating. Spend 5 minutes on one butt cheek and then stand up and squeeze your glutes as hard as you can. What you'll find is that the side you mobilized contracts with a lot more force than the other. What does that mean? You just got a little bit stronger and more powerful. It's like a free super power.

IMPROVES:

- ▶ Hip External Rotation Capacity
- ▶ Low Back and Hip Pain
- ▶ Hip and Trunk Extension

METHODS:

- ▶ Contract and Relax
- ▶ Pressure Wave
- ▶ Smash and Floss

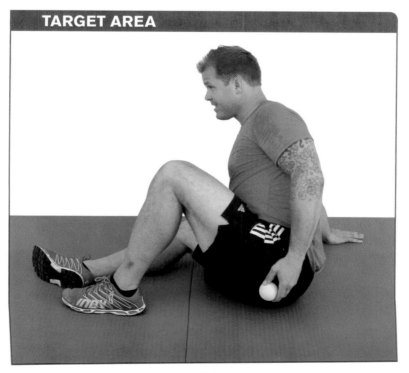

TARGET AREA

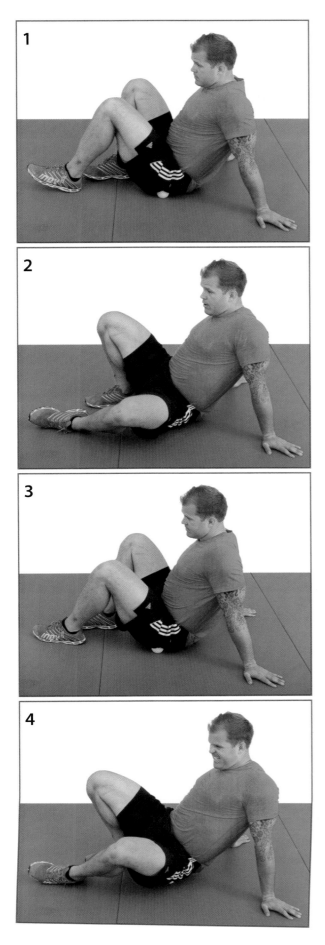

Position a lacrosse ball in the side of your hip.

With the ball tacking down the underlying muscle, move the surrounding tissue around the area by externally rotating your leg and dropping your knee to the mat.

Continue to floss the tacked-down tissue by pulling your knee in toward your center.

In addition to smash and flossing with internal and external rotation of the leg, you can try slowly rolling side to side across your glute. With this you want to really focus on pancaking across the grain of the tissue in a pressure wave fashion. If you stumble across a particularly painful area in the process, you can contract and relax until you get to the bottom of the tissue.

High Glute Smash and Floss

Your glutes are responsible for extending your hips and trunk. When these tissues get tight, generating force through your primary engine becomes difficult. Think about it like this: If you can't open your hips to full extension, the only way to achieve an upright torso is to overextend, forcing the musculature of your trunk and lumbar region to stabilize around your bad position. What happens? You lose your ability to generate force and you end up with low back and hip pain. By simply ungluing the musculature of your high glute and butt region, you can resolve a lot of your positional mechanics and pain up and down stream. In most cases, ten minutes of qualitative smashing allows you to reclaim a neutral posture, create sufficient external rotation torque, and generate force through your primary engine. Not only that, you feed slack to the tissue upstream, relieving low back pain.

For the best results, post your feet onto a box or a bench. This will allow you to capture the high glute region underneath the back and iliac crest of your hip. In addition, elevating your feet allows you to get more pressure through the ball. It also allows you to feather from side to side across the grain of your muscle, which is the best way to break up the tissue and restore suppleness to the region.

Note: This mobilization is often used in conjunction with the single lacrosse ball low back smash.

IMPROVES:

▶ Sliding Surfaces

▶ External Rotation Capacity

▶ Low Back and Hip Pain

▶ Hip and Trunk Extension

METHODS:

▶ Pressure Wave

▶ Smash and Floss

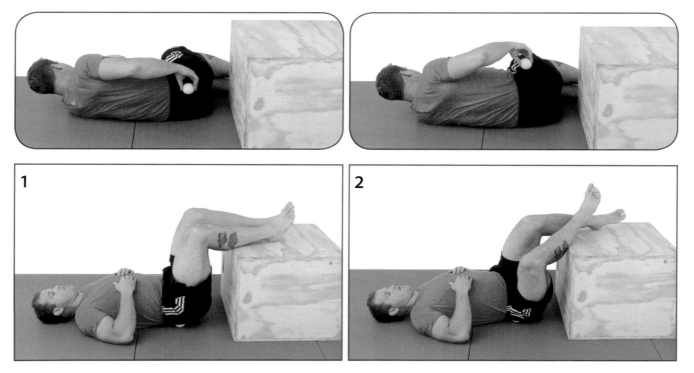

1. Position a lacrosse ball on your upper glute to the outside of your sacrum. To increase the pressure and prevent defaulting into an overextended position, position your feet up onto a box.

2. Curling your left heel into the box, slowly roll toward your right side, smashing all the tissues across your upper glute region. The goal here is to pressure wave across the grain of the tissue. If you find a really sticky spot, floss around the tacked-down tissue by pulling your knee to your chest, and internally and externally rotate your leg.

Side Hip Smashing

The side hip smash is another easy way to restore good hip function, as well as feed some slack upstream and downstream of your primary engine (hip). There are two areas that you're trying to capture with this mobilization. As you can see from the photos, you start on the posterior region of the upper glute, which comes into the top

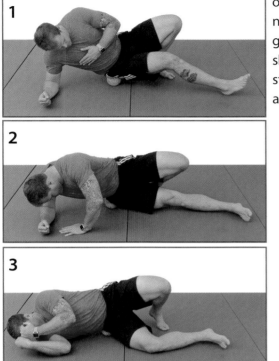

of the hipbone, and rip across that muscle into your hip flexor wad near the front of your hip. This mass ranging from your posterior glute to the front of your hip gets chronically stiff and adaptively short. I'm not going to lie. Smashing a lacrosse or softball across this stiff tissue is horrible. If you're in public, you might need to cover up and hide that pain face.

IMPROVES:

► Hip Function (Flexion, Extension, Rotation)

► Low Back and Hip Pain

METHODS:

► Pressure Wave

► Contract and Relax

1. Position a ball into the outside of your high glute, just below your hipbone.

2. Roll onto your belly—distributing as much weight as possible into the ball—and smash the tissue across the muscle fiber.

3. Continue to roll onto your side. For privacy, you should use both of your arms to cover up your pain face, blocking it from view. Nobody needs to see that.

Single-Leg Flexion with ER Bias–Option 1

This mobilization fits perfectly into our model of mobilizing within the context of movements we're trying to change. If you glance at the photos you'll notice that I'm essentially mobilizing the bottom of the squat one leg at a time. It doesn't need to be any more complicated than that. If I tried describing what's happening in the hip in classic terms, it would hold zero meaning. But if you understand that *I'm just squatting one leg at a time and trying to mobilize the bottom of the squat position*, it becomes very simple and easy to understand. There is purpose and intention that goes along with the mobilization: If I do this, I will squat better.

Here's how to achieve optimal results: First, you have to apply motion to this mobilization by hunting out tight corners and then oscillating in and out of those vectors. Don't just throw your leg up, drop your knee out, and then hang out. If you're tight in that first position, try capturing the tight pieces of your hip capsule by drawing small circles with your elevated hip. Once you feel like you've made some change, turn away from your elevated leg or rotate your belly button toward your knee while shoving your knee out. You can also shoot your hips back and extend your lead leg, which ties in the hamstring and allows you to hit a different corner of the hip. To put it simply, you want to capture all the different pieces of the tissue by moving your hip into different positions, and then "break the paper clip" by moving in and out of end-ranges.

The second key is to consider proper squat mechanics as you hunt around for tight corners. For example, the most common fault with this mobilization is to let your foot come off the ground as you drive your knee out to the side. Although this is a great way to capture some elements of your hip that might be tight (something that I demonstrate later), it doesn't necessarily fit into this mobilization piece. The reason? The moment your foot comes off the ground, you start bleeding torque out of your ankle and biasing a different range, which does not represent proper squat mechanics. Stapling your foot to the ground allows you to tie in your ankle range and most closely represents what you're trying to change, which is a foot flat movement in a weight-bearing squat situation. The same rules apply to other faults like tracking your knee over your foot and breaking at your lower back to hit certain corners. If it doesn't make sense mechanically, don't do it.

IMPROVES:

- ▶ Bottom of the Squat
- ▶ Deadlift Setup
- ▶ Overall Hip Function
- ▶ Hip Flexion with External Rotation
- ▶ Low Back and Hip Pain

METHODS:

- ▶ Paper-clipping (Oscillation)
- ▶ Contract and Relax
- ▶ Smash and Floss

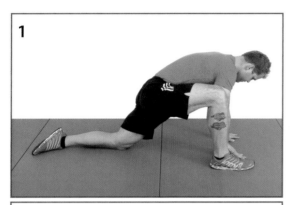

1

Starting on your hands and knees, post your right foot next to your right hand, making sure to keep your right shin vertical.

2

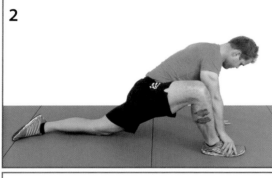

Place your right hand over your right foot, stapling it to the ground, sprawl your left leg back, and drop your knee out to the side. As you do this, actively drive your left hip to the ground and flatten your back. From this position, you can oscillate around by driving your weight into the corner of your butt, going in and out of end-range tension.

3

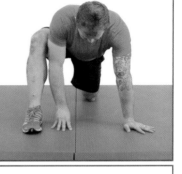

Start hunting for tight corners by rotating your upper body away from your elevated leg.

4

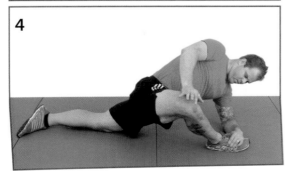

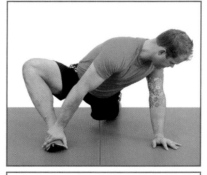

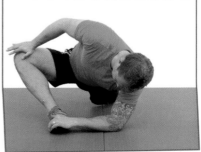

To increase knee-out positioning, drop your left elbow to the mat, cup your left hand over your right foot to keep it pinned to the ground, turn toward your elevated leg, and shove your knee out using your right hand.

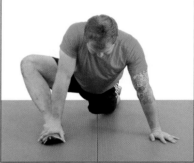

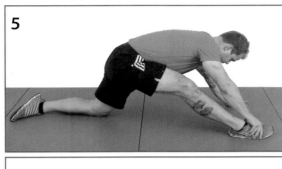

5

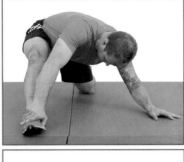

Drive your hips back. This captures the back of your hip and biases your hamstring into the mobilization.

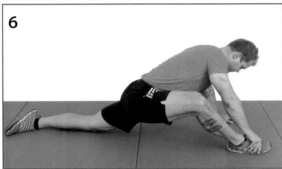

6

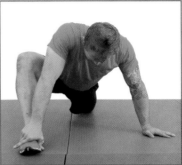

Having loaded your hip into a new position, slide forward and scour for new areas of stiffness.

Banded Distraction

Although this mobilization will provide some radical change without a distraction, it's always better to use a band when possible. Creating a distraction can multiply the effectiveness of the mobilization by a factor of 4 or 5. With this mobilization, you can create a distraction to the hip in two different directions. You can distract laterally, pulling your hip into the side of your capsule, or you can distract toward your posterior end, pulling your hip to the back of your socket. There's no wrong way. The idea is to change the orientation of the distraction so that you can magnify the stretch and clear any impingement that you may have.

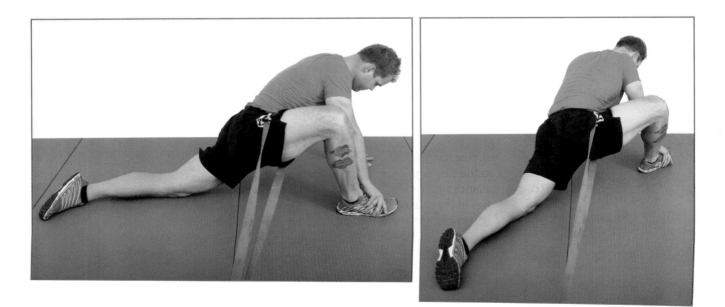

Single-Leg Flexion with ER Bias—Option 2

The single-leg flexion with external rotation bias acts as a two-for-one mobilization: You're capturing a flexion with external rotation piece with the lead leg and an extension piece with the back leg. A lot of athletes, especially powerlifters the size of highway demolition machines, are restricted in extension when executing this mobilization on the floor, which prevents them from dropping into deep flexion in the front. If that happens, mobilizing with your lead foot up on a box will give you a much better outcome.

Aside from elevating the foot, all the same rules apply: Mimic the mechanics of the squat by keeping your lead foot straight and pinned to the box, hunt out your stiff corners by forcing your hip into different positions, and apply the paper clip technique as you scour in and out of tight areas.

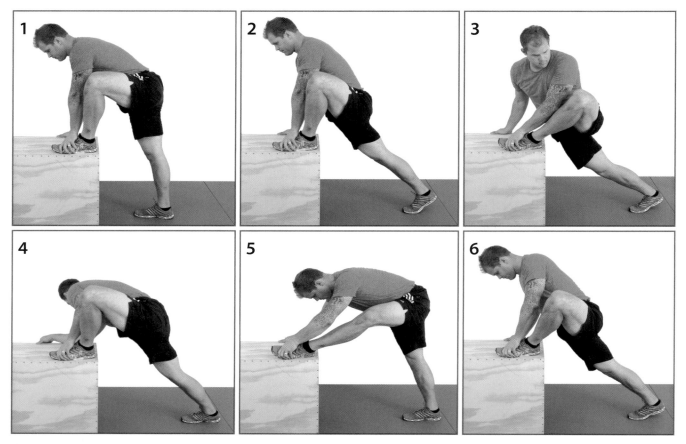

1. Post your left foot on the box and pin it to the surface with your left hand. To mobilize around a good squat stance, keep your lead shin vertical and your foot straight.

2. Keeping your left foot stapled to the box using your left hand, slide your right foot straight back and drop your left knee out to the side.

3. Rotate toward your elevated knee. This forces increased knee-out positioning on your left leg and biases an open hip position on your right hip and leg.

4. To bias more hip flexion, rotate toward your right and drop your chest toward the box.

5. Continue to hunt for stiff corners by driving your hips back. This captures the back of your hip and biases your hamstring into the mobilization.

6. Having loaded your hip into a new position, slide forward and scour for new areas of stiffness.

Banded Distraction

If you have a band, use it! Applying a distraction will dramatically increase the effectiveness of this mobilization. As with option 1, you can distract your hip laterally or toward the back of the capsule.

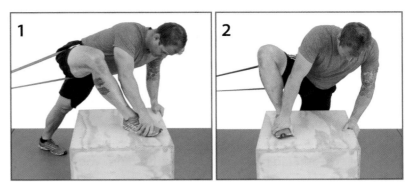

Hip External Rotation with Flexion–Option 1

In the previous mobilization elements, you emphasized flexion first, and then added external rotation as a tensioner. In this series, you do the opposite. If you glance at the photos, you'll notice that I emphasize external rotation first and then load the position with flexion, which provides a slightly different stimulus. As you can see, this mobilization is very similar to the classic yoga pigeon pose, but with a key difference: We're never going to collapse into a flexed, forward-rounded position. In addition to compromising spinal mechanics, the flexed, forward-rounded position doesn't give you the creative leverage to scour into the deep crevices of your stiffness. By placing one hand on your knee and blocking your foot with your opposite hand, you can load forward with a flat back and hunt for tight corners by rotating side to side.

Let me caution you here: If you can't position your leg perpendicular to your body because you're restricted, or you experience knee pain at any point, stop what you're doing and implement one of the subsequent variations.

IMPROVES:
- ▶ Bottom of the Squat
- ▶ Deadlift Setup
- ▶ Overall Hip Function
- ▶ Hip Flexion with External Rotation
- ▶ Low Back and Hip Pain

METHODS:
- ▶ Contract and Relax
- ▶ Paper-clipping (Oscillation)

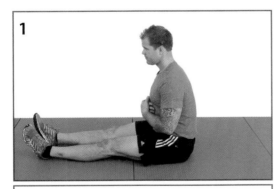

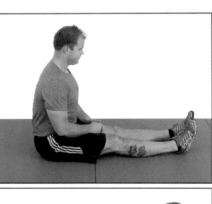

Sit upright with your legs straight out in front of you.

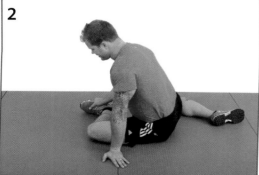

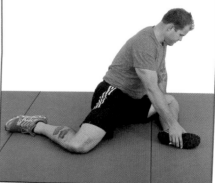

To set up, lean toward your left and post your left hand on the mat for balance. Next, swing your right leg behind you, position your lower left leg perpendicular to your body, and post your right hand on your left foot.

3

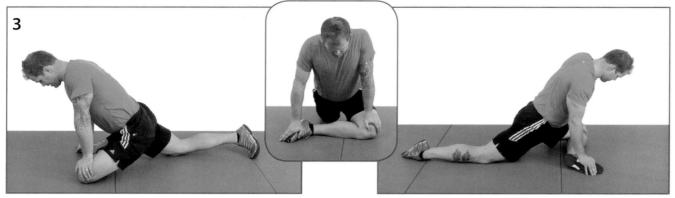

Post your left hand on your left knee, sprawl your right leg back, and lockout your arms, making sure to keep your shoulders back.

4

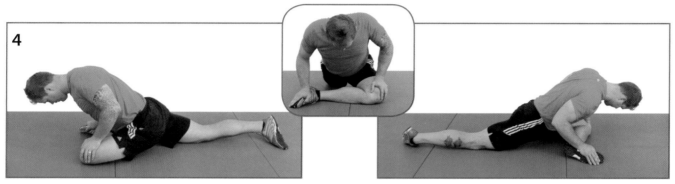

Keeping your back flat, lower your chest toward the ground.

5

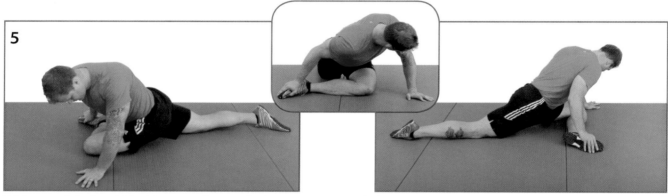

With your right hand blocking your foot—which prevents your left foot from sliding underneath your body and losing tension in the stretch—rotate toward your left side to hit a different corner.

6

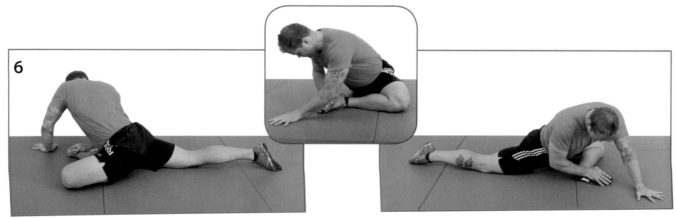

Rotate toward your right side and try to get your belly button over your left foot.

Hip External Rotation with Flexion–Option 2

This is the first mobilization that I recommend to people who experience lateral knee pain in the first position. If you're so tight you're not flexible enough to get your knee to the ground, you end up pulling your lateral knee joint apart as you load your leg into flexion. By posting up on your foot and then letting your knee drop out to the side, it solves a lot of the knee-gapping issues that causes your knee to flare up. Not only that, the position is much easier to get into because you're not as restricted by your back leg in extension.

Note: If you continue to experience pain in your knee or ankle, don't try to be tough and grind through it. There are other ways to approach this same mobilization without blowing out your knee or putting stress on your ankle joint. Consider options 3, 4, and 5.

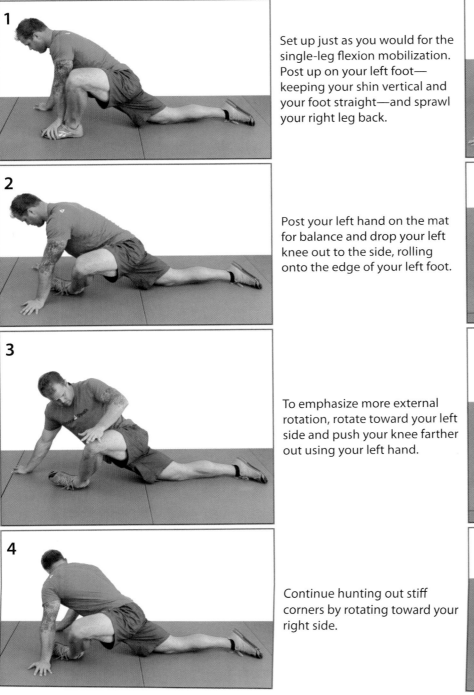

1 Set up just as you would for the single-leg flexion mobilization. Post up on your left foot—keeping your shin vertical and your foot straight—and sprawl your right leg back.

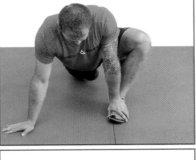

2 Post your left hand on the mat for balance and drop your left knee out to the side, rolling onto the edge of your left foot.

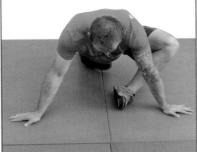

3 To emphasize more external rotation, rotate toward your left side and push your knee farther out using your left hand.

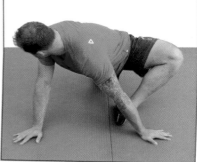

4 Continue hunting out stiff corners by rotating toward your right side.

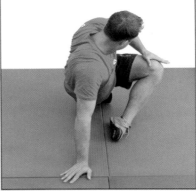

Hip External Rotation with Flexion–Option 3

This is another hip external rotation with a flexion option that you can implement if you experience lateral knee pain, or struggle to get into an optimal position from the ground. Even if you're not limited by range, positioning your lead leg on an elevated surface is a good option. Although it takes on the same shape as the variations previously demonstrated, it provides a slightly different stimulus. With your lead leg elevated, you can get a little bit more hip rotation, and add a more aggressive flexion load.

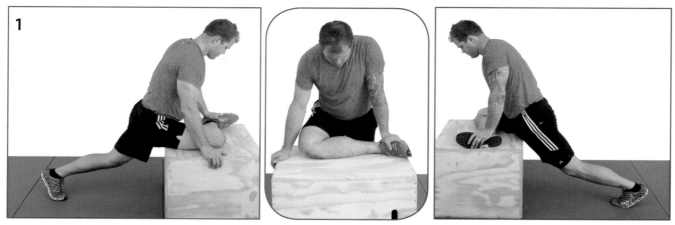

Post your right foot on the left side of the box, sprawl your right leg back, and let your right knee drop to the side, positioning your right leg across the box. With your lower leg perpendicular to your body, post your left hand on your right foot, pinning it in place.

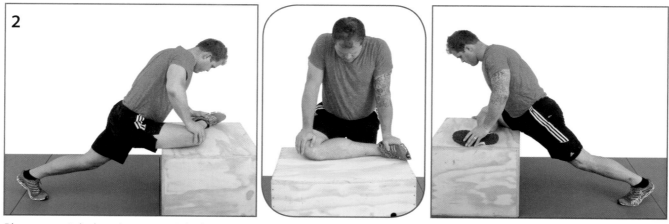

Place your right hand on your right knee. To increase the stretch, flex forward with a level back. From here, you can apply the paper clip technique by oscillating in and out of end-range by folding forward and pushing yourself up.

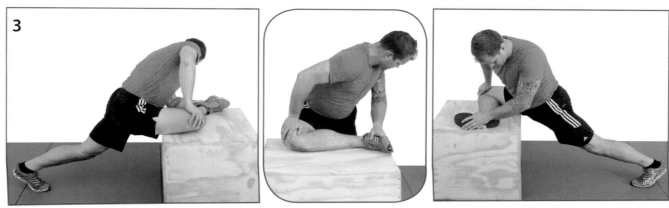

Turn toward your left and try to get your belly button over your foot.

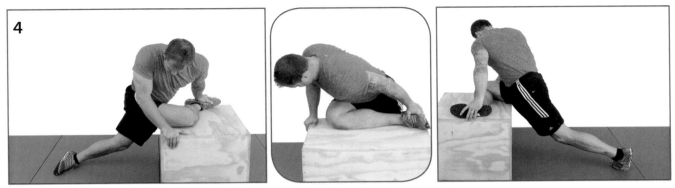

Keeping your left foot pinned, rotate toward your right, positioning your chest over your right knee.

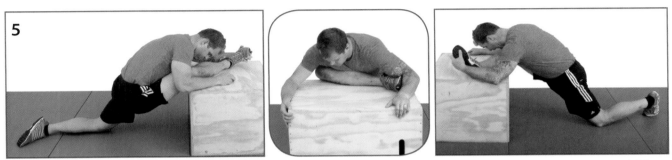

To hit the deep corners of your hip and capture some of that high hamstring, drop your left knee to the mat and fold forward. This position should be reserved for supple ninjas.

Hip External Rotation with Flexion–Option 4

There are a lot of athletes who are so stiff they can't get into any of the previously demonstrated positions without their knee joint ripping apart. If you fall into that category, you need to address the stiffness with some quality quad and hip smashing, and you need protect your knee joint by dropping your foot off a box. This takes some of the rotational torque off your joint so that you can explore your business without pain.

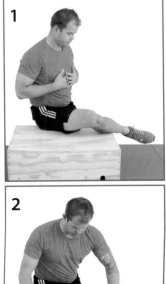

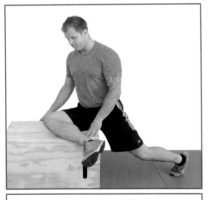

To reduce the load on you knee, sit halfway on the box and drop your right foot off the edge.

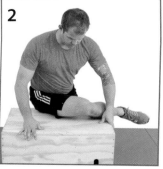

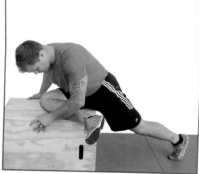

Fold forward from your hips and lower your chest to your right knee, creating a stretch in your right posterior hip.

Hip External Rotation with Flexion–Option 5

Here's the last option in the hip external rotation with flexion series: Cradle your knee to your chest and add a flexion load by leaning forward. This allows you to bias external rotation of your hip without challenging your knee joint.

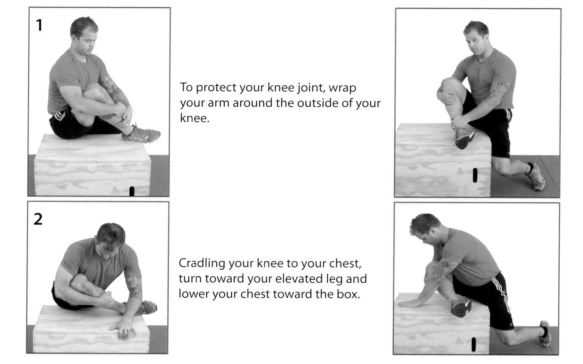

To protect your knee joint, wrap your arm around the outside of your knee.

Cradling your knee to your chest, turn toward your elevated leg and lower your chest toward the box.

Olympic Wall Squat with External Rotation

This is another oldie but goodie hip mobilization that works on flexion and external rotation. Creating a lateral distraction at your hip or wrapping a band around your knees to account for your hip capsule will create a larger impact; something that you'll find is true for the other Olympic wall squat variations.

IMPROVES:
▶ Flexion and External Rotation

METHODS:
▶ Contract and Relax

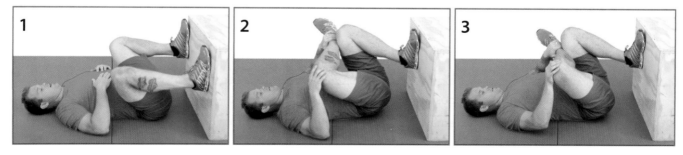

1. Position your butt as close to the box as possible and assume a squat stance with your feet positioned just outside shoulder-width. Your shins are vertical and your feet are straight.

2. Throw your right leg over your left knee.

3. To increase the aggressiveness of the stretch, pull down on your right instep with your left hand and slide your right foot toward your hip. Use your right hand to push on your right knee.

Executive Hip Mobilization

Are you sitting in a chair as you read this book right now? If the answer is yes, you should 1) be ashamed of yourself and 2) at least make the best of a bad situation and get something done (i.e., stick a ball into the side of your hip, underneath your hamstring, or bias some external rotation).

Warriors in the Supple Legion understand the toxic impact that sitting has on their performance and will do all in their power to avoid it. However, sometimes you just can't. If you're trapped at the desk or shackled into a Boston-to-LAX window seat, use the following stretches to work on your hip function and try to reverse the slow pending death to your mobility.

Obviously, there are much better ways to work on your hip mobility than sitting in a chair and trying to stretch! But something is better than nothing, so putting your hip into these positions and applying the contract and relax method is definitely useful if you're stuck in a chair.

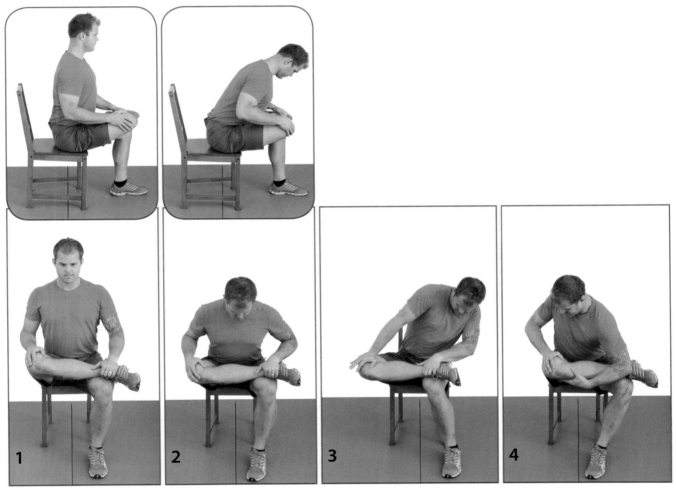

1. Establish a neutral posture sitting position and then cross your right foot over your left knee.

2. With your right leg biased into external rotation, apply a flexion load by folding forward from your hips with your back flat.

3. Using your left hand to keep your right foot from sliding off your left thigh, push your right knee toward the floor and lockout your arm. This helps tie in some of the side abdominal and low back tissues into the stretch.

4. Still pushing your knee toward the floor and keeping your back flat, rotate toward your right hand and lower your chest toward your knee, capturing another piece of your hip.

Executive Hip Workaround

Sometimes crossing your foot over your knee and adding forward flexion will cause lateral knee pain in people who are missing key ranges of motion. If that happens, wrap your arm around your leg and cradle your knee to your chest. This will take strain off your joint and allow you to rotate from side to side and apply load without pain.

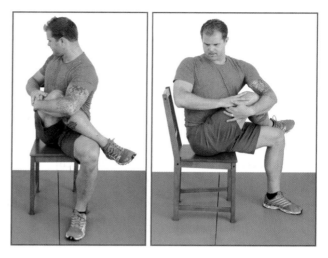

Gentle Hip Distraction

When I treat people with arthritis or work with an athlete who tweaked his hip or knee, I generally start with a simple banded joint distraction mobilization. In these situations, people are dealing with some bone on bone contact (i.e., femur rubbing against the hip joint) and inflamed tissue that causes a lot of pain and discomfort. By wrapping a band around their ankle and adding some tension, you can effectively un-impinge their hip and give joints some room to breathe. With any luck, you will alleviate pain and reset the joint to the normal, ideal position.

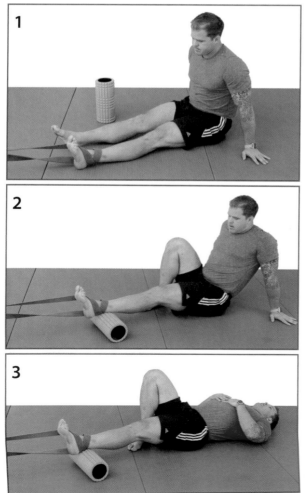

IMPROVES:

- ▶ Hip and Knee Pain
- ▶ Arthritic or Inflamed Knees and Hips
- ▶ Hip Function

1. Hook a band around the top of your foot and then wrap it around the base of your heel.

2. Create tension in the band and then prop your foot onto a foam roller. This will help keep your hip in a neutral position and maximize the distraction force through the ankle.

3. To encourage a neutral pelvic position and help prevent defaulting into an overextended position, curl your free leg in tight to your body, keeping your foot on the mat, and lie back. The idea is to relax your leg and allow the band to pull and decompress your joints, giving your knee and hip some breathing room.

Hip Capsule Mobilization–Option 1

Remember, it's not just your muscles that get tight. Your joint capsule system accounts for a huge chunk of tissue restriction. Here's an example: Say you experience an impingement at the front of your hips when you squat, restricting your range-of-motion. This is what I refer to as a "flexion wall," which is your femur running into the front of your pelvis. In order to reach end-range, you now have to compensate by turning your feet out or overextending.

If that happens, one of the first things you should do is reset the positioning of your hip to the back of the socket. Accomplish this by using the hip capsule mobilization. By aligning your knee directly underneath your hip and loading your weight over your femur, you can drive the head of your femur into the posterior capsule and restore normal hip function. It's a quick and dirty way to improve the efficiency of your hip mechanics without having to go see a physical therapist.

The goal here is to spend at least two to three minutes (or longer if possible), ideally using a band to distract the hip into a good position. To measure your results, you can test and retest by squatting or by lifting the knee you mobilized toward your chest from the standing position. You'll most likely find that simply resetting your hip to the back of the socket dramatically improves your hip flexion.

Note: We secretly call this the Donny Thompson World-Record-Breaking Squat Technique because he was able to reclaim a better position and smash the world record squat simply by mobilizing his hip capsule. He did this after failing in three previous attempts. Implementing this hip capsule mobilization is the only thing he changed as he prepared for his fourth attempt. Amazing.

IMPROVES:

▶ Squat and Pulling Mechanics ▶ Proper Hip Function

▶ Flexion and Extension of the Hips

▶ Intra-Articulation of the Hip
  (Internal and External Rotation)

METHODS:

▶ Paper-clipping (Oscillation)

▶ Contract and Relax

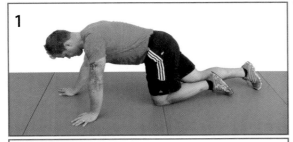

1 Kneel on the ground and shift the majority of your weight onto your left knee, aligning your knee directly underneath your hip.

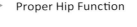

2 Drop your hips toward your left side, keeping your weight loaded over your left knee. Imagine trying to pop the head of your femur out the side of your butt.

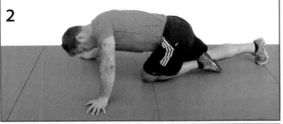

3 Still keeping your weight distributed over your left leg and driving your hips toward your left side, crawl forward and bias the tissues at the front of your capsule.

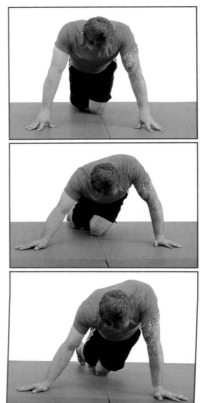

Hip Capsule External Rotation–Option 2

1

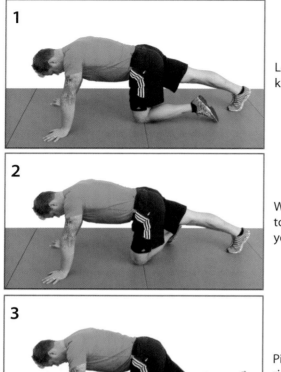

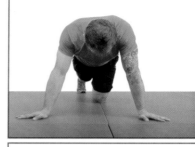

Load your weight over your left knee, keeping your femur vertical.

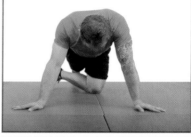

2

With the head of your femur reset to the back of the capsule, swing your left leg across your body.

3

Pin your left leg in place using your right knee.

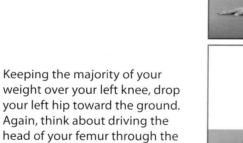

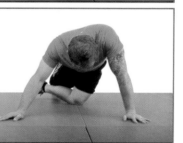

4

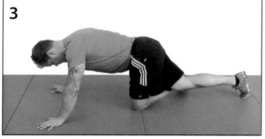

Keeping the majority of your weight over your left knee, drop your left hip toward the ground. Again, think about driving the head of your femur through the side of your butt.

5

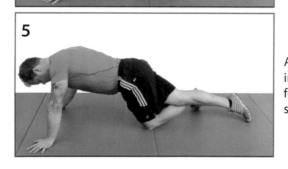

After spending a couple of minutes in the previous position, crawl forward to capture some of the tissues at the front of the capsule.

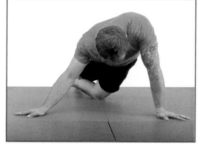

Banded Distraction

A lot of people will feel an impingement in the front of their hip when executing this mobilization. Here's what's happening: The head of your femur is positioned to the anterior edge of the socket, pinching some tissue between your femur and acetabulum (the housing of the hip joint). If this happens, mobilizing without a band is simply a waste of time. To make an impact on the hip capsule, wrap a band around your hip crease and create a lateral or posterior distraction. This will clear any impingement that you may have in the front of the capsule, allowing you to drop your hip to the back of the socket.

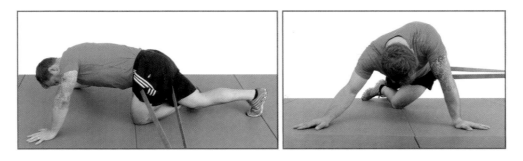

Hip Capsule Internal Rotation

Internal rotation capacity is critical for creating stability when your leg is behind you. It also plays a role in creating torque when your legs are in flexion, like when your knee is in the out position in the bottom of a squat. To help you understand this, think of internal rotation as an expression of your capsular slack. In other words, if you're missing internal rotation range, you won't be able to externally rotate when your leg is flexion, like when you're squatting; or internally rotate when your leg is behind you in extension, like when you're running or performing a split-jerk. Essentially, without this, you won't be able to create mechanically stable positions or generate power through your primary engine.

In this sequence, I demonstrate a very effective way to restore internal rotation capacity using the exact same setup as the hip capsule mobilization. But instead of biasing external rotation by kicking your leg across your body, you swing your leg to the outside of your body and hook your foot on a weight such as kettlebell.

IMPROVES:
- Internal Rotation Torque
- External Rotation Torque
- Capsular Slack
- Hip Function

METHODS:
- Paper-clipping
- Contract and Relax

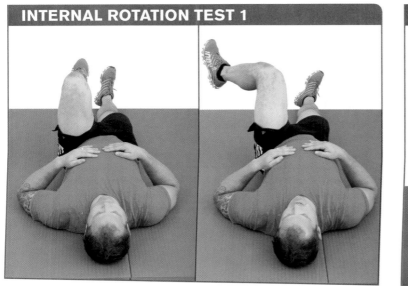

INTERNAL ROTATION TEST 1

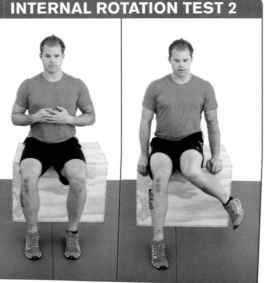

INTERNAL ROTATION TEST 2

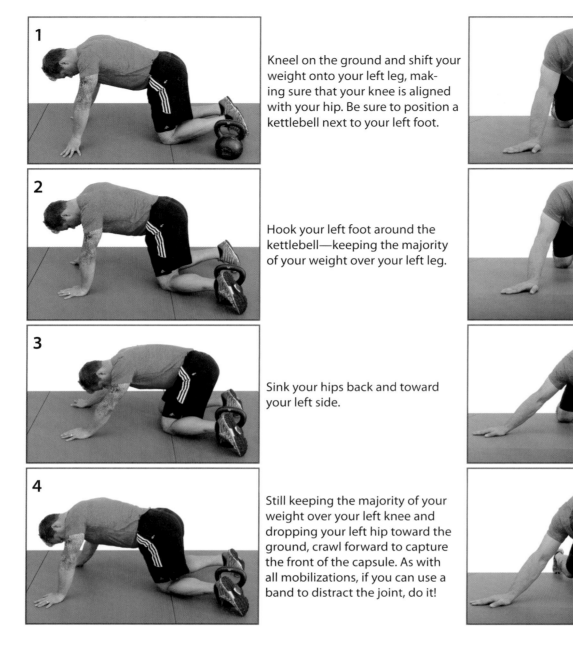

1 Kneel on the ground and shift your weight onto your left leg, making sure that your knee is aligned with your hip. Be sure to position a kettlebell next to your left foot.

2 Hook your left foot around the kettlebell—keeping the majority of your weight over your left leg.

3 Sink your hips back and toward your left side.

4 Still keeping the majority of your weight over your left knee and dropping your left hip toward the ground, crawl forward to capture the front of the capsule. As with all mobilizations, if you can use a band to distract the joint, do it!

Cueing Internal Rotation With Distraction

If the head of your femur is jammed into your hip capsule, it's difficult to work on restoring or improving rotational hip range-of-motion using the hip capsule internal rotation mobilization. For some people, wrapping a band around their hip and applying a lateral or posterior distraction is not enough to un-impinge their femur from their hip socket. They still feel a radical pinch at the front of their hip that prevents them from correctly performing the hip capsule mobilization. If that happens, you need to create space within the hip capsule by pulling the joint apart.

If you glance at the photos, you'll notice that I add a distraction from my ankle, roll onto my stomach, and then actively internally rotate my foot. This is the equivalent of distracting your arm overhead and then actively working on external rotation. But in this case, you're working on improving internal rotation capacities with your leg in extension, which is the stable position for your hip when your leg is behind your body.

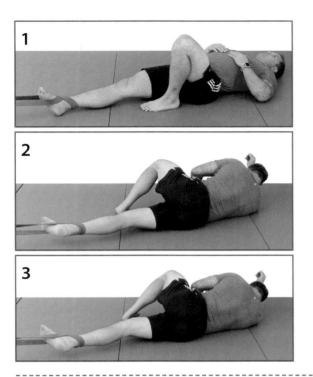

IMPROVES:

▶ Hip Internal Rotation

▶ Hip Pain and Hip Impingement

1. Hook a band around the top of your foot and then wrap it around the base of your heel.

2. Roll onto your stomach. This biases your leg into extension.

3. Keeping your leg relaxed, actively internally rotate your leg.

Olympic Wall Squat with IR Bias

This is another mobilization that improves hip internal rotation. From your back, it's harder to approximate the hip into the back of the socket as you internally rotate, so this mobilization is less effective than the previous technique. However, it's still a very useful idea and something that can be used in conjunction with the other Olympic wall squat variations.

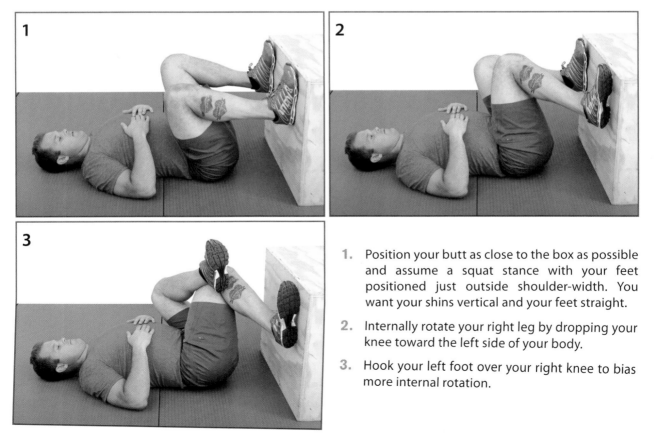

1. Position your butt as close to the box as possible and assume a squat stance with your feet positioned just outside shoulder-width. You want your shins vertical and your feet straight.

2. Internally rotate your right leg by dropping your knee toward the left side of your body.

3. Hook your left foot over your right knee to bias more internal rotation.

Banded Distraction

To improve the effectiveness of this mobilization, create a lateral distraction or wrap a band around your knees to approximate your femurs to the back of the sockets.

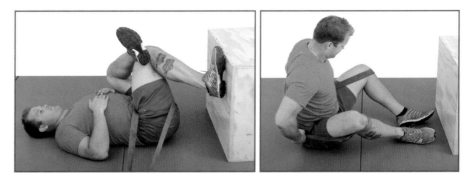

Global Internal Rotation

Although this global internal rotation piece doesn't give you the same impact as the hip capsule mobilization or the Olympic wall squat variation, it's something that you can do when you're relaxing on your back watching TV or just hanging out. As with all the previous techniques, adding a lateral distraction on the hip you're mobilizing is ideal.

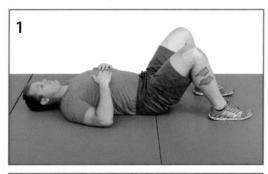

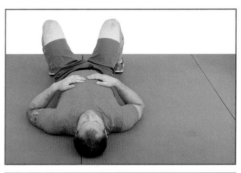

Lay on your back with your knees up.

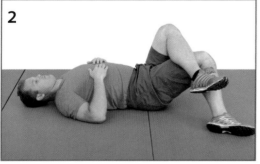

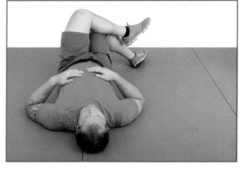

Internally rotate your right leg and cross your left leg over your right knee, anchoring it down to the mat.

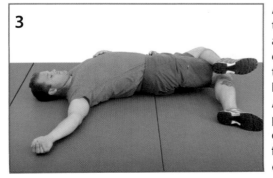

As you drop your right knee to the mat, reach your right arm out to the side. This counterbalances your rotation and ties in the musculature of you lower back. Additionally, it's easy to compensate into an overextended position, so prevent that fault by keeping your butt in contact with the ground.

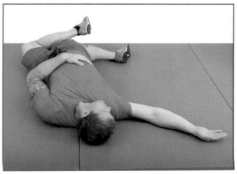

Internal Rotation Workaround

As with the external rotation executive hip mobilization pieces, the internal rotation workaround should not be the first stop when mobilizing your hip. In addition to putting the musculature of your trunk on tension, you can't approximate your hip into a good position, making it easier to compensate into a bad position. However, if you're trapped in a chair and you know you're going to be there for a prolonged period of time, you might as well take a crack at improving internal rotation.

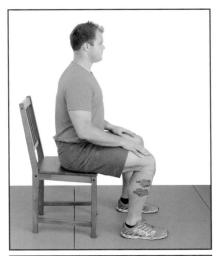

1

Sit upright with a neutral posture.

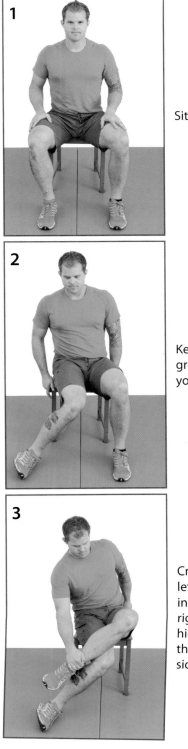

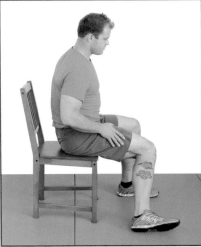

2

Keeping your right foot in contact with the ground, internally rotate your leg by dropping your knee toward the inside of your body.

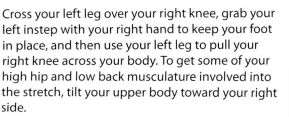

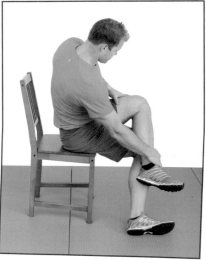

3

Cross your left leg over your right knee, grab your left instep with your right hand to keep your foot in place, and then use your left leg to pull your right knee across your body. To get some of your high hip and low back musculature involved into the stretch, tilt your upper body toward your right side.

AREA 7
ANTERIOR HIGH CHAIN
(HIP FLEXOR, QUADRICEPS)

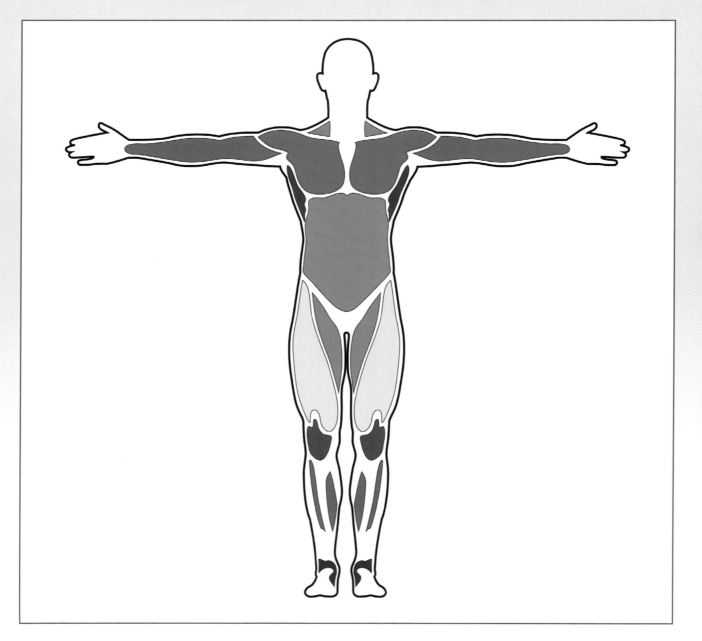

Mobilization Target Areas:

▶ Anterior hip (hip flexors) and quadriceps.

Most Commonly Used Tools:

▶ Single Lacrosse Ball
▶ Rogue Monster Band
▶ Roller

Test and Retest Examples:

▶ Squat and Pulling Position
▶ Top Position

Quad Smash

This is one of my favorite global mobilization pieces because it has broad range application and applies to everyone. CrossFitters, elite level Olympic weight lifters, tactical athletes, and desk-bound workaholics all need tools in their mobility arsenal that address global stiffness in large muscle groups like the quads, hamstrings, and glutes. They are under constant tension, put under tremendously large loads, and get adaptively short from sitting. Yet very little is done to restore suppleness to the stiff tissue. In this sequence, I demonstrate a potent way to smash your quads and restore normal function to this large bundle of hardworking muscle. However, before you delve into the technique, it's important to revisit some general rules.

Rule #1: Go against the grain of the tissue. Whenever you're dealing with global smashing elements, focus on slow, qualitative, back and forth smashing. As with the T-spine smash, rolling up and down the length of the muscle fiber with zero intention or purpose is a waste of time. You might as well just do some classic static '70s-style stretching and calisthenics, because you're not going to change anything. To produce significant change, create large pressures across the tissue, applying the big three mobilization techniques: contract and relax, smash and floss, and pressure wave.

Rule # 2: Stay on the tissue until you make change. The key is to clear a section until it normalizes (meaning it's not painful) before you move up or down the length of the muscle. When I treat athletes in my practice, I will smash one leg for no less than 10 minutes before I switch to the other leg. The point is you need to commit at least 20 minutes (10 minutes per leg) to unglue the tissue. If you can't clear the entire leg in 10 minutes, remember where you left off and switch to equal out the other side, then go back and attack the rest of the leg later.

Rule #3: Use a mobility tool that will make change. To penetrate into deeper layers of the tissue, you have to apply large blunt pressures. If you've never smashed your quad before, starting out with a foam roller is not a bad idea. However, if you're a monster athlete, a foam roller will impact you about as deeply as a bag of marshmallows. If you fall into this category, use a pipe, barbell, or have a Superfriend stand on your quad. Be warned, smashing your quads is very painful. You will catch a lot of people hiding in the deep crevices of the pain cave. It may take twenty rolls back and forth before you can take the full pressure of your weight (or friend's weight) before it stops hurting. So pony up and get some work done.

IMPROVES:
▶ Hip Function
▶ Knee, Hip, and Low Back Pain
▶ Intra Muscular Stiffness
▶ External and Internal Rotation

METHODS:
▶ Pressure Wave (Side to Side)
▶ Smash and Floss
▶ Contract and Relax

1

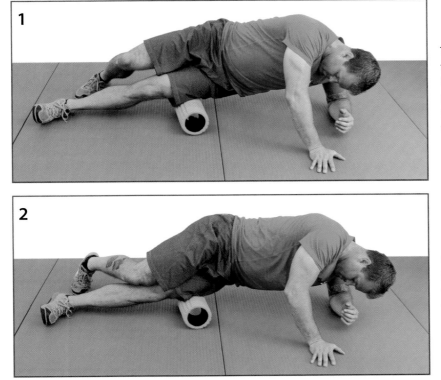

To set up, lay over the foam roller, positioning the roller directly under your left leg. Notice that I'm on my side. To keep my weight distributed over my leg, I plant my left foot down while supporting the weight of my upper body with my arms.

2

With your weight distributed over your left leg, create a pressure wave across the grain of your tissue by slowly rolling toward your right.

3

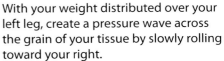

As you roll onto your stomach, plant your right foot on the opposite side of your leg. From here, you can contract and relax and oscillate on and off of tight spots.

4

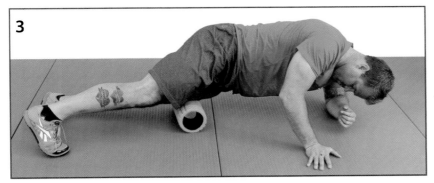

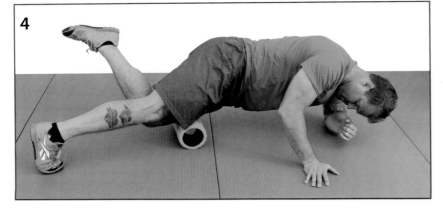

Floss around tacked-down tissue by pulling your heel toward your butt. The idea is to stay on the tight area, using the smash and floss and the contract and relax techniques until you no longer feel pain. Once you clear the area, progress up your quad to clear another chunk of your muscle.

Barbell Quad Smash

Next to having a buddy stand on your thigh, the barbell quad smash is probably the second most effective way to tap into the deep tissue stiffness of the quad. As I said, you need large blunt forces to effect change; this is easily done using a barbell. However, going against the grain of the muscle fiber is difficult using this technique. To restore sliding surfaces to the underlying tissue, be sure to go very slowly, clearing one small area at a time. Think about pressure waving back and forth over stiff muscle bundles until something changes or until you stop making change. You can also try rolling your leg from side to side to get the full smashing effect or as a way to tap into different corners.

Note: The barbell quad smash is particularly effective for clearing upper quad stiffness near the hip.

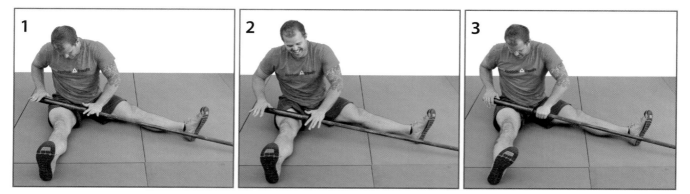

1. Position the sleeve of the barbell over your upper quad. To create pressure, lean forward with a flat back and push the barbell into the meat of your thigh.

2. Slowly roll the barbell down the length of your muscle, maintaining as much downward pressure as possible. Remember to focus on small chunks and go as slowly as possible. The goal is to create a large pressure wave through the tissue. If you encounter a really stiff spot, you can roll your leg from side to side as well as use the contract and relax technique.

3. Pull the barbell back up your thigh, internally rotate your leg, and prepare to attack a new line. For optimal results, only create pressure through the barbell going down the length of your leg.

Superfriend Quad Smash

The Superfriend quad smash is the most efficient way to effect global stiffness change in your quads. While using a barbell, Rumble Roller, or PVC pipe on yourself is certainly a good idea, the simple fact is you will never create the same amount of torturous pressure that someone else will. No one is that sick.

To perform this mobilization, have your training partner step on your quad with the arch of their foot and create large downward smashing pressures back and forth across your muscle. If it's you who is doing the smashing, avoid using pinpoint, lacrosse-ball-like pressures by driving your heel or ball of the foot into the meat. Uncool at the least. The goal is to create a shear force across the muscle so that you can restore sliding surfaces to the underlying tissue, as well as make it a little bit more tolerable for the guy getting smashed.

If you're on the bottom end of the smash, fight the urge to overextend. Raising your hips is not going to reduce the pain. Also, don't tap out in submission. It's not a grappling match. However, you probably need to pick out and agree on a "safe" word that will get your training partner to ease up when the pain gets to be too much.

Note: This is a great mobilization to drop into a large group of athletes. In fact, the Chinese weightlifting team has been reported to put on large smashing parties before and after training.

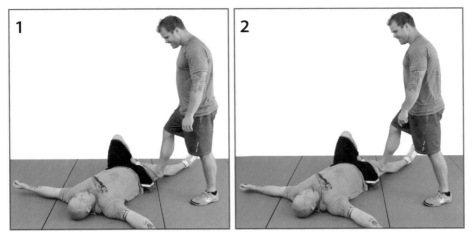

1. As you'll see in the photo, I position the arch of my foot on Jesse's quad. Notice that Jesse posts up on his left leg. This helps him keep a flat back and reduces some of the extension forces (overextending his back) as I mash into his leg.

2. I shift my weight forward and create a large shear force across the top of Jesse's quad.

Suprapatella Smash and Floss

If you're doing a lot of jumping with shins that aren't vertical—rather your knees are tracking forward when your hips are in flexion—or you're performing some sketchy squats where your knees cave in, not only will you experience knee pain, but you're burning through duty cycles at an insanely accelerated rate. Don't wait until your knee explodes to do something about it. First, feed some slack to the kneecap system so that you can reclaim good knee positions and reduce pain. Second, revisit the load-order sequence and fix your faulty mechanics. To address the former, snuggle a lacrosse ball into the area just above your kneecap (the suprapetalla pouch), then apply some pressure and smash and floss until something changes. To address the latter, flip back to the chapters devoted to movement mechanics. By opening up the area right above your kneecap, you can effectively alleviate joint pain, as well as resolve a lot of the knee dysfunction that occurs in deeper ranges of flexion.

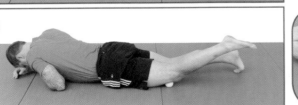

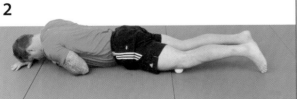

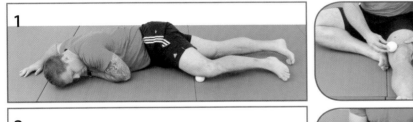

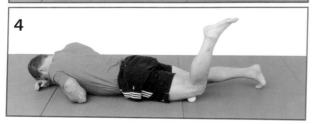

IMPROVES:
▶ Knee Pain
▶ Knee Mechanics and Function

METHODS:
▶ Smash and Floss
▶ Pressure Wave
▶ Contract and Relax

1. Position a lacrosse ball on the inside of your leg, just above your kneecap.

2. Create a pressure wave across your patellar pouch by internally rotating your knee.

3. Continue to smash across your suprapatellar pouch and quad tendon until you reach the lateral part of your knee.

4. If you encounter a hot spot, floss around the stiff tissue by curling your heel toward your butt.

Voodoo Knee Mobilization

Guess what? Your kneecap does not stretch. The ligaments and tendons that make up the knee structure are a fixed length. The best way to improve knee mechanics (knee out-ness) and reach deeper ranges of flexion is to feed slack to the knee structure by opening up the suprapetallar pouch. In that area, you have the common quad insertion, which shares a large, common tendon sheath entering into your knee. When this area gets matted-down and stiff, it pulls on your knee structure, causing pain and faulty mechanics.

Although the lacrosse suprapatellar smash and floss works, you're limited to a tiny spot and can't get the entire target area. That is why I prefer the voodoo band variation as the first step in dealing with upstream and downstream stiffness. It tears open that big common tendon sheath and clears up the entire area in a very short amount of time.

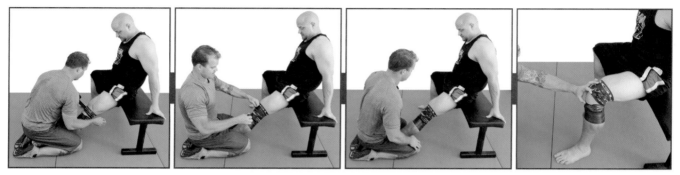

I've wrapped Jesse's knee with a voodoo band. Notice that I've wrapped below and above the knee using two separate voodoo bands. **Note:** You can also wrap the entire knee using one band. To learn how to properly voodoo wrap, revisit the chapter introduction (page 219).

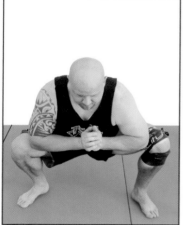 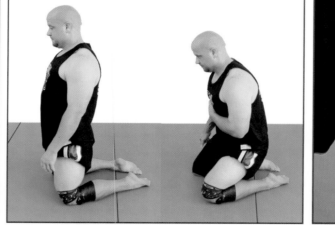 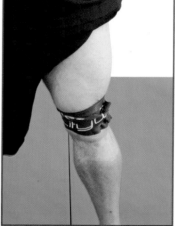

With his knee wrapped, Jesse looks to floss some of the stiffness away by squatting and biasing some knee-out positions. It's important to perform a number of squats, hang out in the bottom position, and force your knee into end-range flexion positions.

Jesse continues to force his knee into flexion by kneeling on the ground and sitting his butt to his heels.

Banded Hip Extension

Opening up the front of your hips while kneeling on the ground is not a new idea (photo 1A). People have been doing this for thousands of years. But there's just one problem: The classic kneeling hip opener does not account for the joint capsule, leaving a huge piece of tissue restriction on the table. What's the solution? Simple: Hook your leg through a band, pull it up to your butt crease, and create a forward distraction. With a large tension force pulling your femur to the front of your hip socket, you idealize your joint position, which not only ties in your anterior hip capsule (y-ligament or iliofemoral ligament), but also makes it easier to mobilize all the musculature at the front of your hip structure.

As you will soon see, there are three ways to bias your anterior hip into extension: banded hip extension, banded hip extension lunge, and the infamous couch stretch. In this sequence, I start with the most basic of these elements, the banded hip extension. To correctly perform this mobilization, create tension in the band and then slowly shift your body forward while keeping your back flat. A lot of athletes mistakenly arch the back and hyperextend their back as they open their hip. To avoid this fault, shift your weight over your grounded knee while keeping your posture straight and your butt squeezed.

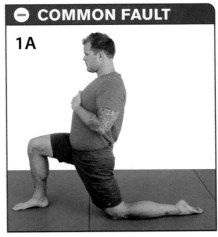

● COMMON FAULT

1A

Note: To capture some of the stiffness in your high anterior hip, put your left arm over your head (if your left knee is on the ground), lean back, and then come back to center. The key is to oscillate back and forth, in and out of end-range. As with the classic hip extension, you *must* keep your butt squeezed to support your lumbar spine. This is just another option that you can infuse into this mobilization. It is a nice way to tear open that high front hip region, which tends to get very nasty.

IMPROVES:

▶ Hip Extension

▶ Top Position (Squat and Deadlift)

▶ Normal Posture

▶ Low Back and Hip Pain

▶ Knee Pain

METHODS:

▶ Contract and Relax

▶ Paper-clipping (Oscillation)

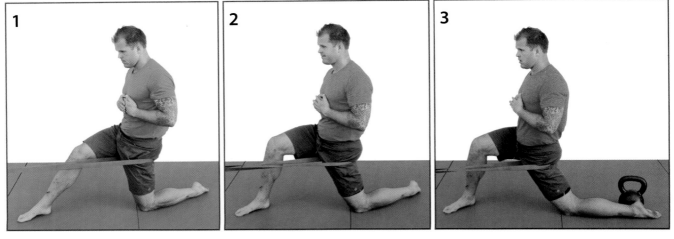

1. Hook your left leg through the band and step back to create tension—keeping your rear foot internally rotated. To avoid breaking into an overextended position, squeeze your left glute and keep your belly tight.

2. With the band distracting your femur into the front of your hip socket, slowly shift your weight forward over your grounded knee. Notice that I move my entire body rather than thrust my hips forward.

3. For optimal results, hook your foot around a weight so that you can bias internal rotation of your hip, which is the stable position for your hip.

Banded Hip Single-Leg Squat

Mobilizing is a way to deal with muscle stiffness. It restores normal ranges of motion to tacked-down tissues. It is not a warm-up to exercise. However, there are some mobilization techniques that are appropriate prior to training and competition. The banded hip extension lunge is a perfect example. As you can see from the photos, the setup looks a lot like a split-jerk, making it a perfect piece to tie into some Olympic lifting, or anything else that requires you to open up your hips into full extension.

IMPROVES:

- ▶ Hip Extension
- ▶ Top Position (Squat and Deadlift)
- ▶ Normal Posture
- ▶ Low Back and Hip Pain
- ▶ Knee Pain

METHODS:

- ▶ Contract and Relax
- ▶ Paper-clipping (Oscillation)

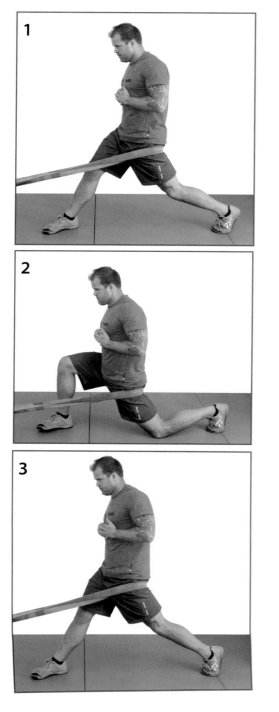

1 Hook a band around your left leg, pull it up to your butt crease, and step back to create a forward distraction on your left hip. To avoid breaking into an overextending position, squeeze your left glute to protect your low back, and brace your trunk.

2 Keeping your left glute squeezed and your belly tight, drop your left knee to the ground. Notice that my lead shin does not go past vertical and my torso is upright.

3 Driving off your lead leg, extend both of your knees and stand up.

Couch Mobilization

The couch mobilization is one of my favorite hip openers and is probably the most famous technique in the movement and mobility arsenal. Athletes have a real love-hate relationship with the couch mobilization because it is both effective and horribly painful at the same time. In fact, it's frack-en gnarly. When I first developed this mobilization, I had to do it on the couch in front of the TV because 1) it's an easy way to get your leg into full flexion and open your hips, and 2) the TV takes your mind off the pain and keeps you from blacking out.

It's important to realize that although the couch mobilization is unique to the Movement and Mobility System, it's not a new idea. People have been doing variations of this for a long time. You'd recognize this as the classic standing quad stretch that you did in elementary school (photo 1), or the traditional yogi pose (photo 2), which requires you to grab your foot and pull it to your butt while kneeling on the ground. The problem with these iterations, aside from being difficult to maintain a stable position, is they do not take you to end-range. To effect change, you need to be able to mobilize in a good position and hit end-range knee flexion and hip extension, which is what the couch mobilization allows you to accomplish.

Whether you're trapped at the airport, hanging out watching a movie, at work in front of your desk, or getting ready to work out, the couch mobilization is a highly effective way to reclaim range-of-motion and reduce muscular stiffness in the front of the hips and quads.

Note: The positions illustrated in the photos are basic physiologic ranges of motion, meaning everyone should be able to get into position 1 and position 2 without pain or restriction. While this is ideal, it's just not possible for the majority of people. So this turns into a really quick diagnostic for athletes and coaches. If you can't get your leg into the pre-start position or pull your back to the wall, you know something is seriously wrong: Your quads and the front of your hips are freakishly tight.

IMPROVES:	METHODS:
▶ Hip Extension	▶ Contract and Relax
▶ Top Position (Squat and Deadlift)	▶ Paper-clipping (Oscillation)
▶ Normal Posture	
▶ Low Back and Hip Pain	
▶ Knee Pain	

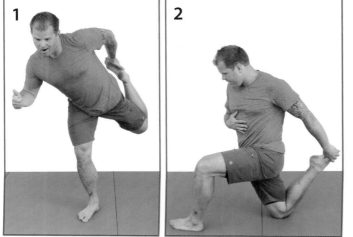

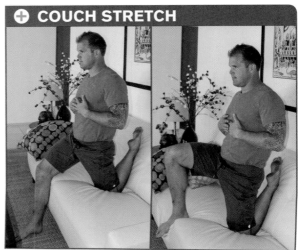

COUCH STRETCH

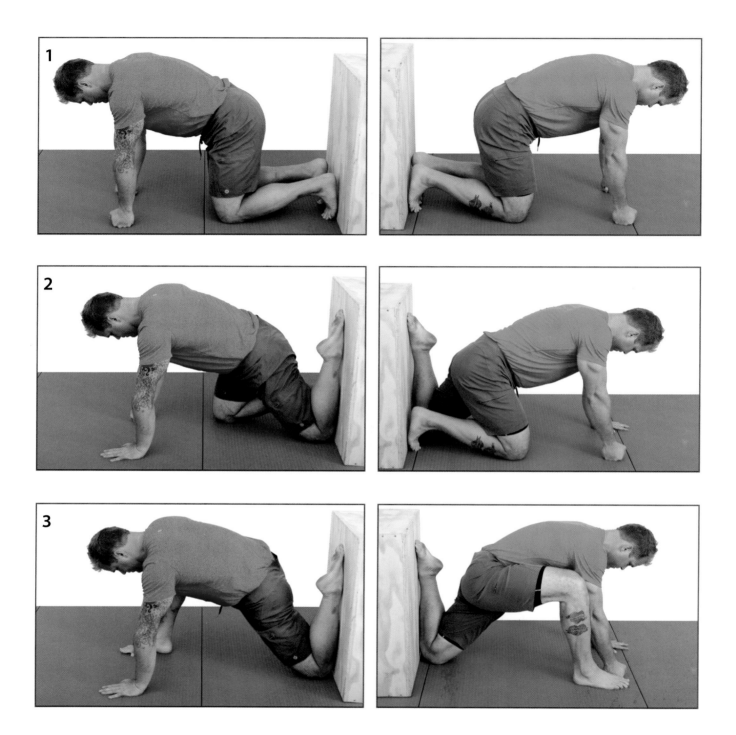

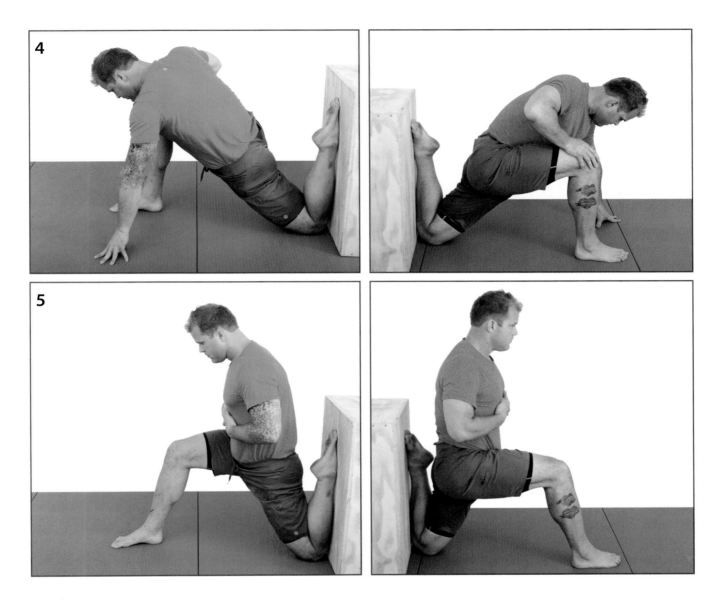

1. Back your feet up to the side of a box.

2. Slide your left leg back, driving your knee into the corner and positioning your right shin and foot flush with the side of the box.

3. Squeezing your butt to stabilize your lower back, post up on your right foot, keeping your lead shin vertical. **Note:** If you're unable to post-up on your opposite leg because you're too stiff, position a small box in front of you for extra stability.

4. Still squeezing your left glute, drive your hips toward the ground. With your lower leg in full flexion (heel to butt), pull the tissue slack to end-range (quad and anterior hip structure), making it extremely difficult and painful to open up the hips. As long as you don't feel hot, burning nerve pain, you're okay.

5. After hanging out in the previous position for a minute or two, lift your torso into the upright position. If you find it difficult to support the weight of your upper body from the upright position, position a chair, box, or bench in front of you for extra stability.

Common Faults

One of the biggest issues people have with the couch mobilization is they can't get into the correct positions because they are too tight. For example, it's not uncommon to see athletes slide their knee out to the side, pull it away from the corner, or overextend as a way to circumvent their mobility restriction. If you find that getting into position 1 or 2 is difficult, keep your opposite knee on the ground and stabilize your weight on a box. For the best results, put

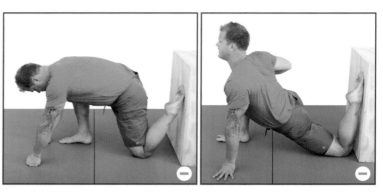

your knee in full flexion so that you can tie in the quads and open up the business at the front of your hips. And remember: If your butt goes off tension a dear friend will probably die, so don't do it.

Super Couch Variation

The super couch is the DEFCON 5 version of the couch mobilization. By adding a band and creating a forward distraction you increase the brutality and effectiveness of this mobilization by a factor of 10. Remember: Anytime you can make a mobilization feel worse, it's probably better. Despite increasing your chances of blacking out, the band opens up your hip capsule and tears into the anterior structures of your quad and hip like nothing else. The results are truly amazing.

Disclaimer: If you don't have full-range in your quads and hips, you should probably stick with the couch mobilization because adding a band is like dropping a nuclear bomb on your quads and hips. This is the favorite mobilization technique of powerlifter Laura Phelps Sweatt—world champion, world record holder, and one of the greatest strength athletes of our generation—so we commonly refer to the super couch as the Laura Phelps.

Note: Wrapping a band around your hip and then positioning your leg against the wall is tricky. Unless you have a $10,000 dollar mobility setup, or you have a large enough box that you can position next to a pole, you have to get a Superfriend to pull on the other end of the band, which is not ideal. Enter the Coach Roop variation.

Coach Roop—San Francisco CrossFit super coach—identified this problem and came up with a solution. In Coach Roop's iteration, you wrap your leg up in a band, pinning your foot to your butt, so that you can implement the super couch anywhere. All you need is two bands and a pole. It's genius.

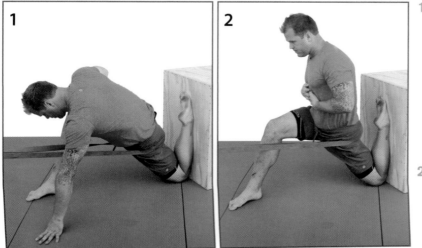

1. To set up for the super couch, hook your left leg through a band and create a distraction by pulling your left leg back. To prevent the band from pulling you forward, post up on your right foot and then force your knee into the corner of the box. With your shin flush and foot flush with the box, squeeze your left glute with all your might and drive your left hip toward the ground.

2. Keeping your butt squeezed and your trunk braced, very carefully lift your torso into the upright position.

Trailing Leg Hip Extension–Option 1

Although the banded hip and couch series is without question the most effective way to mobilize the anterior structures of your hip, you're never really biasing pure hip extension. In other words, if you're always mobilizing with your back leg bent, you never get to open up the hip into full extension. The trailing leg hip extension is a simple way to remove the flexion component so that you can get your hip into pure extension. This is another one of those mobilizations that is only worth doing with a band.

Note: This mobilization can be used in conjunction with the banded hip extension. For example, you can start in the banded hip extension and then, after a few minutes, slide your trailing leg back and open your banded hip into full extension.

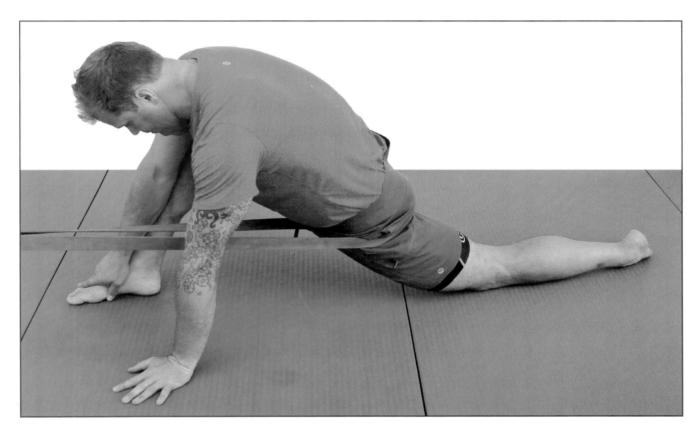

Hook your left leg through the band, positioning the strap around your hip, and sprawl your left leg back. To initiate a stretch, squeeze your left glute and drive your left hip toward the ground. From here, you can hunt around for stiff areas by dropping your hip out to the side and exploring side-to-side ranges. To hit deeper ranges of hip flexion, slide your lead leg out or forward (as if you were trying to do the splits) and lower your left hip toward the ground.

Trailing Leg Hip Extension–Option 2

In this sequence, I demonstrate another trailing leg hip extension option, but add an internal rotation bias by putting my lead foot up onto a box. With your foot off the ground, you can come up onto the ball of your back foot and rotate your knee toward the inside of your body. This internal rotation bias not only accounts for the stable position of your hip (extension and internal rotation), but also takes on the shape of athletic positions and stances (split-jerk, sprinting, combat and fighting stance).

IMPROVES:
- Hip Extension
- Hip Internal Rotation
- Top Position (Squat and Deadlift)
- Normal Posture
- Low Back and Hip Pain

METHODS:
- Contract and Relax
- Paper-clipping (Oscillation)

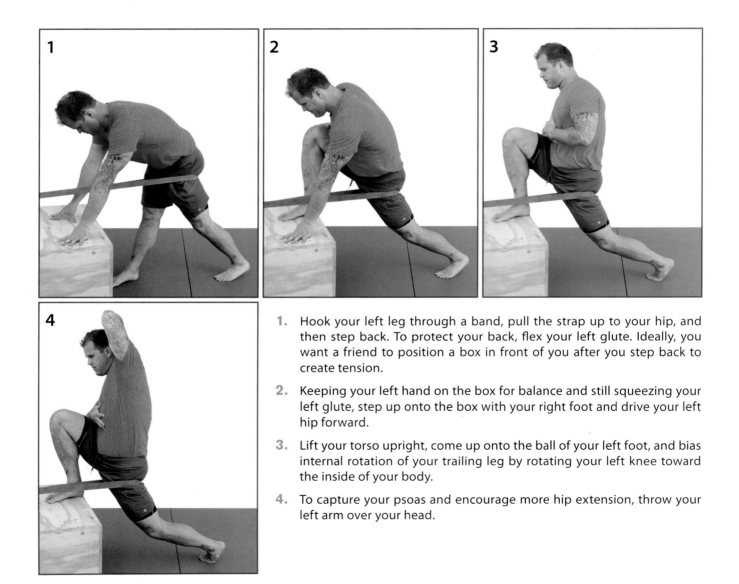

1. Hook your left leg through a band, pull the strap up to your hip, and then step back. To protect your back, flex your left glute. Ideally, you want a friend to position a box in front of you after you step back to create tension.

2. Keeping your left hand on the box for balance and still squeezing your left glute, step up onto the box with your right foot and drive your left hip forward.

3. Lift your torso upright, come up onto the ball of your left foot, and bias internal rotation of your trailing leg by rotating your left knee toward the inside of your body.

4. To capture your psoas and encourage more hip extension, throw your left arm over your head.

Reverse Ballerina

The reverse ballerina mobilization is an easy way to tap into hidden stiffness upstream and downstream of your hip. As you can see from the photos, this technique takes on the same shape as a lot of kicking movements, making it a great mobilization piece for sports that involve any kind of leg swing rotational elements. Think dance, martial arts, and gymnastics.

In addition, the reverse ballerina ties in the adductors (muscles on the inside of your thighs). When these muscles get tight, they pull your pelvis into a bad position in the bottom of the squat (butt wink fault page 91) and limit your capacity to drive your knees out. By throwing your leg up onto a box, bringing your leg out to the side, and rotating away from your leg, you still get to bias extension and internal rotation, but you add an abduction component, which adds another level of gnarly.

IMPROVES:
- ▶ Hip Extension
- ▶ Hip Internal Rotation
- ▶ Flexion and External Rotation (Knees Out Range)

METHODS:
- ▶ Contract and Relax
- ▶ Paper-clipping (Oscillation)

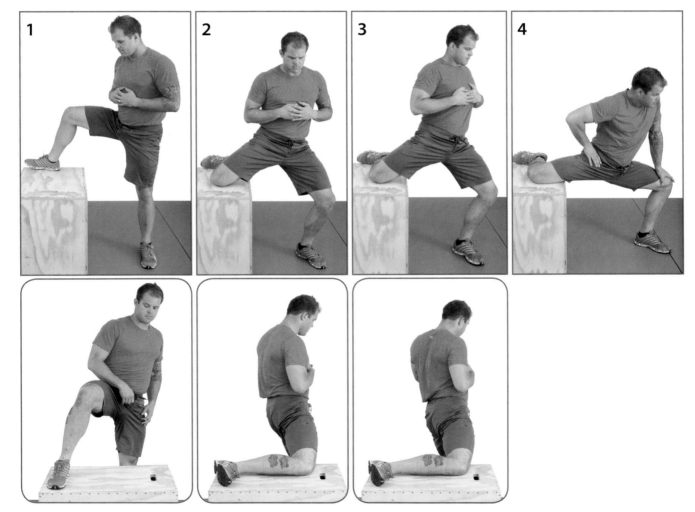

1. To set up, post your right foot up on the far edge of the box.

2. Keeping your right foot open, drop your right knee and ankle to the box and rotate away from your right leg.

3. Driving your knee down into the box, continue to rotate away from your leg. This helps capture some areas in the front of your hip, as well as the musculature running down the inside of your leg.

4. You can hunt for untapped stiff areas by lowering your body while twisting away from your leg. You can also throw your arm over your head, twist around, and scour for some hard-to-reach corners.

AREA 8
MEDIAL CHAIN
(ADDUCTOR)

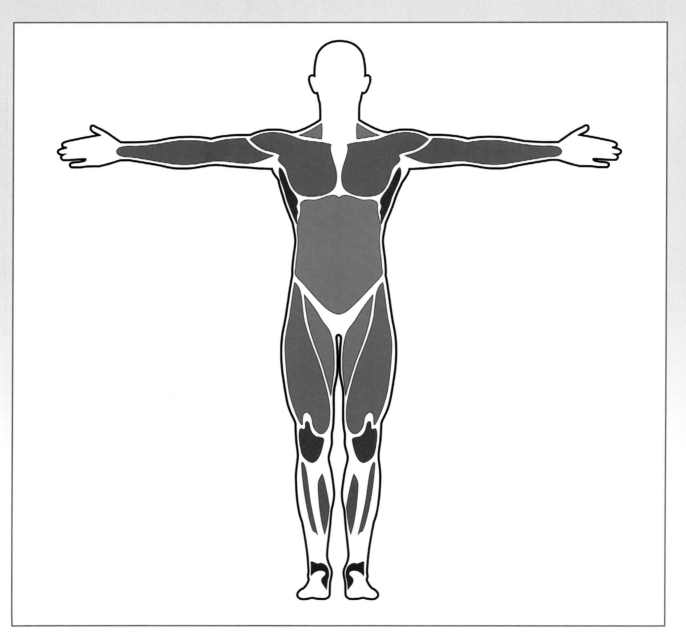

Mobilization Target Areas:

▶ Inside of the leg and hip (adductors)

Most Commonly Used Tools:

▶ Roller

▶ Rogue Monster Band

▶ Barbell

▶ Bumper Plate

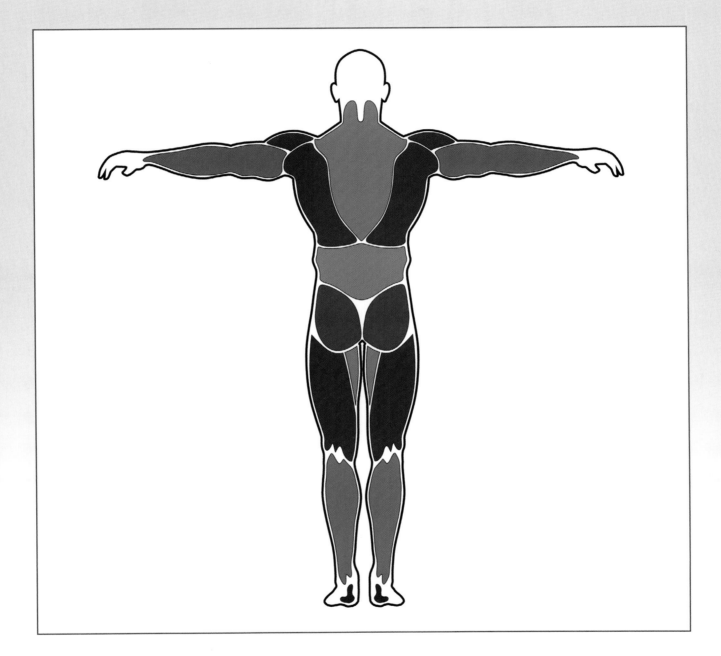

Test and Retest Examples:

▶ Bottom of the Squat   ▶ Top Position

▶ Pulling Position

Adductor Smash

The adductors—big masses of tissue on the inside of your thighs—are like the undervalued stepchildren of your legs. They play a critical role in the family unit, but get ignored and passed over by more important muscles groups like your quads and hamstrings. The fact is your adductors are responsible for stabilizing your back and pulling your knees back to center as you rise out of a squat. They also give you external rotation slack and stabilize your body laterally when you're standing on one leg (i.e. kicking, spinning, or planting).

As I've said, you have to look at your body as a whole and work on solving your mobility issues from all angles. The next time you're having trouble getting your knees out when you squat, don't go straight to your favorite kids—the quads and hamstrings—because there's a good chance that it's the adductors that are limiting your position.

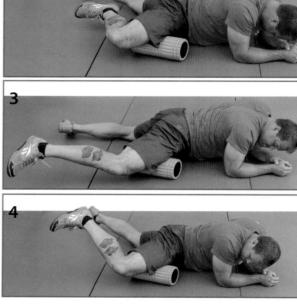

IMPROVES:

- Flexion External Rotation (Knee-Out Position)
- Knee Pain
- Back and Hip Pain

METHODS:

- Pressure Wave
- Contract and Relax
- Smash and Floss

1. To set up for the adductor roller smash, position the inside of your right leg on a roller. Keeping your right leg relaxed, create pressure into the roller by driving your right hip toward the ground.

2. When you roll onto a tight spot, stop, get as much pressure into your leg as possible, and then floss around the tacked-down tissue by pulling your heel toward your butt.

3. Straighten out your leg and then turn your knee toward the mat to create a lateral shear force across the muscle fiber.

4. Staying on the stiff tissue, try moving your leg around in all directions to clear the stiffness.

Adductor Barbell Smash

As with the quad smash, there are several different smashing methods that you can employ. You can use a roller, a barbell, or have a Superfriend step on the inside of your leg. Each has distinct advantages. For example, the roller gives the freedom to smash and floss around tacked-down tissue; the barbell allows you to isolate pockets of knotted-up muscle using the pressure wave and contract and relax techniques; and the Superfriend variation unglues more global stiffness than you can hope to accomplish on your own. Note: The Superfriend variation takes a lot of control and trust, especially if you're a male. And you probably should avoid making eye contact because that would be weird.

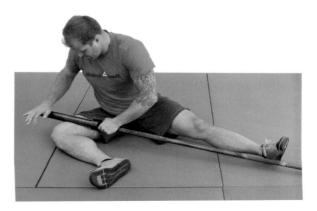

Banded Super Frog

The banded super frog is the most effective and consequently the most brutal medial chain (inside of your leg and hip) mobilization in the movement and mobility arsenal. For the longest time, I only had the adductor smash, the super frog, and a few other mobilizations that hit the medial chain of the high hip, adductor, inner hamstring, and groin area. While all these techniques yielded good results, I struggled to come up with a way to bias the hip into a good position so that I could account for the joint capsule.

Enter the banded super frog. By hooking your leg through a band hanging from a pull-up bar, sliding it up to your groin, and then placing a bumper plate, barbell, or weight over your banded leg, you tap into the deep regions of your hip and hit corners of your high hamstring that you didn't even know were there. As with so many of the great mobilizations, this is not very comfortable. But anything that causes that level of ugly must be good, right? The fact is this mobilization captures multiple systems within one technique, which is always the goal. To keep your hip in a good position and protect your back from large extension forces (bridging the hips and hyperextending the back), keep your butt fully engaged.

You can also have a Superfriend step on the weight for an additional level of gnarly-ness. Make sure you save this for after your workout or maybe after a good warm-up because this is going to create some serious change. Remember, you don't want to monkey around with your pelvic position too much before strenuous activities or heavy lifting.

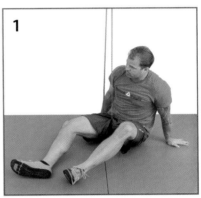

This has also been called the super sumo groin because a lot of our big strong powerlifters have a hard time locking out while maintaining a good hip position. The reason they have such a hard time is because this area of the groin and pelvis is short and stiff.

IMPROVES:
- ▶ Locking Out Your Hips In The Squat
- ▶ Flexion External Rotation (Knee-Out Position)
- ▶ Normal Posture (Neutral Pelvis)

METHODS:
- ▶ Contract and Relax

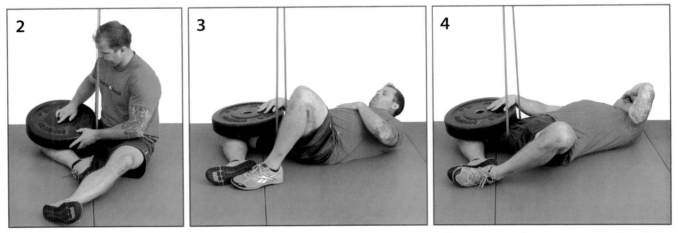

1. Hook your right leg through a (skinny) band and pull it up to your groin. This sets your femur into a good position within the hip socket, allowing you to tap into tightness at your hip capsule.

2. Set a 45-pound bumper plate over your right leg, pinning it to the ground.

3. Squeezing your right glute to support the hip joint and lower back, slowly lie back and bring your left foot next to your right foot.

4. Cover your face using your arms so nobody can see your grisly expression, and then lower your left knee toward the ground to add tension. You can contract and relax by driving your right knee into the weight and continue to lower and raise your opposite knee to control the tension.

Super Frog

If you don't have a band hanging from a pull-up bar, you can still execute the super frog. Realize, however, that it won't have the same impact. The band adds a whole new level of gnarly and allows you to tap into another system of restriction (hip capsule). Still, something is better than nothing.

Remember, you have to take a systems approach when you try to improve position. Failing to account for any one of these pieces—motor-control, sliding surfaces, muscle dynamics, or the joint capsule—will always leave you a little short when it comes to optimizing or restoring function to the movement or the tissues you're trying to change. So if you can use a band, do it. But please do not rip down your ceiling fan; it's probably not worth it.

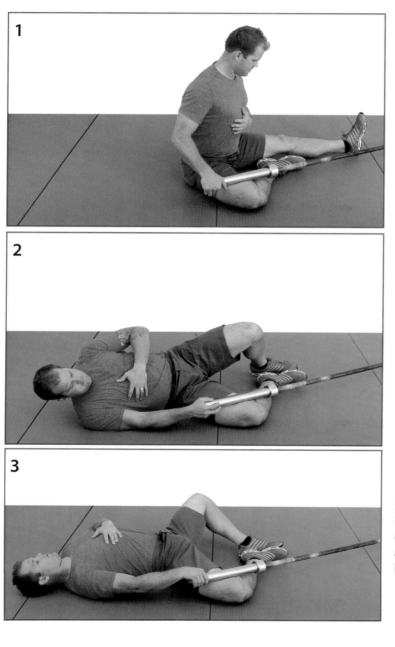

1 Sitting upright, place the sleeve of a barbell over your right thigh, pinning your knee in place.

2 Squeezing your right glute to stabilize your hip and back, lie on your right side and position your left foot next to your right foot.

3 Keeping your right hand on the barbell to keep it positioned over your right leg, lie back and drop your left knee toward the ground to create a greater stretch through your pelvis and medial line (groin).

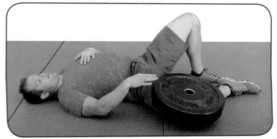

For a more aggressive mobilization, you can also use a large plate.

Olympic Wall Squat

I call this mobilization the Olympic wall squat because if you turn the position upright, it's like being in the sickest, deepest, most upright squat position possible.

To correctly execute this mobilization, get your butt as close the wall as possible and position your feet in your squat stance. With your back supported by the ground and the load taken off your legs, you can really feel the areas that are restricting good mechanics. What most people find is that their adductors are very tight, limiting their capacity to drive their knees out in the bottom of the squat: You can really feel your feet try to spin out as you drive your knees out.

Although this mobilization can easily be performed without a distraction, wrapping a band around your back and hooking it around your knees helps set your femur into the back of your socket, allowing you to tap into some of the hip capsule. This compression also helps clear impingements at the front of the hip.

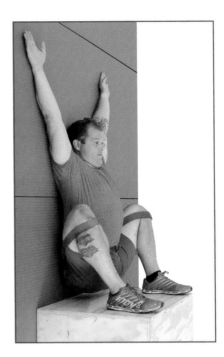

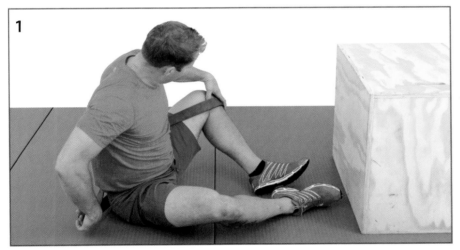

To begin, wrap a band around your back—holding it with your right hand—and hook it around your left knee.

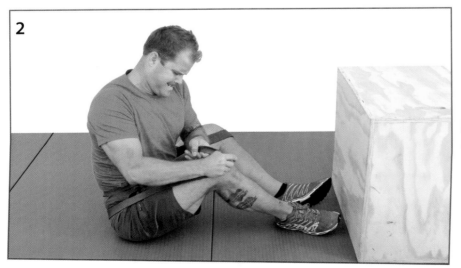

Next, hook the band around your right knee.

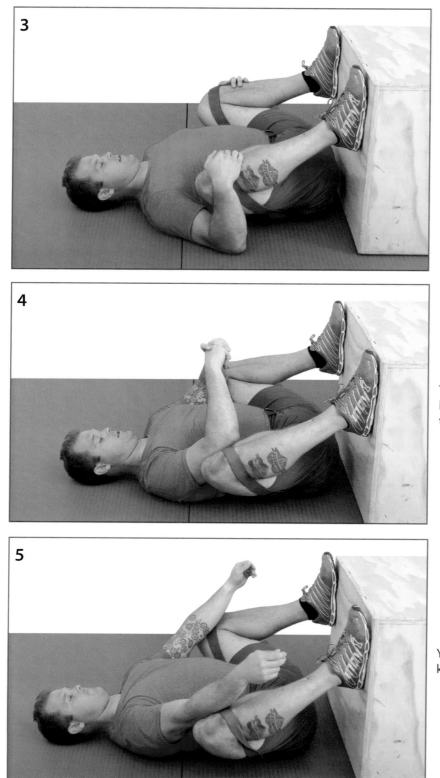

3

Position your butt as close to the box or wall as possible and assume your squat stance, keeping your feet as straight as possible. From here, you can pull down on your knees to increase hips flexion.

4

To tap into you adductors and bias a more knee-out position, drive your elbow into the inside of your knees.

5

You can also spread your arms into your knees.

Happy Baby Test

For reasons readily apparent, this is one of the mobilizations that should be done in the privacy of your own home. What I like about this mobilization is that it has very low stabilization demands, meaning that you don't really have to work that hard to get a good stretch. It's important to realize that it's not as effective as some of the other mobilization pieces, but it's a great technique to throw in when you are just lying around watching television.

Another reason why I like this is because it shows you that when there are low stabilization demands on your back, you automatically adopt a straight foot stance. In other words, no one ever adopts a 30-degree turned-out position because it feels really awkward. Your feet naturally orientate somewhere between 5 and 12 degrees, which is the ideal squat stance.

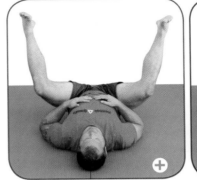 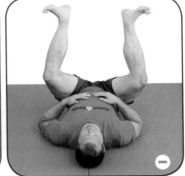

1

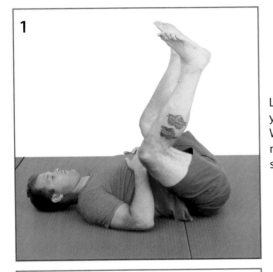

Lie on the ground and bring your knees toward your chest. What you'll find is that you naturally gravitate toward a straight foot position.

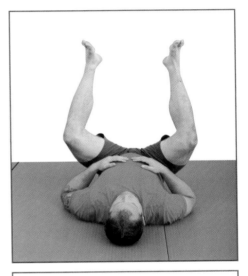

2

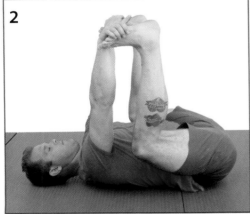

Keeping your back flush with the ground and your shoulders locked into a good position, reach up, grab the inside of your feet, and pull your legs toward your chest.

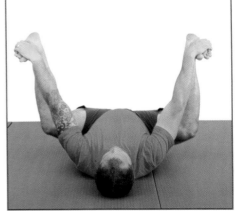

AREA 9
POSTERIOR CHAIN
(HAMSTRING)

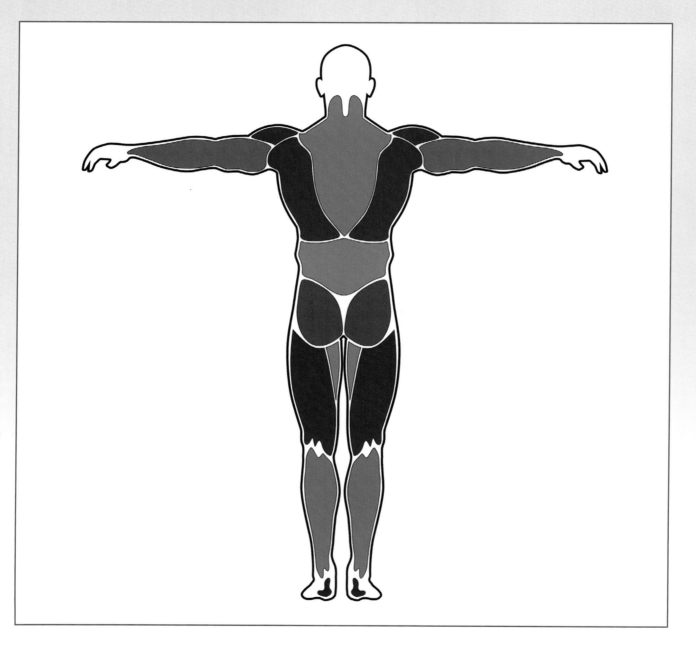

Mobilization Target Areas:

- Hamstrings

Most Commonly Used Tools:

- Roller
- Barbell
- Single Lacrosse Ball

Test and Retest Examples:

- Air Squat
- Bottom of the Squat
- Pulling Position

Posterior Chain Smash and Floss

Most athletes train their posterior chain like it's their job. We're talking glutes and hamstrings here, just so you know what I mean. The problem is they put in a ton of work to get their posterior chain strong, and then put their muscles to sleep by sitting all day, or doing absolutely nothing to restore some of the sliding surfaces in these tissues.

There are three big muscles that make up your hamstring—the semimembranosus, semitendinosus, and biceps femoris—all of which arise from different places in your hip and then snake down on different sides of your leg. For hamstrings to function optimally, you need full-range in all of these tissues. In other words, you need to schedule a smash party for your hamstrings every time you put them to work and especially after long periods of sitting.

If you have some down time at work, you're stuck at the airport, or cooling off from a workout—you get the idea—find a hard surface (a chair or box). Then stick a lacrosse ball or softball underneath your hamstring, get some weight over the ball, and just smash across the tissue. As with most ball smashing techniques, if you hit a hot spot, stay on the area while pumping your leg back and forth. It's quick and easy, and it's time well spent.

IMPROVES:

▶ Hip Extension ▶ Squat and Pulling Techniques

▶ Knee Flexion ▶ Hip, Back, and Knee Pain

METHODS:

▶ Smash and Floss ▶ Pressure Wave

▶ Contract and Relax

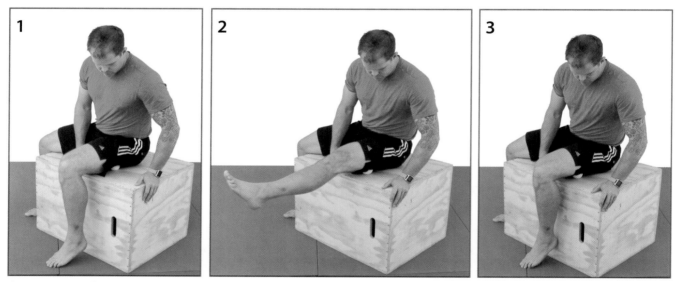

1. Position a lacrosse ball or softball underneath your leg into the meat of your hamstring and distribute as much weight over the ball as you can handle.

2. Hunt around for a tight spot, and then extend your leg. The idea is to bend and straighten your leg and move it from side to side.

3. You can also pressure wave across the length of the muscle by shifting your weight over the ball and oscillating on and off bound-up pockets of knotted-up tissue.

Posterior Chain Smash and Floss:
Monkey Bar of Death Variation

Remember sitting on top of the monkey bar structures as a kid with one leg draped over the bar, just kind of swinging back and forth as if it were nothing? I'd be willing to bet that if you did this now you'd slide into the hellish depths of the pain cave and then scramble away—or worse, black out and plummet off the monkey bars. If you're like the majority of athletes, most of your hamstring stiffness resides near the insertion at your hip, which is a difficult area to target and extremely painful area to mobilize. Let's face it: Nobody is going to get into your personal regions and work around your business, or at least not as effectively as you can do it yourself.

Unless you're looking to get arrested, I wouldn't recommend climbing on the monkey bars where kids play so you can mobilize around your grundle region. That's just creepy. Instead, set a barbell on a rack at about mid-thigh level. This ends up being a much more aggressive and effective way to break up the tissue and get large pressure into the insertion of your hamstring. Again, the idea is to just grind back and forth from side to side against the grain of the muscle tissue.

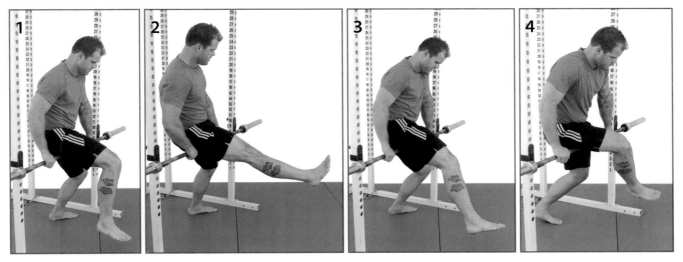

1. Set a barbell on a rack at about mid-thigh level and throw one of your legs over the bar, positioning the bar into your high hip, near the insertion of your hamstring.

2. When you find a piece of matted-down tissue (it shouldn't take long), straighten your leg.

3. As you bend your leg, you can shift your weight to the side, rolling across the length of the muscle.

4. You can also rotate your leg from side to side, and—using your hands—roll the bar into your sit bones and muscle insertion points.

Voodoo Groin and Hamstring Wrap

Mobilizing with a voodoo band offers a few distinct advantages: You can mobilize in the movement or position you're trying to change, you address multiple systems simultaneously—joint mechanics, sliding surface, and muscle dynamics—and you can capture tissues that are otherwise very difficult to target. For example, smashing or getting enough pressure into the high (proximal) hamstring and adductor area or tapping into your groin and hip flexor region is not an easy thing to do using conventional mobility tools like a lacrosse ball or roller.

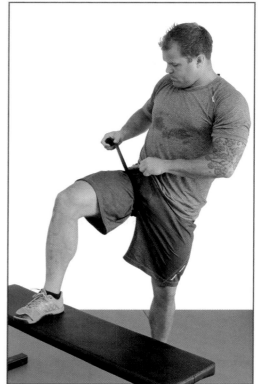

The fact is people spend a lot of time sitting on their high posterior chain, turning the high hamstring, glute, and groin area into a nexus of junky, matted-down tissue. And when the tissues around the insertion of these muscles get tight, injury follows. As anybody that has strained his or her groin or hamstring can attest, it's a painful and limiting injury that takes a long time to heal. It affects your ability to generate force and causes a ton of funky movement and tissue adaptations. To make matters worse, it's very difficult to get in there and break up the knotted-up scar tissue that starts to form post injury. This is why voodoo flossing is so great. You get a circumferential compression around those hard-to-reach areas. Add some full-range movement into the equation and you have a model for dealing with the scar balls (which restrict and compromise movement) and restoring sliding surfaces to matted-down tissues.

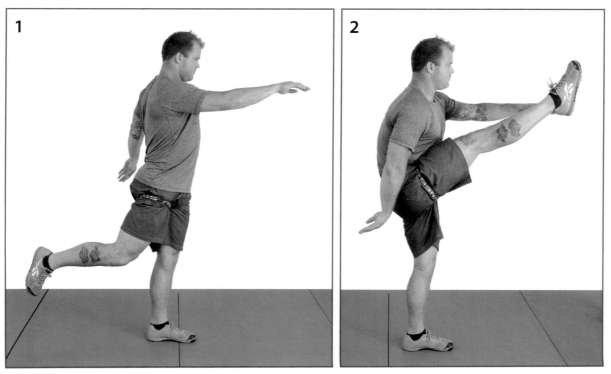

Dynamic leg swings are a great way to safely restore sliding surfaces to the high hamstring and groin region. Keep your knee straight, foot neutral, and swing your leg out in front of you as if you were punting a football.

Posterior Chain Floss

If you're a full grown adult, you're not going to magically grow new hamstrings. To lengthen these muscles, you need to restore shortened and tight tissue back to their ideal ranges. The bottom line is that stretching is not going to do anything to restore normal range to those steel cables running down the back of your legs. If you want to make lasting change, you have to take a systems approach. You have to clear sliding surface dysfunction with some qualitative and aggressive smashing, as well as incorporate end-range mobilization to lengthen the tissue.

One of the key concepts of my Movement and Mobility System is to mobilize tissues into ideal positions, and then use them so that the musculature gets appropriately stimulated for normal range development. To be blatant, the best way to lengthen your hamstrings is to use them in a functional setting. The posterior chain mobilization is a perfect example of a weight-bearing exercise that takes on a very similar shape to something that you'll actually do (deadlift, pick something off the ground). As you can see, you have a few different options. You can post your hands on the ground or a box and floss by bending and flexing your knee (option 1 and 2) or hinge forward from your hip (option 3). Whether you use one or a combination of all, these options provide a fantastic pre-game, pre-workout mobilization that will help restore normal range-of-motion to your hamstrings and hips.

IMPROVES:

- Hamstring Range-of-Motion
- Hip Extension (Top Position)
- Knee Flexion
- Squat and Pulling Techniques
- Hip, Back, and Knee Pain

METHOD:

- Floss

Option 1

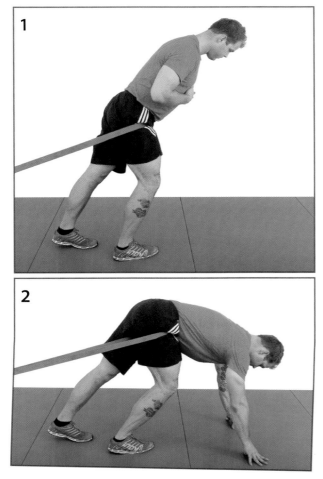

1

Wrap a band around your hip and walk forward to create tension. For this particular option, it helps if your banded leg is positioned slightly in front of your free leg.

2

Fold forward from your hips—keeping your belly tight and back flat—and plant your hands on the ground. If you can't reach the ground without rounding your back, position a box or bench in front of you.

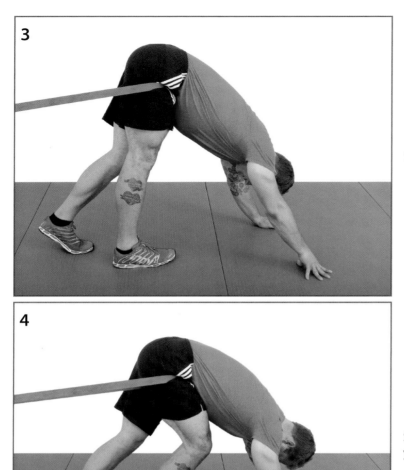

3

Straighten your leg and drive your hips back.

4

Still keeping your back as flat as possible, bend your knee.

5

Keeping your weight on your heel, continue to floss by extending and flexing your knee. The idea is to put in twenty to fifty knee bends. To capture your high hip (glute region), you can also rotate your hips slightly as you lockout your leg and walk your upper body around your planted foot in either direction.

Option 2

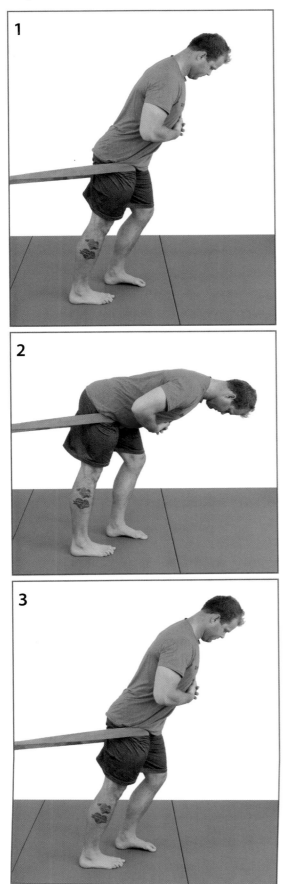

1 Hook your leg through a band, pull it up to your hip, and then walk forward to create tension.

2 Keeping your belly tight, back flat, and leg straight, hinge forward from your hips until you reach your end-range.

3 Pull yourself back to the upright position. From here, you can continue to bend forward and floss in and out of end-range hip flexion. The idea is to keep your spine rigid, your knee locked out, and your weight centered over your heel.

Option 3

Remember, to effect true change, you have to hit your hamstrings from different angles. That means changing your position so that you hunt out hard-to-reach corners of tight muscle. By putting your leg onto a box, you get your leg into a flexed position (think squatting), which allows you to tap into the high hip and hamstring region that is difficult to get.

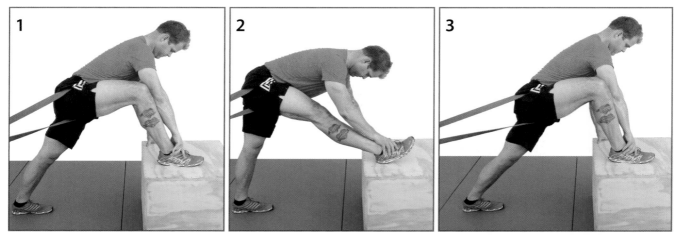

1. Wrap a band around your hip and plant your foot on a box. Try to keep your foot flat to the box. You'll probably feel a good stretch in this position so feel free to scour around for tight corners in this position.

2. Straighten your leg and shoot your hips back. To really capture your high hip region, keep your foot flat on the box until your reach end-range and then allow the ball of your foot to come up as you lockout your knee.

3. Slowly bend your knee and shift your weight forward. From here, you can continue to floss by bending and flexing your knee.

Banded Classic Posterior Chain Mob

As you know, I'm a big fan of mobilizing in positions that reflect the realities of life and sport. For example, I prefer to mobilize my hamstrings from the standing position because it has a weight-bearing element that reflects the movements that I use in my day-to-day training, like deadlifting. More importantly, it seems to yield better results. However, that is not to say that you can't apply this same method while lying on your back. In fact, this classic approach has real value, especially for our Jiu-Jitsu leopards or MMA fighters who utilize this range while lying on their back, fighting from their guard.

What's great about this option is there's no weight-bearing element on your spine—so you don't have to work as hard to keep your back in a good position. The key is to approach the stretch just as you would when setting up for a deadlift: Load your hip into flexion and then apply tension at your knee by straightening your leg. As I've mentioned, this allows you to capture the tight corners of your hip and high hamstring, which is where most people are tight. If you straighten your leg first and use your whole leg as a tensioner, which is very common, you tend to lose some of the effectiveness.

Another key aspect with this mobilization is to add a posterior distraction. As with the previously demonstrated techniques, this clears impingements at the front of your hip and helps tie in the musculature of your high hamstring. You can do this one of two ways. The first is to distract from a pole. This allows you to put a lot of tension into the band, offering a really aggressive distraction. The problem is hooking a band around a pole isn't always a viable option. The second option addresses this issue. To set yourself up, loop a band around your foot a couple of times, hook it around your hip, and then use your banded foot to create a posterior distraction—see photos on the next page. This not only allows you to mobilize with your hip in a good position, but also allows you to control the tension with your banded foot. Plus, you can execute this in the comfort of your living room or office.

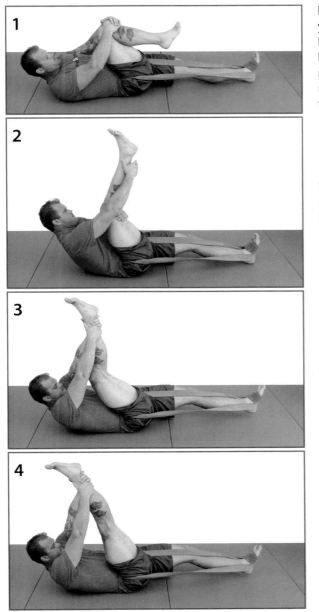

1 Loop a band around the center of your left foot (if it's a thin band you may need to wrap it a few times), hook it around your right hip, and then pull your knee to your chest. Try to keep your left leg straight. By adding this posterior distraction, you pull your femur to the bottom of the capsule, which will clear any impingement you may have at the front of your hip. It also allows you to tie in the musculature of your high hamstring.

2 With your hip loaded into a flexed position, wrap your left hand around the back of your right knee, sit up, and grab the back of your right ankle.

3 Grab the back of your ankle with both of your hands.

4 Next, apply tension by straightening your knee. From here, you can continue to floss by bending and straightening your leg, contract and relax by resisting into your arms, and scour around for tight corners by manipulating your leg to either side of your body.

If you can't reach your foot because you're missing hamstring range-of-motion, wrapping a band or rope around your foot is certainly a valid idea. In other words, don't flex into a weird position just to grab your foot. That goes against everything I've been trying to teach you. This is also a good option if you're sweaty from a workout or your grip is blown, making it difficult to grip your calve.

The key: Keep your foot in a neutral position by hooking the band around the center of your foot. A lot of people mistakenly wrap it around their toes and pull their foot into flexion, creating a big stretch at the back of their knee.

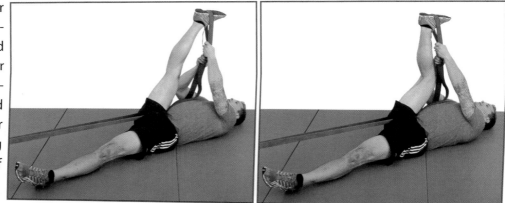

Super P-LATIES

As I mentioned, I prefer weight bearing mobilization techniques because they're a closer correlate to what we're trying to change. That said, you need options. And what works for some doesn't necessarily work for others. In any case, you can still make a positive impact on your posterior chain musculature using mobilizations like the one demonstrated below. This is a great pre-game, pre-workout option that doesn't put a lot of structural demand on your body. By moving your leg through a full range-of-motion under tension, you can relieve some muscle stiffness as well as prep your hamstrings for any kind sport activity.

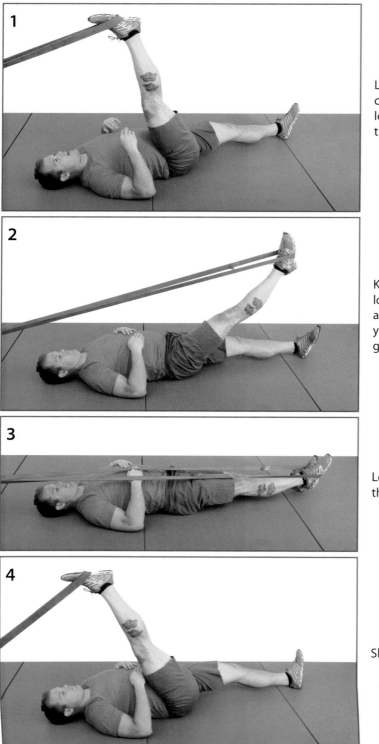

1 Load your hip into flexion, hook a band around the center of your foot (arch), and then straighten your leg. Note: Make sure you wear shoes when doing this mobilization.

2 Keeping your foot slightly pointed and your knee locked out, drive your heel toward the ground. To avoid breaking into an overextended position, keep your abs braced and your lower back flush with the ground.

3 Lower your leg until your heel makes contact with the ground.

4 Slowly, pull your leg into end-range flexion.

Banded Distraction

Adding a posterior distraction to this mobilization is tricky, but if you can pull it off, I encourage you to do it. The key is to keep your hands on the band so it doesn't snap off your leg.

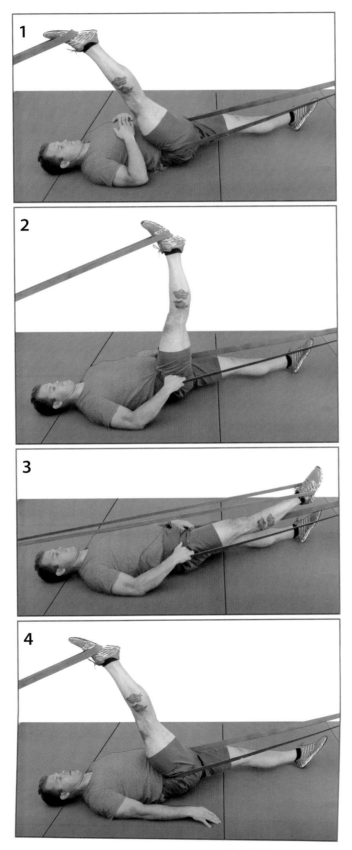

AREA 10
KNEE

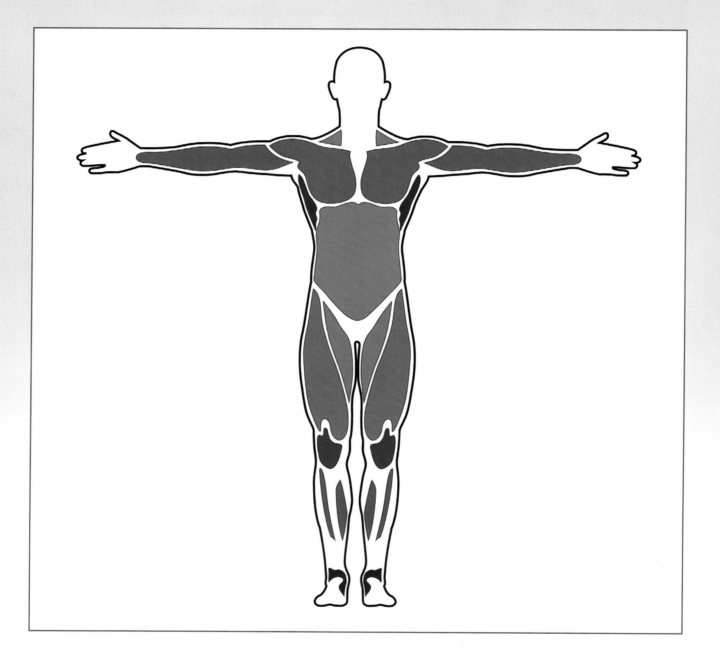

Mobilization Target Areas:

▸ Knee and surrounding musculature

Most Commonly Used Tools:

▸ Single Lacrosse Ball
▸ Voodoo Band
▸ Rogue Monster Band

Test and Retest Examples:

▸ Bottom of the Squat
▸ Terminal Knee Extension Test

Terminal Knee Extension (Knee Tweak Fix)

When I evaluate athletes for knee pain, one of the first things that I check is terminal knee extension. What I'm looking for is whether or not they have full knee range-of-motion.

An easy way to test this is to sit with your legs out in front of you and then extend one of your knees by flexing your quad. If you have full knee range-of-motion, your heel will lift up off the ground and you will see a little bit of hyperextension at the knee joint. If you have a slight bend in the knee or you can't lockout the joint, it's a good indication that you're missing the capacity to achieve terminal knee extension.

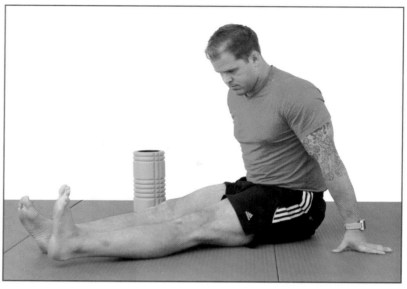

When your knees are stuck in a bent or flexed position, they are under constant tension while standing. It's the equivalent of not being able to extend your arm and then doing a handstand. Add 10,000 steps a day and heavily loaded movements into the equation and you have the smoking gun for knee pain and lost potential. In addition, every movement starts in a pre-loaded, biomechanically-compromised position.

Consider driving your knees forward as you initiate the squat. It's impossible to unload that tension once you've entered the tunnel. It doesn't matter how much tension you have in your hips and hamstrings in this situation, your knees will remain fully loaded. This is why driving your knees forward when you squat, or bringing your elbows back when you bench press, dip, or do pushups, is a faulty mechanic. These secondary joints are not designed to handle the load. This is a job for the primary engines of your hips and shoulders. You will continuously load your knee and quad instead of your hips and hamstrings every time you hinge from your hips, placing an insane amount of strain on your knee, quad, quad ligament, patellar tendon, and more.

To restore function and normal range-of-motion to the joint, you need to pull the joint surfaces apart so that you can reset your knee into a good position. When athletes are missing knee extension, in most cases their knee is unlocked and twisted inside the knee structure. Put simply, there's a kink in the joint that prevents them from opening up their knee. This often stems from a knee fault or knee tweak of some kind. It's like a door that doesn't swing correctly or open all the way because one of the hinges has a twist in it.

To realign the joint, the first thing you need to do is create some space within the knee joint, which is accomplished by applying a distraction at the ankle. Next, grab your shin and internally rotate your lower leg bone, the tibia. This will realign your knee into an idealized position. To restore extension range, apply downward pressure and flex your quad.

IMPROVES:
▶ Terminal Knee Extension

▶ Knee Pain

METHODS:
▶ Band Distraction

▶ Voodoo Band

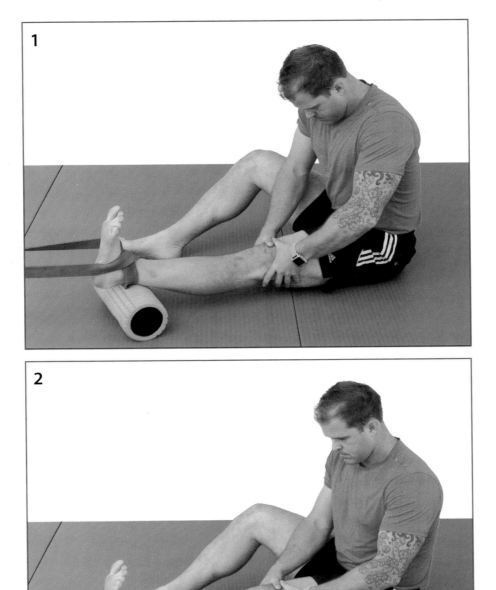

1. Hook a band around the top of your foot and then wrap it around the base of your heel. Once that's done, create tension in the band and prop your foot onto a foam roller.

2. Grab above your knee and press down. You're not trying to break your knee in half. Apply just enough pressure to achieve full extension and hold it in position for a couple of seconds. If you still can't lockout your knee, grab your shin, internally rotate your tibia, and then apply downward pressure in the same manner. Repeat this process until you restore normal function to the joint or experience some kind of positive change.

Voodoo Variation

If possible, wrap a voodoo band around your entire knee (a couple inches below and a few inches above) before executing this mobilization. This will not only help reset the joint in a good position, but the compression forces will create a gapping effect. This gives you a little bit more breathing room within your knee structure, which allows you to press and rotate your knee into newly challenged ranges. Anytime you can use a distraction in conjunction with compression, it is a win.

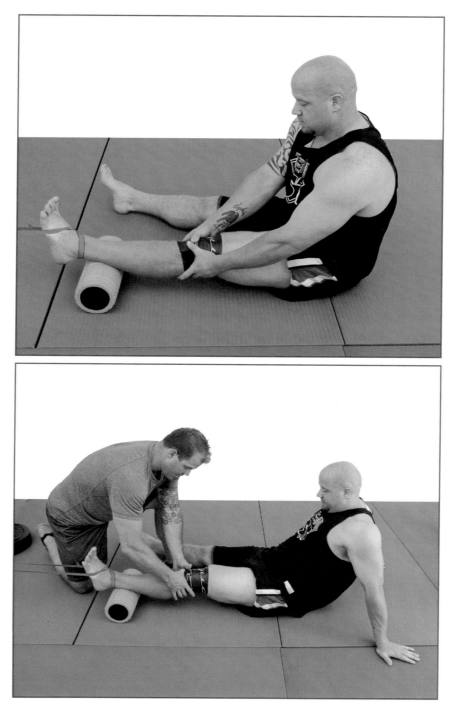

Grab your shin, internally rotate your tibia, and then apply downward pressure, encouraging your knee into full extension. Having a Superfriend facilitate this motion is ideal.

Gap and Smash

If you have knee pain, think this: "I need to mobilize the tissues surrounding my knee joint." Then get to work.

The gap and smash mobilization is a fast way to hit the areas just behind your knee where your hamstring and calf cross the joint. It's kind of a two-for-one because you hit upstream and downstream of the knee with a single mobilization.

This is also a great technique for addressing tight calves. Most people spend tons of time working on their calves at the ankle level. What they forget is the calf crosses two joints, the ankle and the knee. By getting into the high gastrocnemius, you can effectively deal with these tight tissues and feed slack to your knee and ankle.

The idea is to sandwich a ball behind your knee—either on the inside or outside—creating a large compression force. From there you can implement one of two strategies. You can floss around by moving your foot in all directions, pulling on your shin with both of your hands; or you can plant your foot on the ground and scoot your butt into your leg. The key is to work the inside and outside of the knee, smashing both sides of the gastroc.

IMPROVES:
- ▶ Terminal Knee Extension
- ▶ Knee Pain
- ▶ Tight Calves
- ▶ Ankle Range-of-Motion

METHODS:
- ▶ Smash and Floss
- ▶ Contract and Relax

Inside Line

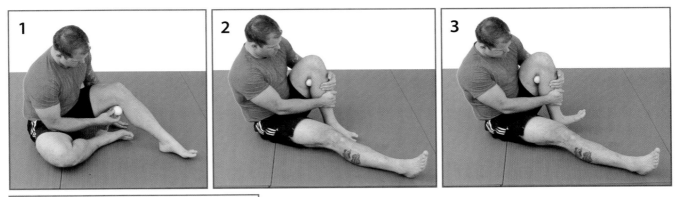

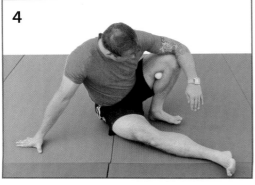

1. Place a lacrosse ball behind your knee on the inside of your leg.

2. With the ball in place, curl your heel toward your butt and pull your leg tight using both of your hands. This creates a large compression force that targets your lower hamstring and upper calf.

3. Still pulling on your shin with both of your hands, start moving your foot around in every direction.

4. To increase pressure, plant your foot on the ground and scoot your butt toward your heel.

Outside Line

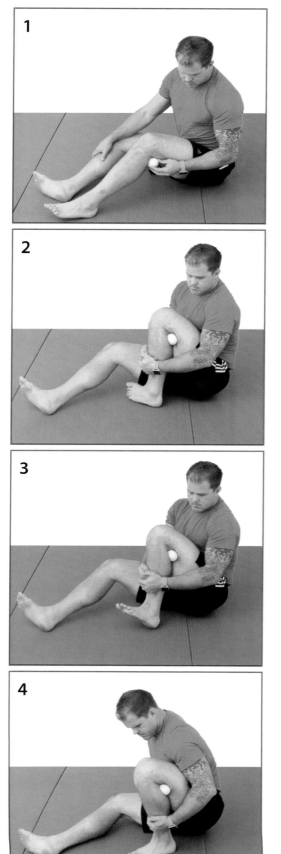

Position a lacrosse ball behind your knee on the outside of your leg.

Curl your heel toward your butt, cup your hands around your shin, and pull your leg in tight to your body, sandwiching the ball behind your knee.

Pulling on your shin to create a large compression force, start moving your foot around in every direction. Tacking down the tissues of your distal hamstring and upper calf will help restore suppleness to the tight tissues that cross the knee.

To increase pressure, plant your foot on the ground and scoot your butt toward your heel.

Flexion Gapping

When I teach seminars and work with athletes, I encourage people to think about treating the issues in and around the area that is giving them trouble. You don't need a background in anatomy to address your business. For example, if you're having knee problems, it's conceivable that one of the structures around the knee is tight or not working correctly. When people have arthritic knees or a really stiff joint for example, hinge dust starts to accumulate below the knee. Flexion gapping is a simple way to blow away that hinge dust and restore normal function to the joint.

A simple way to screen for knee flexion problems is to sit butt to ankles. You should be able to smash your calves into your hamstrings without pain or restriction. If you're unable to achieve this range, it could be quad stiffness, poor ankle range-of-motion, or a stiff knee capsule. This technique is an easy way to deal with the latter issue. If the joint capsule is restricted, achieving full hip or knee flexion is difficult because there is not enough space in the front of the knee to accommodate for the rotation of the femur on the tibia. Like the banded distraction iterations, this is an easy way to restore that passive accessory motion and restore normal range-of-motion to the knee.

IMPROVES:
▶ Knee Extension
▶ Knee Pain

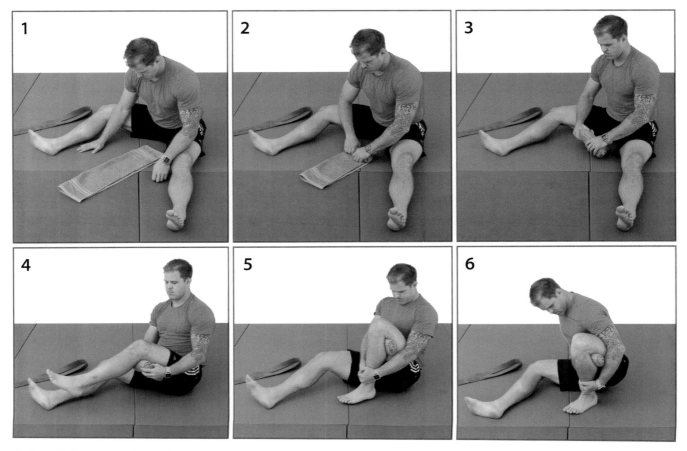

1-4   Roll up a small towel and place it behind your knee.

5-6   Grab your shin, pull your heel toward your butt, and then scoot your butt towards your foot, creating as much pressure as possible. Try to keep the foot straight while oscillating in and out of peak compression.

AREA 11
MEDIAL AND ANTERIOR SHIN

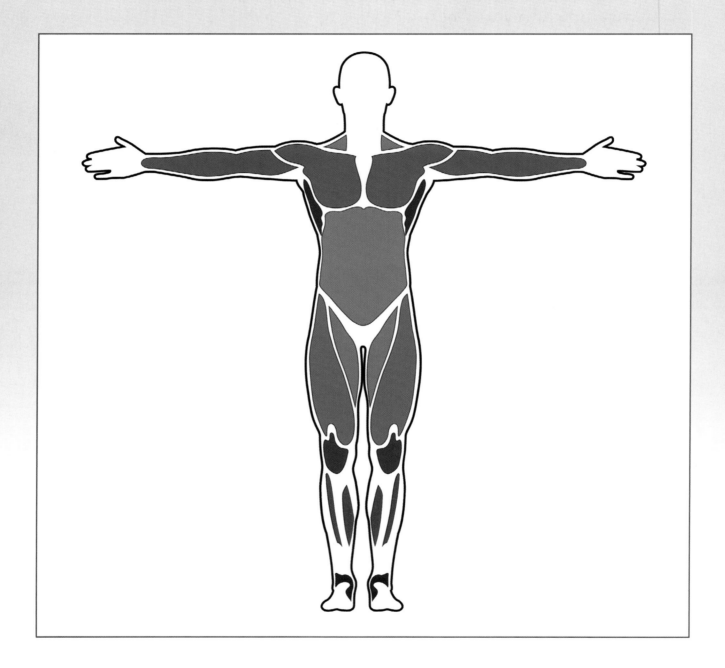

Mobilization Target Areas:

▶ Inside and outside areas of the shin, from your knee down to your ankle

Most Commonly Used Tools:

▶ Single Lacrosse Ball

Test and Retest Examples:

▶ Bottom of the Squat (Pistol)
▶ Dorsiflexion and Extension

Medial Shin Smash and Floss

If you run a lot, or you're on your feet all day, there is a good chance that the tissues of your lower leg are brutally tight and in need of some serious love. The musculature extending from your knee to your ankle on the inside of your shin—specifically the soleus, posterior tibialis, and gastrocnemius muscle—is responsible for giving your foot arch support. Anytime you stand, walk, or run you are putting demand on these tissues. As the calf musculature becomes tight and locked up, people start defaulting to an open foot position. This causes the ankle to collapse and places stress on the upstream tissues.

To restore good positions and normalize those tissues, take a ball and smash it into the inside of your shinbone. Work from the base of the knee down to the anklebone. The idea is to create large pressures and work all the elements. You can pressure wave, contract and relax, and smash and floss by moving the foot through various ranges. People will find areas of high pain and areas of low pain. The key is to skip over the low pain and stay on the hot, grody areas behind the shin.

This mobilization should be your first stop if you have plantar fascia problems, posterior tibialis tendonitis, if you can't get your foot into a good arch, or if you're someone who does a lot of running—especially Pose-centric running.

IMPROVES:

▶ Neutral and Straight Foot Position

▶ Foot and Ankle Problems

▶ Knee Pain

METHODS:

▶ Contract and Relax

▶ Smash and Floss

▶ Pressure Wave

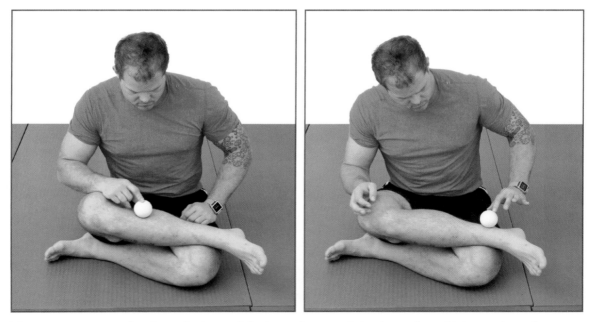

The target area stretches from the base of the knee down to right above the anklebone along the inside of the shin.

Medial Shin Tack and Floss–Option 1

There are a few different ways to approach this mobilization. Personally, I like to sit on the ground with my legs crossed, but not everyone can comfortably get into this position. If you are physically restricted, you can cross your leg over your knee from the sitting position (Option 2) or implement the double lacrosse ball variation (Option 3).

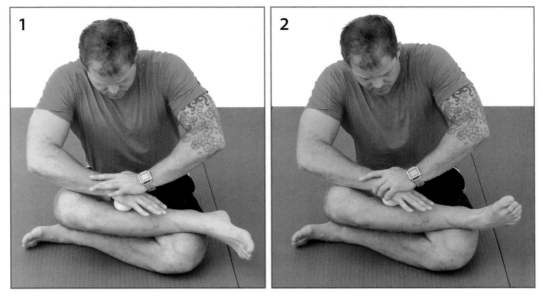

1. Pin a lacrosse ball on the inside of your shin and apply downward pressure using both of your hands.

2. Once you find a hot spot, tack the tissue down and move your foot around in all directions. You can also apply a pressure wave or implement the contract and relax technique.

Executive Medial Shin Tack and Floss–Option 2

This is a fantastic option for the less flexible. It also serves as a perfect lower body maintenance strategy for the desk-bound athlete. It's a win any time you can work on improving your position and mobilizing stiff tissues while trapped at work or in a chair. It's kind of like you're getting paid to mobilize.

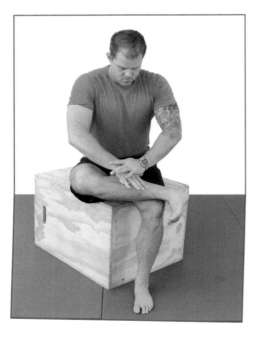

Cross your leg over your knee, wedge a lacrosse ball between your shin-bone and calf, and apply downward pressure with both hands. From there, you can contract and relax, roll your foot around in different directions, or apply the pressure wave technique.

Double Lacrosse Ball Medial Shin Smash and Floss–Option 3

This option is attractive because it's easy to get into the position, plus it allows you to target both sides of your leg. If you're an endurance athlete with tacked-down tissues, or you have foot pain or a weird ankle pain, consider this a gold star technique.

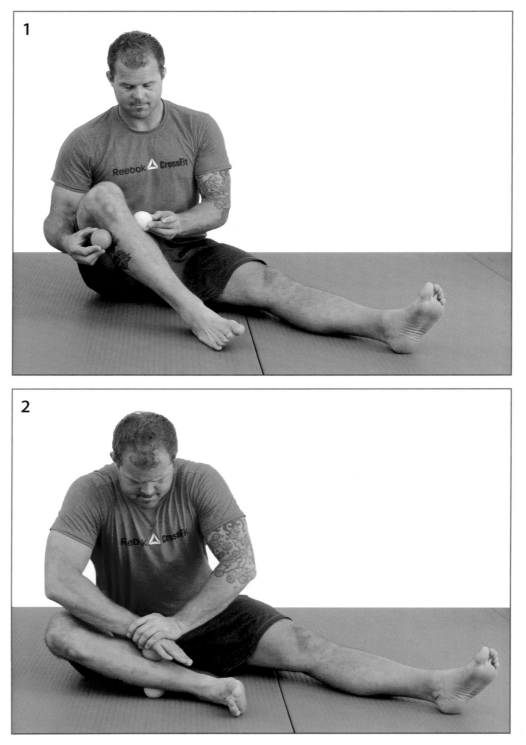

1. Position a lacrosse ball on the bottom and top of your leg.

2. Align the top ball over the bottom (on a tight area) and apply downward pressure using both of your hands.

Lateral and Anterior Compartment Smash

If you have foot problems or strange downstream pain, you have to look at the shin and calf. All of the tissues that run and control your feet are housed in your lower leg. The calf and shin are the master of puppets pulling the strings to your feet.

The problem is people tend to forget about the front of the shin because all the meat is on the back of the leg, which is where most people focus their attention. However, if an athlete does a lot of running, walking, and standing—especially if he heel strikes and stands with his feet turned out—those peroneal muscles that run down the outside of the lower leg are on constant tension and will get extremely tight. This is precisely how people get shin splints.

When I treat athletes who have shin splints, I'll ask them, "What are you doing for those tissues?" They'll pause, think about it for a second, then say, "Nothing." It's odd because those tissues are stiff and being pulled off the bone, but more often than not the athlete isn't addressing the area of localized pain. Obviously, working upstream and downstream of the problem is part of the conversation, but to restore those tissues to their normal function, the athlete has to get in there and give those stiff tissues some love.

It's important to realize that when this anterior compartment of the shin gets tight, the muscles don't contract very well, limiting dorsiflexion range-of-motion. It also inhibits your ability to point your toes. For this reason, the test and retest is to simply flex and point your foot back and forth. If your shin is working efficiently and the sliding surfaces are actually sliding, you will be able to pull and point your toes farther with less discomfort.

If you have strange knee or ankle pain, you're struggling to get your foot into a good position, or the front of your shins hurt—meaning that you have shin splints—this mobilization should be at the top of your list. Know that there are a couple different ways you can attack these tissues. You can use a rolling pin or stick massager, or you can pressure your weight over a lacrosse ball or roller as demonstrated here. The tools that you use are not important as long as you can get the job done.

IMPROVES:

▶ Neutral and Straight Foot Position

▶ Anterior Compartment Pain (Shin Splints)

▶ Knee and Ankle Pain

METHODS:

▶ Smash and Floss

▶ Pressure Wave

▶ Contract and Relax

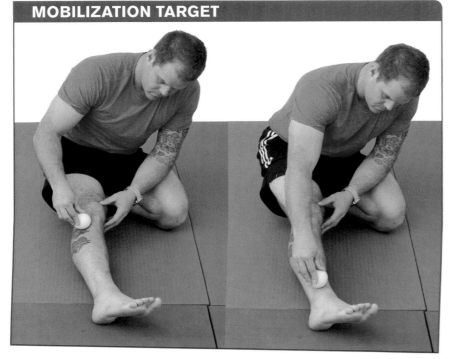

MOBILIZATION TARGET

The goal is to work the anterior compartment and the lateral compartment (the peroneals) along the front of your shins and outside of your leg from your knee to your ankle.

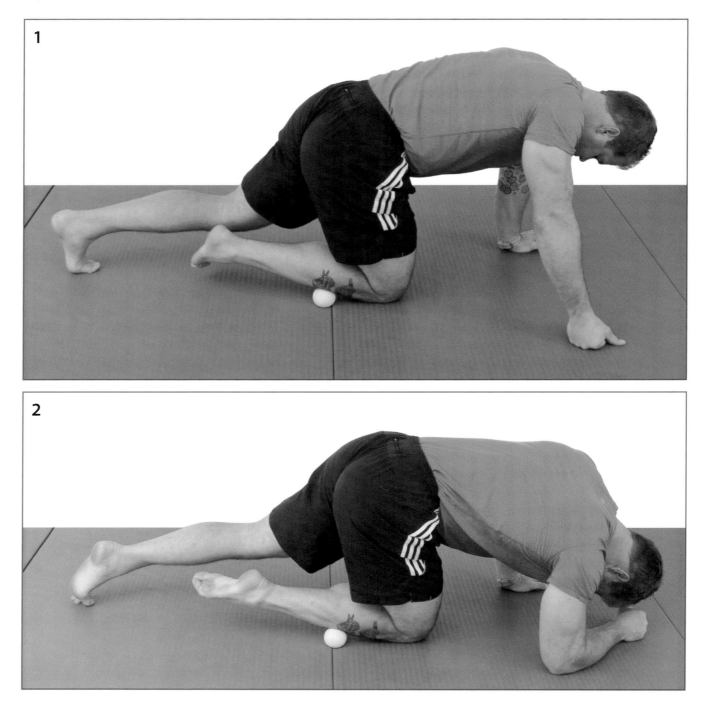

1. Kneel on the ground and position a lacrosse ball to the outside of your shin. To add more pressure, you can sit your butt back, or reposition your center of mass over the ball.

2. Work across the tissue, pressure waving from the outside to the inside of your leg. If you stumble across a painful spot, stop and move your foot around in all directions. You can also contract and relax to penetrate deeper into the tight tissues.

Roller Variation

You can also use a foam roller—ideally a Rumble Roller. Work up and down the length of the tissue hunting out tight areas. When you find a hot spot, rock back and forth from side to side across the tissue while moving your foot around in every direction.

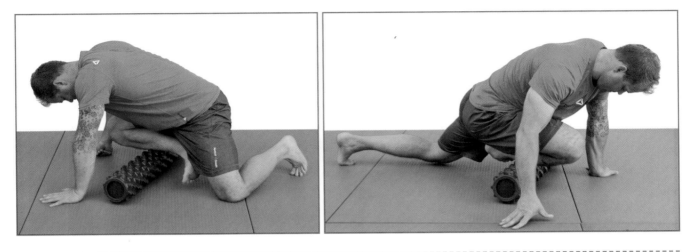

Global Plantar Flexion

This is a sweet and simple global dorsiflexion mobilization and a low-budget way to stretch the front of your shins. It's a powerful counter mobilization to the previous technique that puts the anterior compartment into an end-range position. You can stretch both legs at a time as demonstrated here or stretch one leg at a time by posting up on your foot.

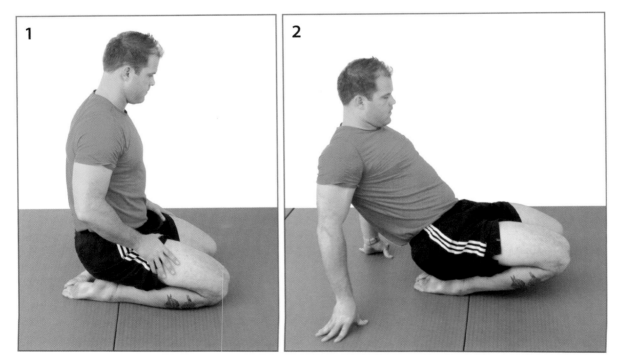

1. Kneel on the ground with the tops of your feet flush with the ground, positioning your big toes right next to each other. **Note:** If you want to isolate one leg, plant one foot on the ground. For example, if you want to stretch your right shin, you would post up on your left foot and plant your right hand on the mat to counterbalance your weight.

2. Keeping your back flat and knees straight, lean back and allow your knees to come up off the ground.

AREA 12
CALF

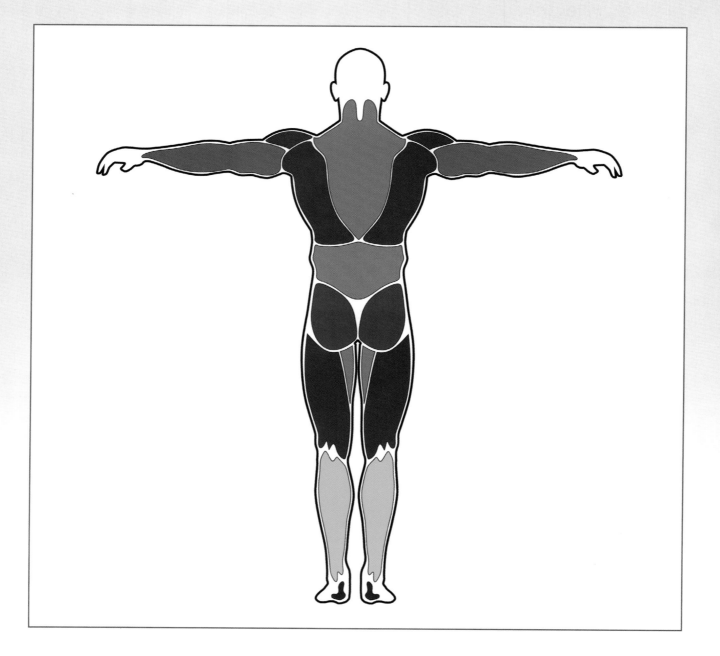

Mobilization Target Areas:

▶ Back of lower leg, from your knee down to your Achilles tendon

Most Commonly Used Tools:

▶ Single Lacrosse Ball

▶ Barbell

▶ Roller

Test and Retest Examples:

▶ Bottom of the Squat (Pistol)

▶ Dorsiflexion and Extension

Calf Smash

Calf muscles have a serious job. An athletic person takes an average of ten thousand steps per day while walking. That is 5,000 loads per calf over the course of a single day, and 70,000 over the course of a week. This doesn't even include going up and down stairs, running, working out, and playing sports. If you have bad foot positioning, whether you're walking with your feet turned out or wearing shoes that compromise position, the insidious calf tightness that accumulates is insane. It's no accident that people's calves are in a state of constant stiffness and their heel cords are like a couple of steel cables.

If you're missing ankle range-of-motion, you have no choice but to compensate into an open foot position. This means that you stand, walk, run, and move with an open knee and collapsed ankle. When this happens, you can't expect everything to be okay. It's the same issue when people are missing wrist extension; they turn their hands out and wonder why their shoulders hurt. If you're missing foot extension or dorsiflexion, you're going to turn your foot out to solve that range-of-motion problem and buffer the issue. Do this and ultimately say hello to bone spurs, Achilles tendonitis, Achilles ruptures, and a slate of other ankle problems. You can avoid all of this if you have full ankle range-of-motion and understand good positioning. You have to make sure that the large drivers of your ankles are full range and supple.

Although the chief problem is usually in the heel cords, the tightness transmits upstream. The gastroc, which is a powerful lower-leg muscle that makes up your calf, is responsible for controlling your ankle. If those tissues get stiff, ankle and knee pain generally follow.

What you have to remember is that you have a lot of musculature controlling your feet, and all that tissue is running through a very small space. This is why you need to prioritize some of the smashing effects as a first step when you're trying to deal with knee pain or trying to improve ankle range-of-motion. You can't just roll aimlessly around on a foam roller. You must smash.

There are several smashing techniques that you can incorporate, ranging from the horribly painful to the mildly uncomfortable. Depending on your level of stiffness and pain tolerance, you may have to start with the most basic, which is the roller calf smash, and work your way up. Just remember, the more uncomfortable the mobilization, the more change you will see, feel, and realize.

IMPROVES:

▶ Neutral and Straight Foot Position

▶ Ankle Range-of-Motion

▶ Ankle and Knee Pain

▶ Calf Tightness

METHODS:

▶ Contract and Relax

▶ Pressure Wave

▶ Smash and Floss

Roller Calf Smash

This is the most basic calf-smashing technique that we use. It's usually reserved for athletes that are extremely sore. As you know, tight calves are very sensitive, making it tough to mobilize without passing out or vomiting on yourself. This is why it's good to have low-level mobilizations that you can throw in as a warm-up to the more aggressive techniques. Remember, in order to make observable and measurable change, you need large acute pressures, which is difficult to get using a foam roller or pipe.

To execute this technique, position your calf and heel cord on a roller or pipe, cross your opposite leg over your shin to add pressure, and then roll your leg from side to side. You can also contract and relax and point and flex your toes.

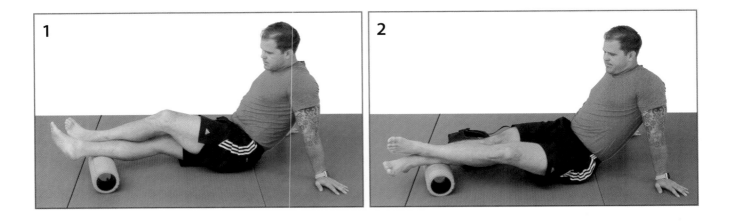

Weighted Calf Smash

Placing a heavy sandbag over your shin to add additional compression force is another good option. Although having a Superfriend apply pressure to your leg or doing the bone saw calf smash yourself (see coming techniques) are more effective, this one is certainly valid.

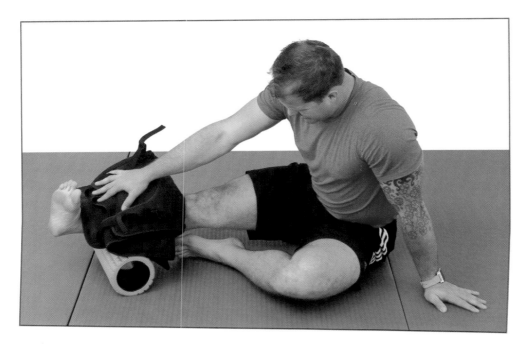

Superfriend Calf Smash

The Superfriend calf smash is great for two reasons: You can get a ton of pressure into your calf, and you are more likely to tolerate higher compression forces than you ever would on your own. The bottom line is there are not too many people out there who will apply the same kind of tortuous pressure as a Superfriend.

Have your training partner apply downward pressure and slowly roll your leg from side to side, clearing one section of tissue at a time. As with the Superfriend quad smash, you probably need to agree on a "safe" word that will cue your partner to ease up.

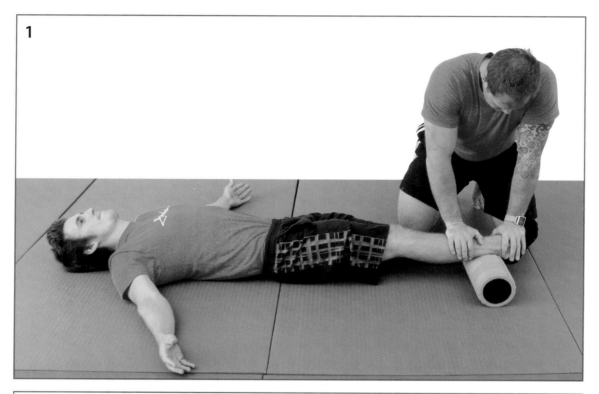

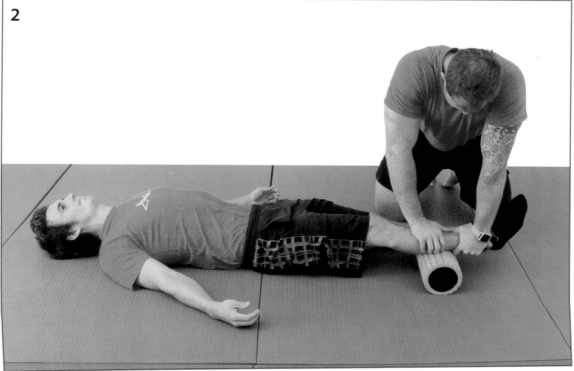

Barbell Calf Smash

The barbell calf smash offers more acute pressure, which is what you want when dealing with tight heel cords because it allows you to restore superficial sliding surfaces to the tissues near the base of your heel and ankle. You can roll your foot from side to side or twist the barbell up your lower leg to get a pressure wave effect. Crossing your opposite leg over your foot and leaning forward is a great way to add more compression force.

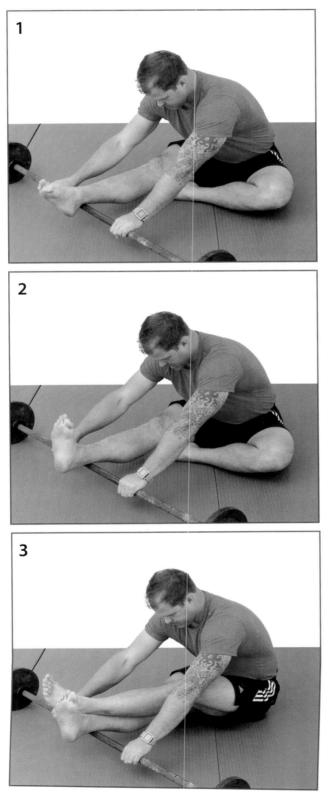

Bone Saw Calf Smash

This is my favorite calf smash mobilization and the first one I use when I have calf and heel cord tightness or ankle or knee related issues. But I'm not going to lie: It's pretty nasty.

By placing your instep over a foam roller and positioning your shin over your leg, you can get large pressures working through the back of your calf. The idea is to slice the blade of your shin into the areas that are tight, oscillating from side to side, as if you were playing a fiddle. What's great about this technique is that your foot is off the ground, so you can mobilize with a relaxed leg, allowing you to smash and floss tight areas. The contract and relax technique also works here.

It's important to note that you can control the pressure by adjusting your weight. Sitting your weight back will increase compression, while shifting forward will take pressure off your leg.

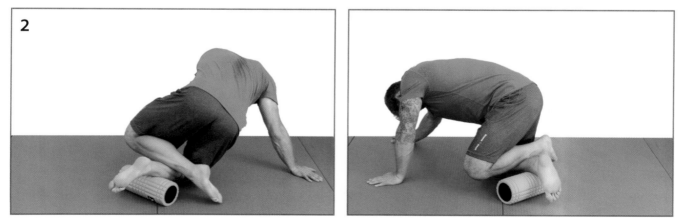

Kneel and place your instep over a foam roller, keeping your foot neutral.

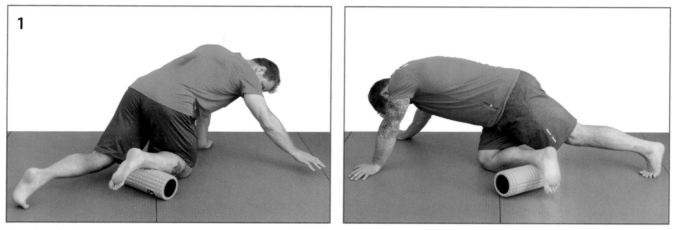

Using your arms to support the weight of your upper body, bring your opposite leg up and place your shin or instep across the tissue you're trying to change.

3

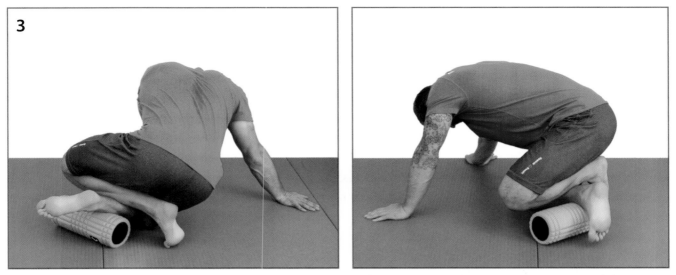

To add a compression force, sit your butt back and shift your weight over your top leg. **Note:** You can control the amount of pressure by shifting your weight forward and backward. The more you sit back, the more aggressive the pressure.

4

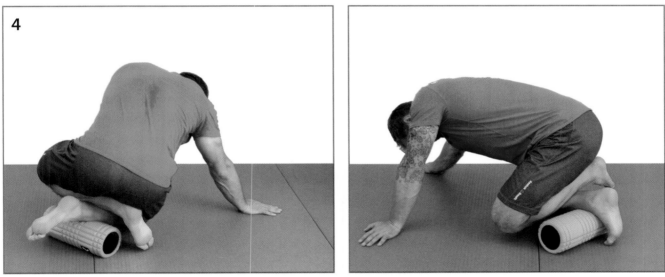

Keeping your weight centered over your leg, slowly smash your shin across the back of your calf. The idea is to shear back and forth across the back of your calf. You can also hang out on a tight spot and apply the contract and relax and smash and floss techniques.

Voodoo Calf Mobilization

If you had to consume a human being (not that you ever would), the calf muscle would be one of the worst pieces to eat. It is so thick and fibrous that you would have to literally boil it for eight hours to break down the grisly muscle tissue. As I said, your calf undergoes an intense number of loading cycles: Walking, playing sports, lifting, wearing high heels, and running all add up. Not to mention that most people spend very little time undoing all that insidious, accumulated stiffness.

The bottom line is this: Your calf is prone to sliding surface restrictions. Left untreated, that stiffness aggregates into intramuscular adhesions and knotted-up scar balls that compromise mechanics and increase potential for injury.

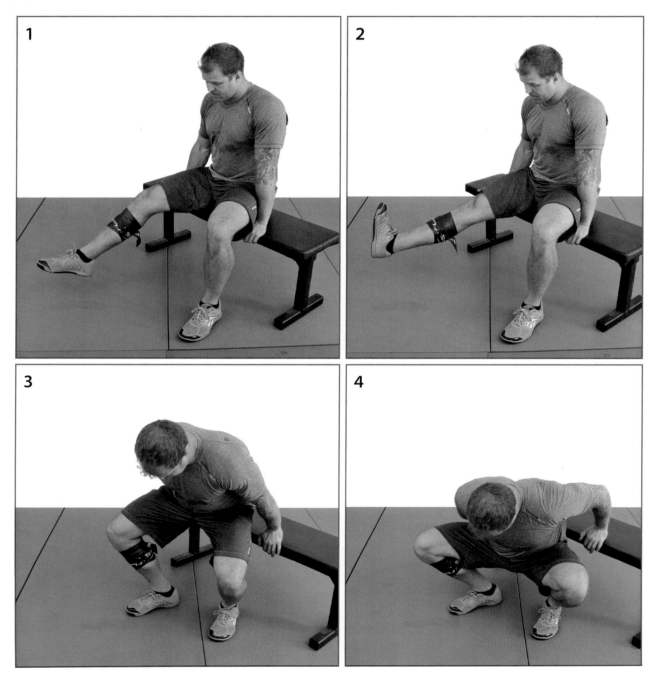

Wrap a band around the area that you are trying to change and then move your foot through as much flexion and extension range as possible.

Classic Calf Mobilization

When people have tight calves, generally their first thought is to just throw their foot on a wall or curb. It's a classic approach that you can do anywhere, anytime, and with zero equipment aside from shoes. (The shoe helps support your foot and provides traction on the wall so that you can keep the ball of your foot in place). However, there are a couple of problems worth noting with this kind of classic calf stretch.

The first problem is that it's difficult to change tissues by simply hanging out in a static position. These muscles are very, very strong and can handle large loads for extended periods of time. It's like hanging on a piece of steel cable hoping that it will stretch.

The second issue is it doesn't take a systems approach. That is, you're only addressing muscle dynamics and not your ankle capsule or sliding surfaces. You are putting yourself into a physiologic range and then hoping that you can get enough pressure to make change. For these reasons, it's imperative that you prioritize the previous mobilizations and, if possible, attach a band around your ankle to tie in the joint capsule.

What is great about this classic mobilization is that it challenges your heel cord and calf at full range and serves as an excellent supplement or counter mobilization of the previous techniques. You can also focus on the tissues at the base of your heel by bending your knee and loading the soleus complex. Just be sure to keep your foot in a good position and maintain a good arch as you hunt around for tight areas.

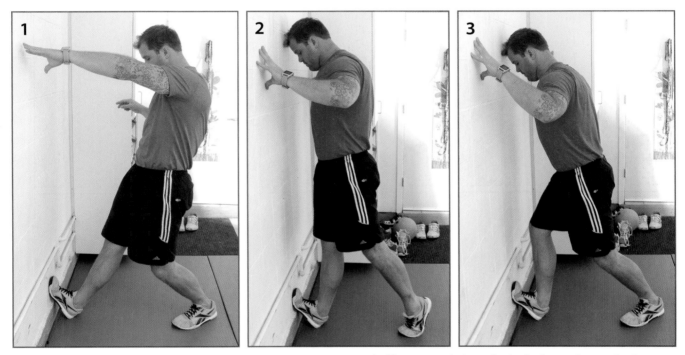

1. Standing a few feet away from a wall, lower into a quarter or half squat and place the ball of your foot as high up on the wall as possible—keeping your heel in contact with the ground, your foot neutral, and your glute squeezed. Sometimes it's easier to start high up on the wall and slide your foot down until your heel touches down. Once your foot is in position, straighten your knee. Don't try to bend your foot.

2. Keeping your foot pinned in place, stand tall and drive your weight toward the wall or pole. With your leg straight, mobilize both your heel cord and calf (gastroc). Remember to keep your glute engaged and your belly tight as you move your hip toward the wall.

3. To explore different ranges of stiffness, lower your elevation by bending your leg and scour around for tight areas by externally and internally rotating your knee.

Banded Distraction

It's a bit tricky, but if you can rig a band and apply a posterior distraction, you will increase the effectiveness of this mobilization twofold. Any time you take a classic stretch and apply a distraction to tie in the joint capsule, you turn a good stretch into a great stretch.

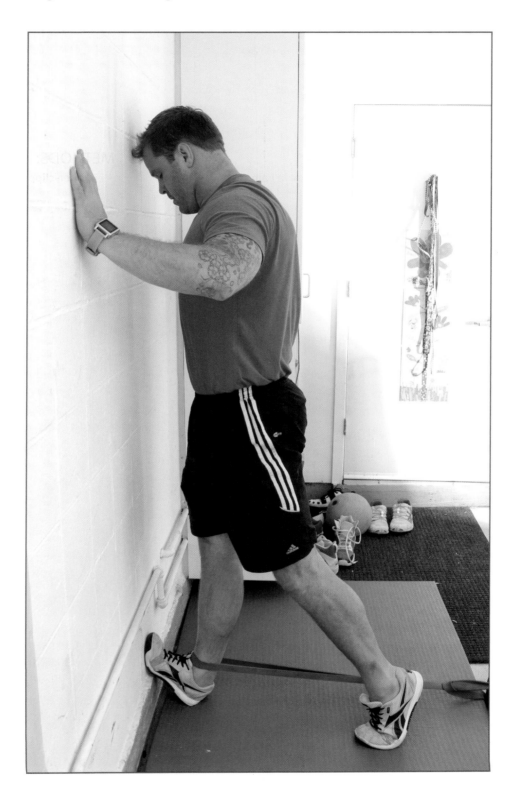

Banded Heel Cord: Anterior Bias

A lot of people report an impingement at the front of their ankle when they perform a classic calf stretch or pull their toes toward their knee. This is the equivalent of an anterior hip impingement. When your femur is resting at the front of your hip socket (usually from too much sitting), it runs into your acetabulum during deep flexion-based movements like squatting. It's the same idea here, but in this situation the bones of your ankle are resting at the front of your joint capsule, causing that familiar pinch at the front of the socket. As with the banded hip distraction, this is a simple way to clear that impingement and restore normal function and range-of-motion to the joint.

For the best results, create as much posterior tension as you can handle, drive your knee forward and out to the side—keeping your entire foot in contact with the ground—and oscillate in and out of end-range until you experience some kind of change.

IMPROVES:

▶ Neutral Foot Position

▶ Clears Anterior Ankle Impingement

▶ Ankle Pain

▶ Increases Ankle Range-of-Motion

METHODS:

▶ Paper-clipping (Oscillation)

1. Hook a band around the front of your ankle at the base of your foot and create as much tension in the band as possible. You want your entire foot in contact with the ground and your foot straight. This allows you to generate a little bit of external rotation force to stabilize your ankle in a good position.

2. Drive your knee forward. The idea is to oscillate in and out of end-range until you experience some kind of positive change.

3. You can also prop the ball of your foot onto a weight to challenge more end-range dorsiflexion.

Banded Heel Cord: Posterior Bias

The banded heel cord will tack-down the tight tissues at the base of your heel and restore sliding surfaces to the area. If this region gets tight, the skin will literally adhere to the underlying tendon. This restricts range-of-motion and causes an onslaught of other problems. This is a simple yet cogent way to unglue that matted-down tissue and help restore normal range-of-motion to your ankle.

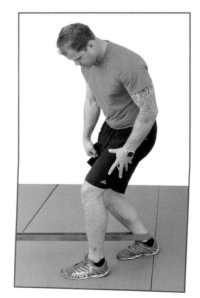

Hook a band around the base of your heel and create as much tension in the band as possible. Keeping your entire foot in contact with the ground, drive your knee forward and toward the outside of your body, oscillating in and out of end-range. The idea is to maintain a slight external rotation force to prevent your ankle from collapsing inward.

AREA 13
ANKLE AND PLANTAR SURFACE

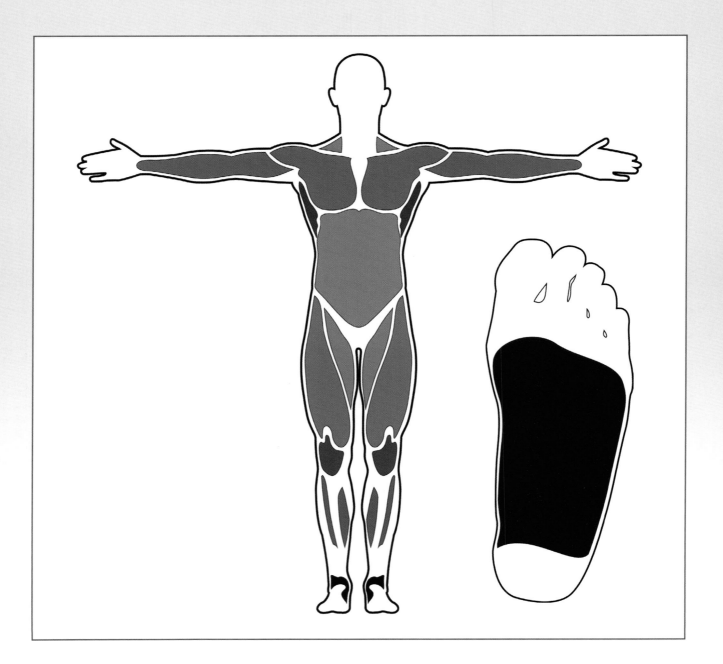

Mobilization Target Areas:

▶ Ankle, heel cord, and the bottom of your foot (forefoot)

Most Commonly Used Tools:

▶ Single Lacrosse Ball

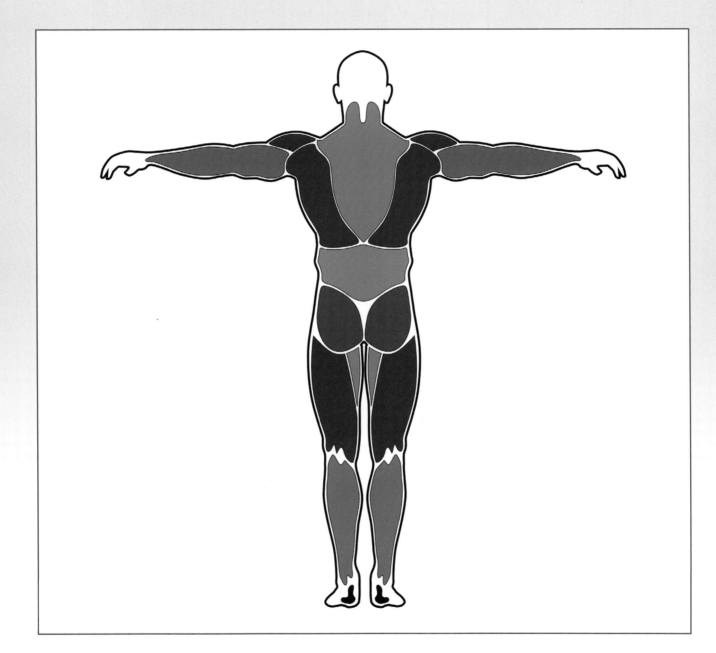

Test and Retest Examples:

- ▶ Bottom of the Squat
- ▶ Dorsiflexion and Extension

Ball Whack

When I see someone in my physical therapy practice that is missing ankle range-of-motion, this is the first technique I use. It's cheap, easy, fast, and yields freakishly good results. The best part is you don't need a Ph.D. in anatomy to figure out where your skin slides over your bones. Bend your knee. Does your skin slide smoothly over the iliotibial (IT) band? Flex your elbow. Does your skin slide over your elbow without restriction? Flex your foot. Does your skin slide over your anklebones and tendons? If it doesn't, you should immediately recognize that as a problem and work on restoring sliding surfaces to that tacked-down skin. To use the ball whack to restore sliding surfaces to the skin over the bony prominence and tendons of your foot, pin a ball on the inside and outside of your anklebone and around the areas of the heel cord and give it a firm whack. This momentarily stretches the skin, peeling it off the underlying surfaces.

Although you can do this mobilization on your own, it's difficult to generate sufficient force. For this reason, I advocate employing the help of a Superfriend.

Note: This technique can be applied anywhere you have skin stretched over a body structure—specifically your elbow or the IT-Band at your knee.

IMPROVES:
- ▶ Sliding Surface Dysfunction
- ▶ Ankle Range-of-Motion
- ▶ Ankle Pain

Inside Ankle

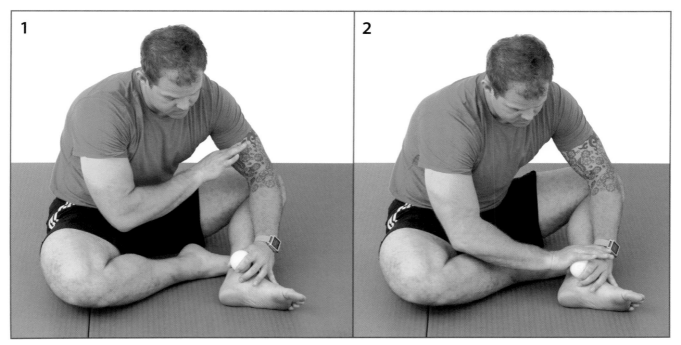

Heel Cord

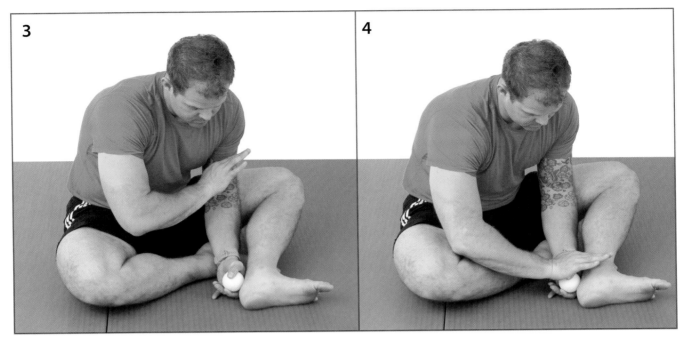

Outside Ankle

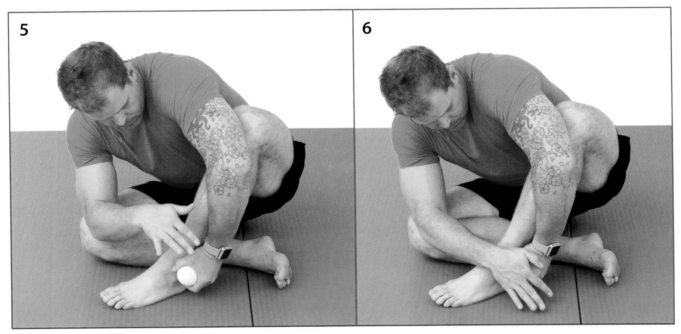

1-6 Pin the ball on an area of tacked-down tissue—focusing your attention on the anklebone, heel cord, and surrounding areas—and then give the ball a firm smack. You can also try applying pressure with the ball and then rapidly pushing it. Don't just limit yourself to one direction, either. To restore sliding surfaces, you need to hit or push the ball in every direction. Do this until the skin starts to slide smoothly over the underlying surfaces. It doesn't take too many whacks to do that.

Voodoo Ankle Mobilization

Voodoo wrapping your ankle is one of the most effective ways to restore sliding surfaces to your heel cord, ankle, and forefoot. As I mentioned before, you can approach this mobilization from a couple of different angles. If you're treating a swollen (sprained) ankle, start near the toes and cover the entire foot, keeping about 50 percent tension in the band. If you're dealing with sliding surface dysfunction and trying to improve ankle range-of-motion, you don't necessarily have to wrap your entire foot. Instead, just focus your attention on restricted areas, which for most people is around the ankle and heel cord. The key is to keep around 75 percent tension in the band and force your foot through a full range-of-motion. You can do this by propping your foot onto a bumper plate, implementing one of the calf stretching techniques, or by simply hanging out in the bottom of the squat.

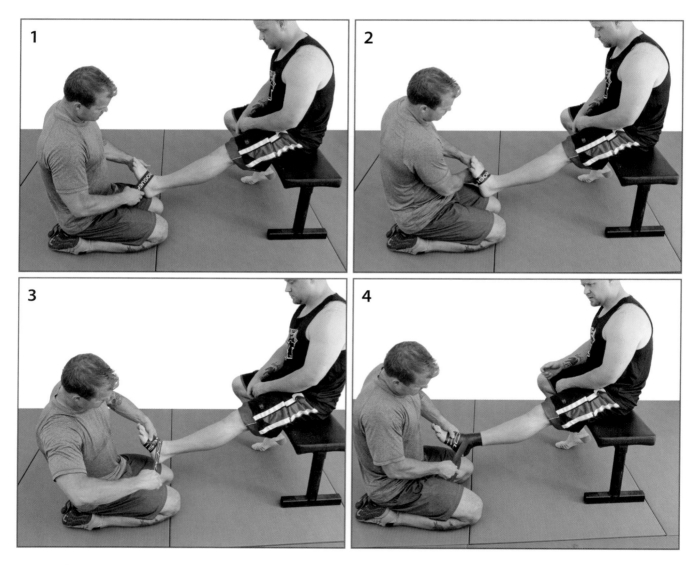

1-4 Whether you're trying to clear inflammation or restore sliding surfaces, start on the forefoot and wrap up the leg. Keep about a half inch (or half of the band) overlap and cover all the restricted areas of the foot.

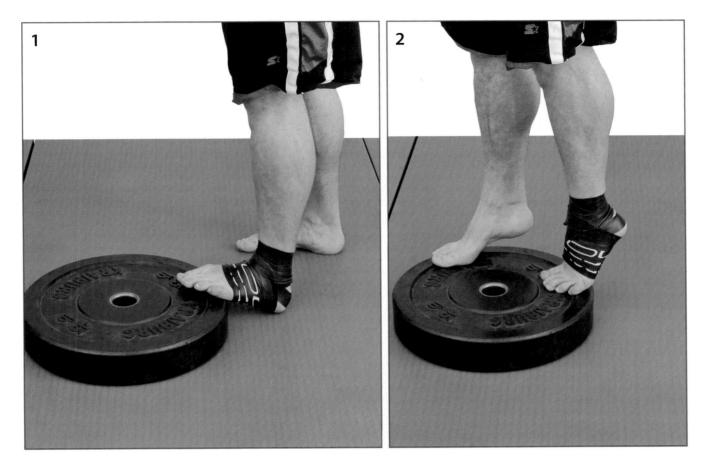

1-2 Move your ankle through as much range-of-motion as possible. You can implement the previous calf mobilization techniques (the banded heel cored is a great option), or prop your foot on an elevated surface like a bumper plate. An even better option is to perform the movement you're trying to change (run, squat, etc.).

Plantar Surface Smash

This is a great mobilization for the common and dreaded foot disease plantar fasciitis. Although there are other mechanisms that can trigger plantar surface problems—posterior tibialis, caught nerve endings, etc.—plantar fasciitis is the catchall term used to describe any kind of pain on the bottom of the foot. The people most susceptible to plantar fascia issues are modern athletes, especially those who gravitate toward barefoot and Pose-centric running practices, and people who move with their feet turned out and stand with their arches collapsed.

The plantar fascia is a big sheet of connective tissue that runs along the bottom of your foot, from the ball of your foot to your heel. As anybody who has had plantar fascia problems can attest, when this area gets inflamed or stiff, it causes a ton of pain and discomfort.

One of the best ways to resolve pain and restore suppleness to the plantar surfaces is to roll your foot over a lacrosse ball. The idea is to put in some qualitative smashing by slowly pressure waving up and down the length of your plantar fascia. You can also think about strumming the musculature of your feet by moving from side to side. If you hit a hot spot, stay on it, contract and relax, and pressure wave into the ropey tissue. You can do this while you're at work sitting at your desk, or you can stand up and get some pressure into your foot. Either way, don't wait until your foot hurts to address the issue. Fix your foot position and make sure your skin slides and glides over your plantar fascia and that the bottom of your foot is supple.

IMPROVES:
- ▶ Foot Pain (Plantar Fasciitis)
- ▶ Ankle and Foot Range-of-Motion

METHODS:
- ▶ Pressure Wave
- ▶ Contract and Relax

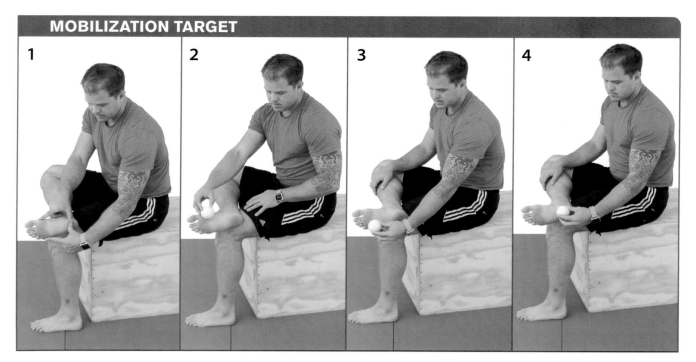

MOBILIZATION TARGET

The mobilization target area encompasses the plantar surfaces of the bottom of your foot, from the ball of your foot to your heel.

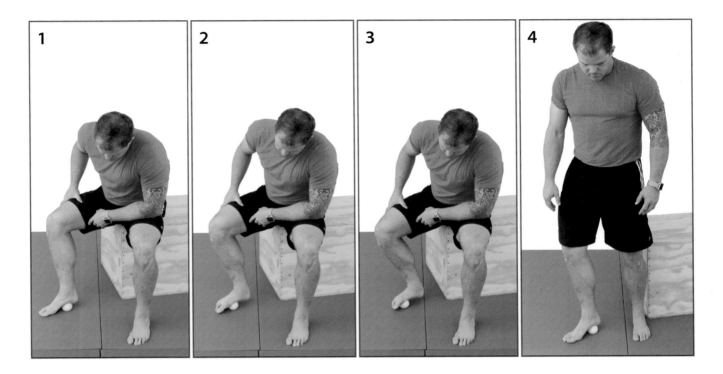

1-3

Step on a lacrosse ball, positioning it anywhere on your plantar surface, and apply as much pressure as you can handle. You can contract and relax on stiff areas and pressure wave up and down or across the tissue. The key is to take your time and focus on qualitative smashing. One of the biggest mistakes that people make is to roll their foot over a ball with zero intention or purpose. It should take you at least a minute to traverse the length of your foot.

4

To get more weight over the ball and increase pressure, do this mobilization while standing.

Forefoot Mobilization

This is another effective foot mobilization that can be used in conjunction with the plantar surface smash.

There is a big joint right in the middle of your foot that is responsible for giving your foot arch support. When this mid-joint gets ropey and stiff—either from bad foot mechanics or barefoot running—it limits your ability to externally rotate and create a good arch. This is one of the reasons why people's feet pop up when they squat. They don't have rotational capacity in their mid-joint so when they try to create external rotation by screwing their feet into the ground, their whole foot rolls up on the outside.

IMPROVES:

▶ Neutral Foot Position

▶ Foot Pain (Plantar Fasciitis)

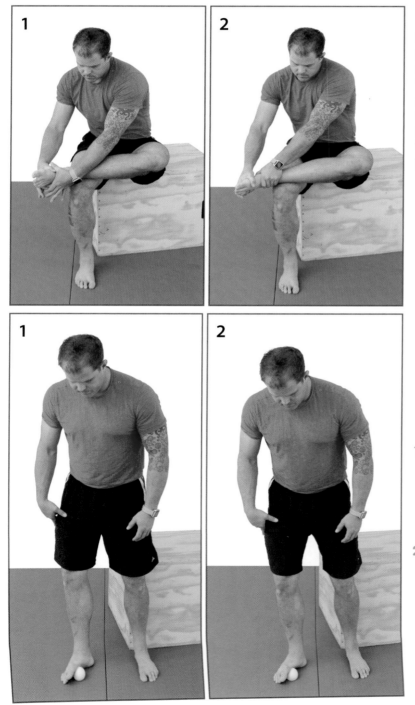

If you grab your forefoot around the base of your toes, you should have slight independent rotation from your heel. Think about like this. Your hand is pretty flexible, right? Well, if the palm of your hand is really stiff, you won't be able to mold and shape it to gripping and grabbing. All we're doing here is making sure that your foot is a little bit moldable so that you can create a good arch.

1. Step on a lacrosse ball with the inside of your forefoot. Notice that the outer edge of my foot is flush with the ground. The idea is to block the front of the foot towards the ball and try to collapse down on it. Block the joint and shear past it.

2. Applying downward pressure, create a shear force across the inside of your foot. Think about collapsing your foot over the ball.

Roller Forefoot Strumming

Unlike the forefoot mobilization, which is more of a pinpoint-targeted smash, the roller forefoot strumming captures the entire arch. Put simply, it's a non-accurate global smashing technique that captures all the structural layers of your foot. For the best results, slowly collapse your foot over the roller as if you are trying to peel off the edge of the roller with your foot.

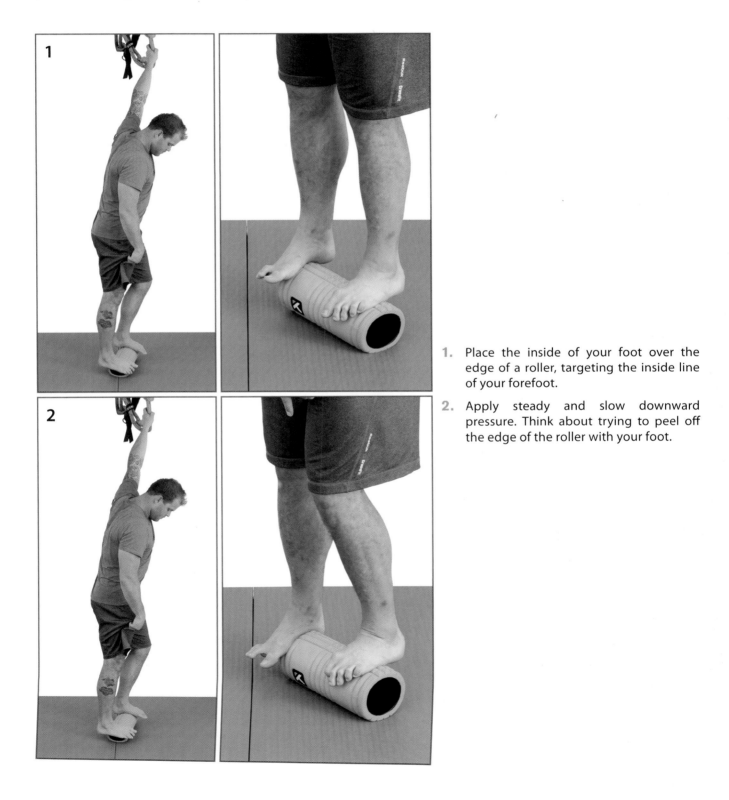

1. Place the inside of your foot over the edge of a roller, targeting the inside line of your forefoot.

2. Apply steady and slow downward pressure. Think about trying to peel off the edge of the roller with your foot.

TO CHECK OUT THE LATEST MWOD TOOLS AND GEAR, AND FOR MORE INFORMATION ABOUT THE STARRETT SYSTEM OF MOVEMENT AND MOBILITY, VISIT:

WWW.MOBILITYWOD.COM

GLOSSARY

Adduction: Describes moving a limb closer to the centerline of the body.

Banded Distraction: To pull the joint surfaces apart using a band, or to try and influence the intra-articular motions of the joint by creating more usable space by manipulating the joint capsule.

Bias: Emphasizing a certain position or movement, such as in a hip flexion with external rotation bias.

Buffer: Refers to the capacity of the body to withstand poor movement or positioning. Theoretically, healthy normal tissues that have their full ranges of motion can withstand more compromised mechanics than their stiff and restricted counterparts.

Extension: The opposite of flexion. This is a movement that opens the angle of a joint, as you do, for example, each time you walk and your back leg straightens out.

Extension Force: Describes either a force vector that facilitates further extension, like lying on a roller and arching back, or the forces on the body consistent with extension-related movements.

External Rotation: Rotation of a limb or joint away from the center or midline of the body. Sitting in lotus pose in yoga, for example, requires both the shoulder and hip to externally rotate.

Flexion: Used to describe a movement that decreases the angle of a joint, such as when you bring your elbow to your face.

Global Extension/Flexion: Refers to spinal movement patterns that occur through more than one functional region (lumbar and thoracic spine, etc.). Athletes use a global spinal position, for example, when doing a forward summersault, blocking a ball at the net, throwing a baseball, or bench pressing.

Internal Rotation: Rotation of a limb or joint toward the midline or center of the body. When you bring your hand to your face, for example, your shoulder has to internally rotate to allow that movement.

Intra-Relate: How tissues relate to themselves. For example, stiff muscle tissue does not "intra-relate" to the muscle tissues within the same muscle. This is different than when tissues inter-relate between different tissue systems.

Load-Order Sequence (Sequencing) and Load-Ordering: A basic principle of tissue loading in the body. In other words, tissues that are moved first during movement are loaded maximally in that movement. The body's tissues are not perfectly self-equalizing in nature. If the knee moves first during the squat, the quads and kneecap will load first and maximally.

Local Extension: Refers to movements in the spine that occur at a few of the spine's motion segments rather than globally throughout the spine. Examples of this include hinging at the neck during a deadlift, or overextending at the bottom of the ribcage during a press.

Missing Corner: An imprecise catchall term used to describe a missing arc, ray, vector or aspect of a range-of-motion. Full shoulder flexion also includes full external rotation of the joint when the arm is over the head. If the athlete cannot externally rotate here, it is said that he or she is missing this "corner."

Motion Segments: The functional moving units (vertebra segments) of the spine.

Passive Accessory Motion: Describes the small intra-articular movements that happen inside a joint during normal range-of-motion.

Posting up: Refers to loading an entire limb in weight bearing during a mobilization.

Shear Force: Describes trying to restore normal sliding surface interaction with a specific, usually oblique force or load. If you were trying to pull apart a grilled cheese sandwich, for instance, you would bring shear force to the sandwich to separate the slices of bread from each other.

Sliding Surfaces: Describes any surface of the body where tissues should normally slide over one another like skin over bone. This term can include skin, nerves, fascia, and muscles.

Superfriend: A trusted confidant who helps you to overcome your crappy mechanics. A Superfriend always knows the safe-word you have both agreed upon and never pushes you beyond the pain threshold you set. Sometimes you just need a Superfriend to smash your quads.

Tacked-Down and Matted-Down: Slang for stiff, unsupple tissues that do not behave like normal human tissue. Sitting in a chair all day will result in matted-down glutes.

Tensioner: When I say, "use the whole leg as a tensioner," I am describing the specific movement of a limb to apply tension to a mobilization. If you were mobilizing your hamstrings and pulled your knee to your chest, for instance, you'd extend your lower leg as the "tensioner."

ABOUT THE AUTHORS

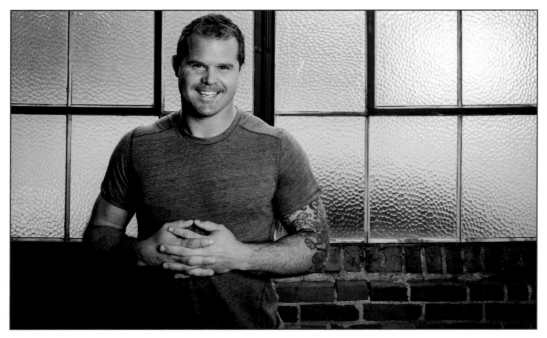

Dr. Kelly Starrett is a coach, physical therapist, author, speaker, and creator of MobilityWOD.com, which has revolutionized how athletes think about human movement and athletic performance.

Kelly received his Doctor of Physical Therapy in 2007 from Samuel Merritt College in Oakland, California. He and his wife Juliet own San Francisco CrossFit—one of the first 50 CrossFit affiliates—where Kelly runs a performance-based orthopedic sports medicine clinic. Kelly's clients have included Olympic gold medalists, Tour de France cyclists, world and national record holding Olympic Lifting and Power athletes, CrossFit Games medalists, ballet dancers, military personnel, and competitive age division athletes.

Since 2009, Kelly has been traveling the country teaching coaches and athletes that good mobility and proper movement are the keys to optimal performance and that all humans should be able to perform basic maintenance on themselves.

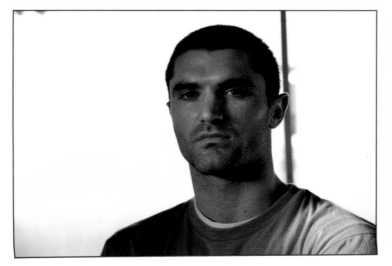

Glen Cordoza is one of the most published authors in the world on the topics of MMA, Brazilian Jiu-jitsu, Muay Thai kick-boxing, and fitness, with over seventeen books to his credit. These works include co-authorship with such martial art luminaries as Randy Couture, BJ Penn, Anderson Silva, Fedor Emelianenko, Lyoto Machida, Eddie Bravo, Cung Le, Antonio Nogueira, and Marcelo Garcia. In addition to Glen's accomplishments as an author, he is a strength-and-conditioning coach and has competed as a professional mixed martial artist (MMA) and Muay Thai boxer.